Artificial Intelligence in Medicine

In the ever-evolving realm of healthcare, *Artificial Intelligence in Medicine* emerges as a trailblazing guide, offering an extensive exploration of the transformative power of Artificial Intelligence (AI). Crafted by leading experts in the field, this book sets out to bridge the gap between theoretical understanding and practical application, presenting a comprehensive journey through the foundational principles, cutting-edge applications, and the potential impact of AI in the medical landscape.

This book embarks on a journey from foundational principles to advanced applications, presenting a holistic perspective on the integration of AI into diverse aspects of medicine. With a clear aim to cater to both researchers and practitioners, the scope extends from fundamental AI techniques to their innovative applications in disease detection, prediction, and patient care.

Distinguished by its practical orientation, each chapter presents actionable workflows, making theoretical concepts directly applicable to real-world medical scenarios. This unique approach sets the book apart, making it an invaluable resource for learners and practitioners alike.

Key Features:

- **Comprehensive Exploration:** From deep learning approaches for cardiac arrhythmia to advanced algorithms for ocular disease detection, the book provides an in-depth exploration of critical topics, ensuring a thorough understanding of AI in medicine.
- **Cutting-Edge Applications:** The book delves into cutting-edge applications, including a vision transformer-based approach for brain tumor detection, early diagnosis of skin cancer, and a deep learning-based model for early detection of COVID-19 using chest X-ray images.
- **Practical Insights:** Practical workflows and demonstrations guide readers through the application of AI techniques in real-world medical scenarios, offering insights that transcend theoretical boundaries.

This book caters to researchers, practitioners, and students in medicine, computer science, and healthcare technology. With a focus on practical applications, this book is an essential guide for navigating the dynamic intersection of AI and medicine. Whether you are an expert or a newcomer to the field, this comprehensive volume provides a roadmap to the revolutionary impact of AI on the future of healthcare.

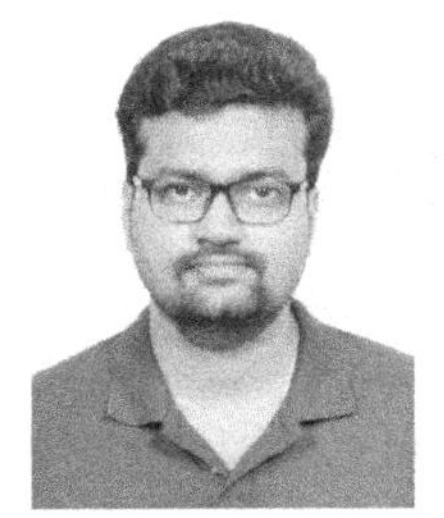

Thompson Stephan earned his PhD in Computer Science and Engineering from Pondicherry University, India, in 2018. Currently serving as an Associate Professor in the Department of Computer Science & Engineering at Graphic Era Deemed to be University, Dehradun, Uttarakhand, India, he achieved recognition among the world's top 2% most influential scientists for 2023, a distinction jointly conferred by Elsevier and Stanford University, USA. Acknowledged for academic excellence during his master's degree, he secured a university rank. Additionally, he was honored with the Best Researcher Award-2020 and the Protsahan Research Award in 2023 by the IEEE Bangalore Section, India. His research interests primarily focus on implementing and applying artificial intelligence techniques in practical settings. He has authored numerous technical research papers published in renowned journals and conferences by IEEE, Elsevier, Springer, and others. Actively serving as a reviewer for esteemed international journals and working as a book editor, Thompson Stephan is dedicated to advancing the field.

Artificial Intelligence in Medicine

Edited by
Thompson Stephan

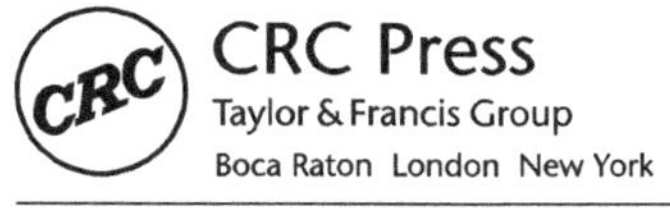

CRC Press is an imprint of the
Taylor & Francis Group, an **informa** business

Designed cover image: © Shutterstock

First edition published 2025
by CRC Press
2385 NW Executive Center Drive, Suite 320, Boca Raton FL 33431

and by CRC Press
4 Park Square, Milton Park, Abingdon, Oxon, OX14 4RN

CRC Press is an imprint of Taylor & Francis Group, LLC

Library of Congress Cataloging-in-Publication Data
Names: Stephan, Thompson, editor.
Title: Artificial intelligence in medicine / edited by Thompson Stephan.
Other titles: Artificial intelligence in medicine (Stephan)
Description: First edition. | Boca Raton : CRC Press, 2025. | Includes bibliographical references and index.
Identifiers: LCCN 2024002758 (print) | LCCN 2024002759 (ebook) | ISBN 9781032438344 (hbk) | ISBN 9781032438351 (pbk) | ISBN 9781003369059 (ebk)
Subjects: LCSH: Artificial intelligence--Medical applications.
Classification: LCC R859.7.A78 A778 2025 (print) | LCC R859.7.A78 (ebook) |
DDC 610.285--dc23/eng/20240503
LC record available at https://lccn.loc.gov/2024002758
LC ebook record available at https://lccn.loc.gov/2024002759

ISBN: 978-1-032-43834-4 (hbk)
ISBN: 978-1-032-43835-1 (pbk)
ISBN: 978-1-003-36905-9 (ebk)

DOI: 10.1201/9781003369059

Typeset in Sabon
by MPS Limited, Dehradun

Contents

List of contributors

Poonguzhali A
Department of Electronics and Communication Engineering
Sri Sairam College of Engineering
Bangalore, Karnataka, India

Shubhashree A
Department of Computer Science and Engineering
M S Ramaiah University of Applied Sciences
Bangalore, Karnataka, India

Jyoti Agarwal
Department of Computer Science and Engineering
Graphic Era Deemed to be University
Dehradun, Uttarakhand, India

Joe Arun
Professor of Marketing
Loyola Institute of Business Administration (LIBA)
Chennai, Tamil Nadu, India

Karthikeyan B R
Department of Computer Science and Engineering
M S Ramaiah University of Applied Sciences
Bangalore, Karnataka, India

Divya B S
Department of Computer Science and Engineering
M S Ramaiah University of Applied Sciences
Bangalore, Karnataka, India

Anbumani Bala
Medical Consultant Paediatrician and Child Psychiatrist
St Thomas Hospital
Chennai, Tamil Nadu, India

Ashwin Balasubramanian
Department of Computer Science and Engineering
Loyola-ICAM College of Engineering and Technology
Chennai, Tamil Nadu, India

Ronit Bali
Amity School of Engineering and Technology
Amity University
Noida, Uttar Pradesh, India

Sumukha Bhat
Department of Computer Science and Engineering
M S Ramaiah University of Applied Sciences
Bangalore, Karnataka, India

Vinoth Kumar C N S
Department of Networking and Communications
SRM Institute of Science and Technology
Kattankulathur, Chennai, Tamil Nadu, India

Rishi Chauhan
Amity Business School
Amity University
Noida, Uttar Pradesh, India

Karthik G
Department of Computer Science and Engineering
M S Ramaiah University of Applied Sciences
Bangalore, Karnataka, India

Shubham Garg
Amity School of Engineering and Technology
Amity University
Noida, Uttar Pradesh, India

Radhika Goyal
Amity School of Engineering and Technology
Amity University
Noida, Uttar Pradesh, India

Shelly Gupta
Department of Computer Science and Engineering (Artificial Intelligence)
KIET Group of Institutions
Ghaziabad, Uttar Pradesh, India

Christina J
Department of Computer Science and Engineering
Loyola-ICAM College of Engineering and Technology
Chennai, Tamil Nadu, India

Limsa Joshi J
Department of Computer Science and Engineering
Loyola-ICAM College of Engineering and Technology
Chennai, Tamil Nadu, India

Arvind K S
Department of Computer Science and Engineering
Jain (Deemed-to-be University)
Bangalore, Karnataka, India

Ranjitha K V
Department of Computer Science and Engineering
M S Ramaiah University of Applied Sciences
Bangalore, Karnataka, India

Kalaivani Kathirvelu
Department of Computer Science and Engineering
Vels Institute of Science, Technology and Advanced Studies
Chennai, Tamil Nadu, India

Vaishali R Kulkarni
Department of Computer Science and Engineering
Graphic Era Deemed to be University
Dehradun, Uttarakhand, India

Piyush Kumar
Amity Business School
Amity University
Noida, Uttar Pradesh, India

Remegius Praveen Sahayaraj L
Department of Computer Science and Engineering
Loyola-ICAM College of Engineering and Technology
Chennai, Tamil Nadu, India

Yashaswini L
Department of Computer Science and Engineering
M S Ramaiah University of Applied Sciences
Bangalore, Karnataka, India

Kanchana M
Department of Computing Technologies
SRM Institute of Science and Technology
Tamil Nadu, India

Sathya Sundaram M
Department of Computer Science and Engineering
Paavai Engineering College
Namakkal, Tamil Nadu, India

Supriya M S
Department of Computer Science and Engineering
Jain (Deemed-to-be University)
Bangalore, Karnataka, India
and
Department of Computer Science and Engineering
M S Ramaiah University of Applied Sciences
Bangalore, Karnataka, India

Aditi Mahadware
MIT School of Engineering, Computer Science Department
MIT ADT University
Pune, Maharashtra, India

Shuchi Mala
Amity School of Engineering and Technology
Amity University
Noida, Uttar Pradesh, India

Abhishek Mishra
MIT School of Engineering, Computer Science Department
MIT ADT University
Pune, India

Padma Priya Dharishini P
Department of Computer Science and Engineering
M S Ramaiah University of Applied Sciences
Bangalore, Karnataka, India

Pandiaraja P
Department of Computer Science and Engineering
M Kumarasamy College of Engineering
Karur, Tamil Nadu, India

Ram Kumar P
Department of Computer Science and Engineering
Sri Sairam College of Engineering
Bangalore, Karnataka, India

Santhi P
Department of Computer Science and Engineering
Amrita School of Computing, Amrita Vishwa Vidyapeetham
Vengal, Chennai, India

Disha Mohini Pathak
Department of Computer Science
ABES Engineering College
Ghaziabad, Uttar Pradesh, India

Manoranjitham R
Division of Computer Science and Engineering
Karunya Institute of Technology and Sciences
Karunya University
Coimbatore, Tamil Nadu, India

Naresh R
Department of Networking and Communications
SRM Institute of Science and Technology
Chennai, Tamil Nadu, India

Dhyana Sharon Ross
Healthcare and Human Resources Management
Loyola Institute of Business Administration (LIBA)
Chennai, Tamil Nadu, India

Angel Latha Mary S
Department of Computer Science and Engineering
SNS College of Technology
Coimbatore, Tamil Nadu, India

Punitha S
Department of Computer Science and Engineering
Graphic Era Deemed to be University
Dehradun, Uttarakhand, India

Shyni Carmel Mary S
Business Analytics
Loyola Institute of Business Administration (LIBA)
Chennai, Tamil Nadu, India

Tamil Selvan S
Department of Computer Science and Engineering
Saveetha School of Engineering
Chennai, Tamil Nadu, India

Abhishek Saigiridhari
MIT School of Engineering, Computer Science Department
MIT ADT University
Pune, India

Saanjhi Saraogi
School of Computer Science and Engineering
Vellore Institute of Technology
Chennai, Tamil Nadu, India

Sakshi Saraogi
School of Computer Science and Engineering
Vellore Institute of Technology
Chennai, Tamil Nadu, India

Achyut Shankar
Department of Cyber Systems Engineering, WMG
University of Warwick
Coventry, United Kingdom

Anukansha Sharma
Amity School of Engineering and Technology
Amity University
Noida, Uttar Pradesh, India

Jash Singh
Department of Computer Science and Engineering
M S Ramaiah University of Applied Sciences
Bangalore, Karnataka, India

Thompson Stephan
Department of Computer Science and Engineering
Graphic Era Deemed to be University
Dehradun, Uttarakhand, India

Pushphavathi T P
Department of Computer Science and Engineering
M S Ramaiah University of Applied Sciences
Bangalore, Karnataka, India

Reji Thomas
Department of Computer Science and Engineering
Sri Sairam College of Engineering
Anekal, Bangalore, Karnataka, India

Aarya Tupe
MIT School of Engineering, Computer Science Department
MIT ADT University
Pune, India

Surya Tejas V
Department of Computer Science and Engineering
M S Ramaiah University of Applied Sciences
Bangalore, Karnataka, India

Sharmila V J
Department of Computer Science and Engineering
Loyola-ICAM College of Engineering and Technology
Chennai, Tamil Nadu, India

Asnath Victy Y
School of Computer Science and Engineering
Vellore Institute of Technology
Chennai, Tamil Nadu, India

Dhanalekshmi Yedurkar
MIT School of Engineering, Computer Science Department
MIT ADT University
Pune, India

Part I

Foundations of AI in healthcare

Chapter 1

Exploring deep learning approaches for cardiac arrhythmia diagnosis

M S Supriya[1,2], *L Yashaswini*[2], *and K S Arvind*[1]

[1]Department of Computer Science and Engineering, Jain (Deemed-to-be University), Bangalore, Karnataka, India

[2]Department of Computer Science and Engineering, M S Ramaiah University of Applied Sciences, Bangalore, Karnataka, India

1.1 INTRODUCTION

Heart-related issues are becoming more prevalent every day. Heart health is greatly impacted by three main factors: emotional stress, physical stress, and psychiatric stress [1]. Cardiac arrhythmia is crucial. Variation in normal heart beat rhythm that can be a form of irregular wave form of the heart is cardiac arrhythmia [2]. The symptoms of cardiac arrhythmia may include irregular heartbeat, with often associated with other symptoms like dizziness, and weakness. Some cardiac arrhythmia are not life-threatening if diagnosed and treated properly. However, improper or late diagnosis leads to continuous rise in death [3].

The electrophysiological mechanisms responsible for Arrhythmia are i) abnormal impulse formation and ii) Conduction disturbances [4]. The abnormal impulse (focal activity) is formed when the cardiac cells generate spontaneous impulse called as automaticity [4]. The automaticity can be slower impulse formation than the normal, called as Bradycardia and increased automaticity called Tachycardia. Whereas, Conduction disturbances also called reentry is a mechanism where cardiac arrhythmia initiates in cardiac muscle and sustains it [4].

Thus early diagnosis becomes important in saving lives of those suffering from cardiac arrhythmia. DL is based on artificial neural network. It was put forward by studying the neural network scheme of humans and their configurations [3]. DL models usually have the algorithm based on human neural scheme. And the models are fed with sufficient or all possible set of data to accomplish the task [5]. In general, DL models are structured hierarchically to connect layers [6]. The DL approach to representation learning consists of a number of algorithms arranged in various layers. Through DL, the neurons are spread to hidden layers. As a result, each layer's number of neurons decreases while the overall amount of layers increases [3].

Traditional ECGs have a lower accuracy which needs the continuous heart monitoring as there are chances that abnormalities in the heart may not be present during ECG [5]. Also due to continuous checks the usual electrocardiogram can be expensive or in many cases the ECG may not be able to trace the signals of heart quite accurately that is real time diagnosis is difficult [7]. Such manual cardiac annotation is susceptible to errors since it might be challenging and time-consuming for the doctor to manually annotate an ECG signal [8]. Arrhythmia can be detected and classified automatically, allowing quick diagnosis using continuous wireless ECG. Surveillance equipment [9].

Deep neural network can track the rhythm of the heart more accurately, with the long-term track of heart beats and give the sharp result on the presence of arrhythmia symptoms [1] or the type of the arrhythmia present by taking intelligent decisions and making predictions by analyzing intricate pattern using the input data set fed to the network [5].

DOI: 10.1201/9781003369059-2

This technique eliminates the need for medical expertise, cost, and inaccurate results [1] all models are discussed in subsequent sections.

There are different conditions leading to different types of cardiac arrhythmia. Each cardiac arrhythmia can be classified based on whether it is abnormal impulse formation or conduction disturbances [10]. From atrial fibrillation many other cardiac arrhythmia are discussed further with their symptoms.

1.2 BACKGROUND

1.2.1 Electrocardiogram

Two bottom chambers called ventricles and two upper chambers called atria make up the heart. Heart rhythm is ruled by tiny regions of right atrium called SA node or sinoatrial node. This node naturally generates the electrical impulses that result in heartbeat. The rhythm of this impulse is in control of the nerves and hormones. Each propagating wave of bioelectricity produced by SA node will pass through atria and then channeled through the atrioventricular or AV node which carries the pulse to the ventricles and this is the atrial contraction. On the way to ventricles from AV node pulse propagates through specialized conducting bundles called His-Purkinje fibers. These fibers transport the pulse all the way to ventricles and thereby facilitates ventricular contraction.

The series of periodic impulses produced by the electrical stimulation of the heart is known to be electrocardiogram [11]. It is an inexpensive, affordable, clear diagnostic tool to monitor the heart activities [11]. Voltage between electrodes positioned on the body's surface computes the heart's electrical activity (usually on chest, sometimes on wrist, feet) [7].

Figure 1.1 shows a typical ECG. The different ups and downs of ECG are named as: P wave, Q wave, R wave, S wave, and T wave. The combination of Q wave, R wave and S wave forms (Ventricular complex), S and T wave together forms (ST segment), P and R waves together to form (PR interval), The three most crucial components of an ECG are the RR interval, PR segment, and QT interval serves detecting various heart disorders, including arrhythmias [12].

P wave represents the excitation of atria (when the new pulse is formed by SA node), QRS represents the ventricular excitation (when the impulse travels through AV node to ventricles) and T wave signifies the relaxation of the ventricles [10].

The usual amplitude range for the ECG signal is between 10uV and 5 mV, and its normal frequency range is between 0.05 and 100 Hz. [1]. Any variations in the signals' amplitude or

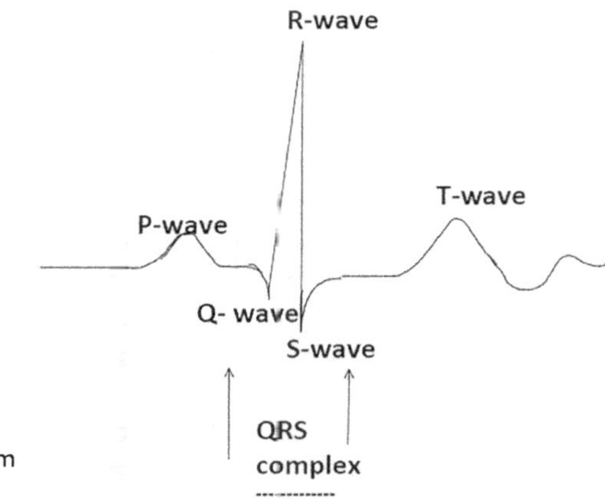

Figure 1.1 Representation of normal electrocardiogram (ECG).

frequency than normal can be considered as abnormality in the heart [1]. Electrocardiograms (ECGs) are commonly used to diagnose cardiac arrhythmias in patients (CAs) [13].

Deep neural networks have shown promise in the classification of ECGs because they can learn intricate representative qualities directly from the data, doing away with the necessity for human feature extraction and generates the accurate outcome [14] (Table 1.1).

1.2.2 Types of cardiac arrhythmia

Table 1.1 Various types of cardiac arrhythmia

Arrhythmia name	*Definition*	*ECG characteristics*	*Symptoms*
Atrial fibrillation	When the heart's natural sinus node pacemaker malfunctions, it causes atrial fibrillation that is due to fast functioning of various regions of upper regions of heart [15].	Eg: End-to-End CNN and RNN model is mostly used to extract the features of ECG [16]	Severity of symptoms for somatization disorders, sadness, or anxiety [17]
Atrial tachycardia	It include abnormal automaticity, triggered activity, and reentry [18]	Abnormal P wave morphology [18]	Palpitations, faintness, chest pain [18]
Atrioventricular nodal reentrant tachycardia (AVNRT)	All tachycardia that develop above the bundle of His bifurcate [19]	Long RP interval characterizes AVNRT [19]	"shirt flapping" and "neck pounding" [19]
Pre-Excitation Syndrome	The condition where prior excitation of ventricles results in hemodynamic disturbances [20]	Short PR interval and delta wave [20]	Dizziness, shortness of breath, chest discomfort [21].
Ventricular fibrillation	It is a condition where there is a rapid impulse formation by from a single reentry [22].	Greater QRS complex [22]	Sudden cardiac death [23]
Ventricular tachycardia	A nodo-ventricular fiber insertion into the right ventricle or a slowly conducting right-sided accessory AV channel are both used for AV conduction [24].	Wide QRS complexes [24]	Loudness in heartsound, change in systolic blood pressure [24]
Torsades de pointes	A prolonged first cycle brought on by the compensatory pause following the premature ventricular beat [25].	Prolonged QT interval [25]	Emotional stress, cardiac arrest [25]
Brugada syndrome	An autosomal dominant mode of inheritance is used to transmit the Brugada syndrome [26].	ST segment elegation [26]	It is mostly asymptotic, or leads to sudden death due to cardiac failure [26]
Sick sinus syndrome	Inability of the natural pace maker of heart to create approximate heart rate that the body needs [27].	Electrocardiogram show abnormal heart rhythms [27]	Lightheadedness, palpitations [27]

1.3 DEEP LEARNING MODELS AND ITS APPLICATION IN CARDIAC ARRHYTHMIA

There are many datasets proposed based on the test result, theoretical results, and hybrid model. But there should be an efficient data set processing models to process the data sets [7].

1.3.1 Multilayer perception (MLP)

MLP is based on feed-forward artificial neural network, this model of DL distinguishes data that are not linearly separable. It works on the principle of back propagation technique, which is a part of the supervised learning method for its training [28].

The algorithm written for the model includes labels which are the features extracted from the data sets by the network, For MLP, the labels will read "arrhythmia" and "normal sinus." That is, MLP uses the normal sinus and unusual heart activity to classify the arrhythmia. Then the labels are encoded and they act as a dependent variable for deep network. Integer encoding, which assigns an integer value to each label or feature, or one-hot encoding, which adds a binary value for each distinct integer value, are two possible types of encoding. In order to eliminate integer coding conflicts, the presented technique employs one-hot encoding, which also makes it possible to divide the data sets into three categories: training, testing, and validation. In the stage after Labels, middle layers, layer of activations, layer of filter, size of filter, placeholders for input, and expected yield placeholders are all created and stored in Tensor Flow data structures. It also has a second tensor defined to hold the results of the trained model after which the model is implemented and trained using the training set of data. [28]. Figure 1.2 depicts the abstract model of MLP.

1.3.2 Convolutional neural network (CNN)

Network of convolutional neurons is the basic methodology in the deep learning algorithm. It is an approach that shows promise for extracting and categorizing arrhythmia features

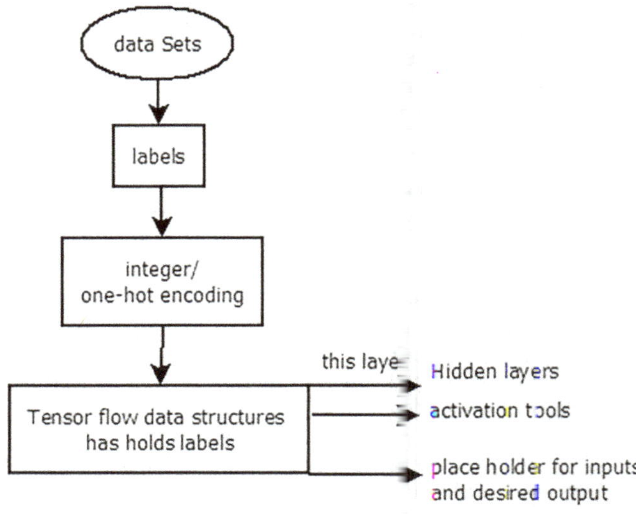

Figure 1.2 MLP model.

from raw time-series data. When connected to a massive data collection, this approach performs faster and more effectively than others [1]. This technique detected the normal and MI (myocardial infarction), a serious type of arrhythmia, with an accuracy of 95.22% [6]. The CNN model works on the architectural design that has INPUT-CONV-POOL-FC stages. The algorithm's input consists primarily of data organized in the sequence of successive time instants, such as one-dimensional time series input data for an ECG [5]. that is the input is a single dimension vector that can be denoted by p = (p1, p2, p3, pn-1, pn) where $p_{n\ belongs}$ to class label either normal or abnormal and denotes features of ECG [6].

Also, it is observed that variations in ECG graph corresponds to unique arrhythmia, in this regard a greater number of sample points of the curve are extracted and fed as an input for the extractor based on DL by calculating the difference of curve from the data-set fed and the test result [29]. The Convolution ID constructs map feature map when the incoming data is put through a convolution process that belongs to class either normal or abnormal and a fresh set of capabilities is again fed to the next block, integrating all feature map the network produce its output [6].

The output after the mapping is given to pooling layer. On each feature map, a max-pooling procedure is carried out. The down-sampling operation thereby selects the features with highest values [6]. These high-value features in pooling extracted are given to the fully connected layer, the last step of convolution neural network. The Soft-Max function, that offers the probability distribution across each class, is contained in this layer [6]. It indicates that the fully connected layer will determine the type of arrhythmia for the CNN's final output [6]. Figure 1.3 depicts the abstract model of CNN.

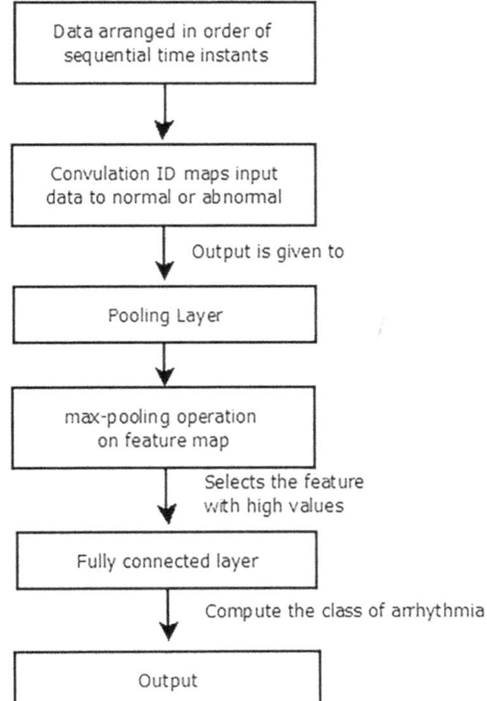

Figure 1.3 CNN model.

1.3.3 Recurrent neural network

This is an illustration of the enormous achievements achieved by sequence-to-sequence models in applications for neural machine translation, which are comparable to manual performance by humans [8]. A cyclic graph is produced by this kind of network, which is actually extended by a forward-looking network with feedback channels. Unlike others, it is not generalized on the ECG curve and may handle temporal sequences of any length.

Then, each heartbeat in an ECG recording is separated into its many features [30]. The normalized ECG is concatenated for the hidden layers and the SoftMax layer results this into one projection vector [30].

The level 2 or the next loop combines the predictions of level 1 models. On the scale of dropout and the recurrent dropout of 60% to 512%, amount of units for each hidden layer and 1 to 5 recurrent layers grid search is performed and is used to choose the hyperparameters of level 1 [30]. To sum up, RNN are models that can well learn temporal behaviors that are dynamic for arbitrary length of input-output.

RNN is used notably, especially for lengthy upright AI obligations in the discipline of machine translation, language modelling, and speech recognition [6].

Figure 1.4 depicts the abstract model of RNN.

1.3.4 Long short-term memory (LSTM)

LSTM was proposed for the language model and well-known for its property of memorizing long-term dependencies [31]. It is the later version of RNN. Instead of RNN components, LSTM uses memory blocks. It works on the INPUT-OUTPUT model. The memory block in

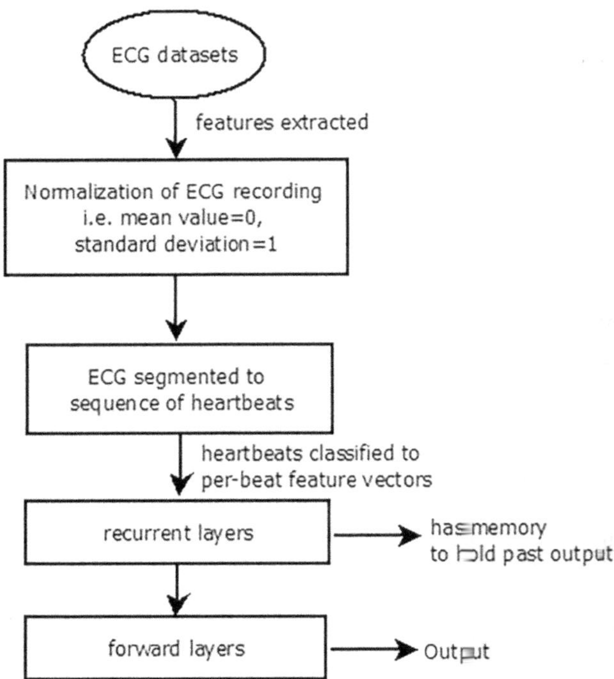

Figure 1.4 RNN model.

this is made of a processing unit which has one or many memory cells. It has included with two multiplicative gates to start for input and end for output. The start gate let input data flow. Input in this network is the series of input data which is of undefined length, such as p = (p1, p2, p3 ... pn-1,pn), taken as input data for LSTM model. And the end gate performs the last status of one node to other; the output data of arbitrary length is given by o = (o1, o2, o3 ... o_{n-1},o_n). A group of adaptive multiplicative gates would be responsible for managing all of the memory block's operations. The forgotten gate and peephole connections, which are new network improvements, are also included in the model's design. The constant error carousel uses this gate. One memory cell is connected to each gate via those peepholes [6].

Among LSTM's traditional models, LSTM NN has reported the high performance [31]. Figure 1.5 depicts the abstract model of LSTM.

With the help of the three adaptive multiplicative gating units, the memory cell stores the records over a wide range of time steps. Input and output gates modulate the input and output, going with the flow of a cellular activation of a reminiscence cell. The project of the forget gate is to reset the self-recurrent fee, whilst it will become inappropriate. By multiplying with a memory cell, the forget gate employs the values 0 to erase and 1 to keep value for the next step. Memory, cellular, and all gates have peephole connections which are used for getting to know the best timings of outputs [6].

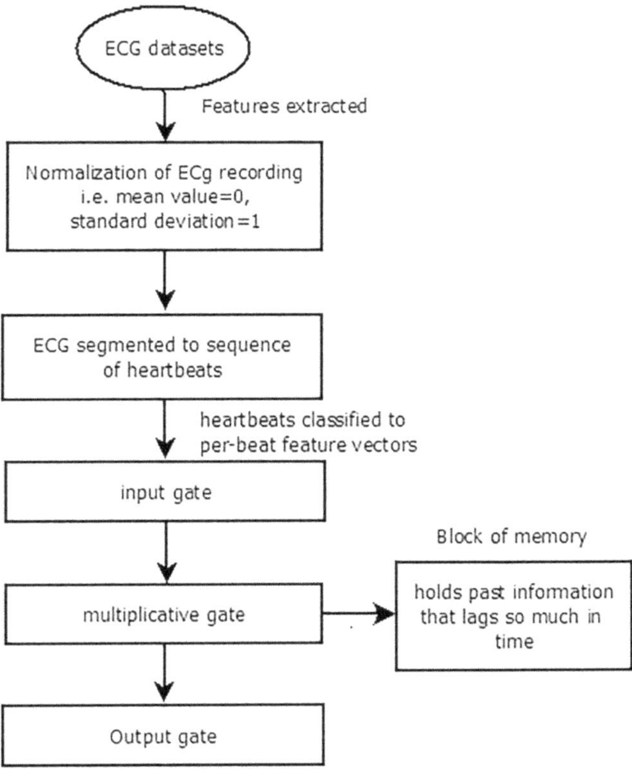

Figure 1.5 LSTM model.

1.3.5 Deep belief network (DBN)

DBN consists of a single visible layer with various hidden layers. The Boltzmann machine (BM) was first proposed by Hiton and Sejnowski. A BM as stochastic neural network version may be used for unsupervised research of crucial elements of an unknown probability distribution based totally on samples, at the same time as the studying process is hard and time consuming. So as to conquer these issues, Smolensky proposed a restrained BM (RBM) in 1986. [38] The RBM is just like the classical BM. Without visible-visible or hidden-hidden links, all viewed units are linked to all hidden units. In line with the value types of seen and hidden units, RBM may be separated into BBRBM and GBRBM [32–34].

Bernoulli-Bernoulli and two different types of limited Boltzmann machines are stacked in DBN. The salient feature of this network is that it can learn automatically from raw ECG signals without the intervention of an expert. To modify the RBM parameters, many techniques are employed, such as contrastive divergence and persistent contrastive divergence [32].

Generally, four steps are included in ECG arrhythmia classification systems i) Preprocessing; ii) Heartbeat Segmentation; iii) Feature Learning; and iv) Classification. In preprocessing, heartbeat datasets are filtered for a particular characteristic or segment. Segmentation steps look for QRS complex in ECG for segmenting the heartbeat with particular characteristics. After layer-via-layer pre-training of DBN, a Softmax regression layer may be extra on top of the resulting hidden illustration layers to achieve classification. Softmax regression is a supervised and multi-magnificence learning set of rules [32]. Figure 1.6 depicts the abstract model of DBN.

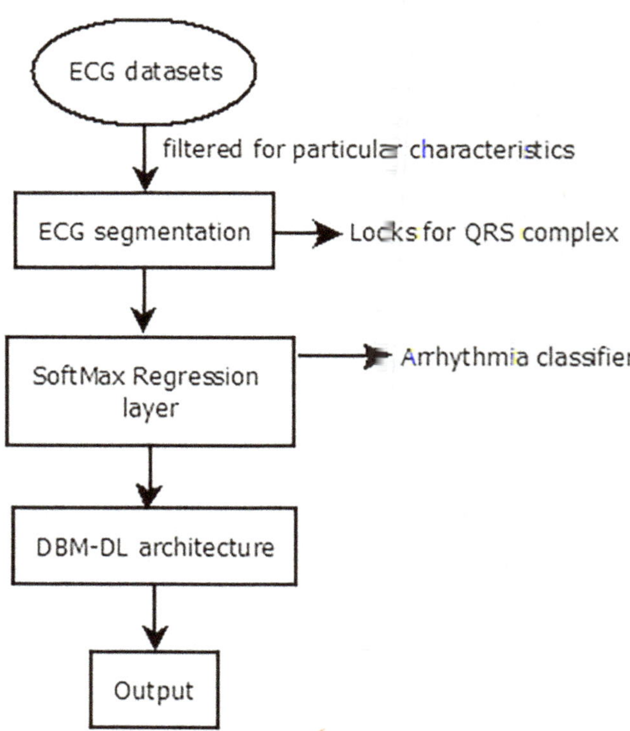

Figure 1.6 DBN model.

1.4 ADVANCE RELATED WORK

Convolutional Neural Networks (CNNs) have recently achieved state-of-the-art results in popular pattern/object recognition challenges, outperforming most conventional pattern recognition techniques despite the majority of them having previously been successfully applied to the ECG arrhythmia detection tasks. This has inspired researchers to incorporate these techniques into the field of medical imaging and signal processing. Deep learning techniques have been applied to even the most difficult medical pattern recognition tasks, and the results have been state-of-the-art. The most significant impact on the performance of computerized classification/recognition systems is typically caused by the extraction of highly representative features from the available data.

Despite the fact that it takes a lot of time and requires expertise, widely used features lack robustness to changes in the data [35].

One of the most recent studies suggested using an ECG recording to identify premature ventricular contraction (PVC) beats using a deep neural network. To distinguish between normal and PVC beats, six distinct layers from ECGs are fed into a deep neural network with six hidden layers to train it. The authors still chose to manually create their own features from the ECG data, even though a deep neural network was used [35].

A deep convolutional neural network is trained to extract characteristics from unprocessed ECG signals and to distinguish between paroxysmal atrial fibrillation (PAF) and regular heartbeats. The demand for a significant labeled training dataset in order to improve network performance (i.e., increasing the number of convolutional layers) is a drawback of creating a deep convolutional neural network from scratch. Even with a very large dataset available, increasing the network's depth will raise the cost of computation during training since deeper convolutional layers contain more complicated convolutional processes. For these training tasks, powerful GPU-powered computers are therefore necessary [35].

Transfer learning, including its variation that incorporates fine-tuning, provides an effective solution for challenges arising from insufficient training data, limited expertise in model training, and constrained computational resources. This approach involves importing a pre-trained deep Convolutional Neural Network (CNN) to the current task, where it serves as an automatic feature extractor. Furthermore, in transfer learning, one or several layers of the pre-trained network may be retrained (or fine-tuned) with data specific to the targeted task [35].

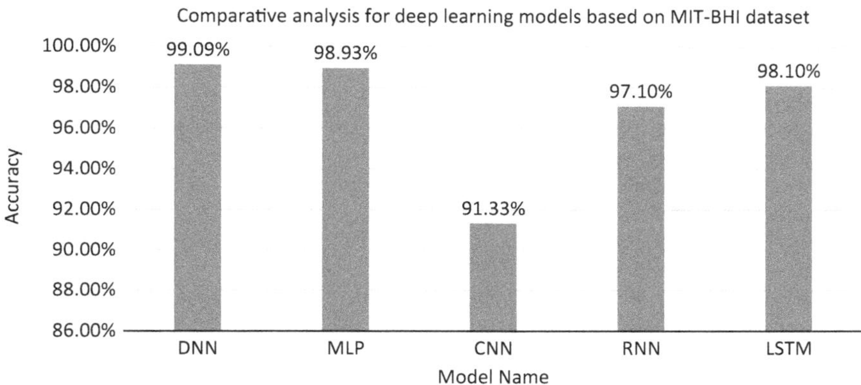

Figure 1.7 Comparative analysis for deep learning models based on MIT-BHI dataset.

1.5 COMPARATIVE ANALYSIS

Each DL model has their own accuracy based on the data set, implementation, and arrhythmia they are classifying or identifying. The comparison chart is depicted in Figure 1.7.

1.6 CONCLUSION

A simple work to pump blood. But, when extra payload is given to the heart such as stress, anxiety it will behave abnormal. This abnormal behavior of heart is called the cardiac arrhythmia.

The traditional approach for this abnormality of the heart does not seem to be successful because the range and kind of arrhythmia recorded are huge.

Hence, by studying the human intricate pattern and designing it as an algorithm for models, that are fed with all the inputs, required to identify or classify the arrhythmia, scientists around the world came up with a variety of efficient models that can process the input according to various algorithm and outputs based on the correct or highly favorable match of arrhythmia for the inputs given.

Usually, inputs are features extracted from ECG, and they are segmented for a particular range of ECG graphs. This will be compared with the data set that the algorithm works on. The data set has the key-value pair of arrhythmia symptoms. On comparison, the model outputs the name of the arrhythmia that has the highest match with the data set.

Hence, the more the features in data set, the more accurate they would be. Also, some of models work best to determine some unique arrhythmias, and each DL model has their own accuracy based on the data set, implementation, and arrhythmia they are classifying or identifying. It can be concluded from the comparative analysis that deep learning models have demonstrated potential for improving cardiac arrhythmia detection and classification.

REFERENCES

1. Rajkumar, A., Ganesan, M. and Lavanya, R., 2019, March. Arrhythmia classification on ECG using DL. In 2019 5th International Conference on Advanced Computing & Communication Systems (ICACCS) (pp. 365–369). IEEE. El-Dahshan, E. (2010). Genetic algorithm and wavelet hybrid scheme for ECG signal denoising. Telecommunication Systems, vol.46, no.3, pp. 209–215.
2. Izci, E., Ozdemir, M.A., Degirmenci, M. and Akan, A., 2019, October. Cardiac arrhythmia detection from 2d ECG images by using DL technique. In 2019 Medical Technologies Congress (TIPTEKNO) (pp. 1–4). IEEE.
3. Assodiky, H., Syarif, I. and Badriyah, T., 2017, September. DL algorithm for arrhythmia detection. In 2017 International Electronics Symposium on Knowledge Creation and Intelligent Computing (IES-KCIC) (pp. 26–32). IEEE.
4. Antzelevitch, C. and Burashnikov, A., 2011. Overview of basic mechanisms of cardiac arrhythmia. Cardiac Electrophysiology Clinics, 3(1), pp. 23–45.
5. Ebrahimi, Z., Loni, M., Daneshtalab, M. and Gharehbaghi, A., 2020. A review on DL methods for ECG arrhythmia classification. Expert Systems with Applications: X, 7, p. 100033.
6. Swapna, G., Soman, K.P. and Vinayakumar, R., 2018. Automated detection of cardiac arrhythmia using DL techniques. Procedia Computer Science, 132, pp. 1192–1201.
7. Sannino, G. and De Pietro, G., 2018. A DL approach for ECG-based heartbeat classification for arrhythmia detection. Future Generation Computer Systems, 86, pp. 446–455.

8. Mousavi, S. and Afghah, F., 2019, May. Inter-and intra-patient ECG heartbeat classification for arrhythmia detection: A sequence to sequence DL approach. In ICASSP 2019–2019 IEEE International Conference on Acoustics, Speech and Signal Processing (ICASSP) (pp. 1308–1312). IEEE.
9. Murugesan, B., Ravichandran, V., Ram, K., Preejith, S.P., Joseph, J., Shankaranarayana, S.M. and Sivaprakasam, M., 2018, June. Ecgnet: Deep network for arrhythmia classification. In 2018 IEEE International Symposium on Medical Measurements and Applications (MeMeA) (pp. 1–6). IEEE.
10. Fenton, F.H., Cherry, E.M. and Glass, L., 2008. Cardiac arrhythmia. Scholarpedia, 3(7), p. 1665.
11. Zhou, S. and Tan, B., 2020. Electrocardiogram soft computing using hybrid DL CNN-ELM. Applied Soft Computing, 86, p. 105778.
12. Warrick, P. and Homsi, M.N., 2017, September. Cardiac arrhythmia detection from ECG combining convolutional and long short-term memory networks. In 2017 Computing in Cardiology (CinC) (pp. 1–4). IEEE.
13. Chen, T.M., Huang, C.H., Shih, E.S., Hu, Y.F. and Hwang, M.J., 2020. Detection and classification of cardiac arrhythmias by a challenge-best DL neural network model. Iscience, 23(3), p. 100886.
14. Salem, M., Taheri, S. and Yuan, J.S., 2018, October. ECG arrhythmia classification using transfer learning from 2-dimensional deep CNN features. In 2018 IEEE Biomedical Circuits and Systems Conference (BioCAS) (pp. 1–4). IEEE.
15. Nattel, S., 2002. New ideas about atrial fibrillation 50 years on. Nature, 415(6868), pp. 219–226.
16. Andersen, R.S., Peimankar, A. and Puthusserypady, S., 2019. A DL approach for real-time detection of atrial fibrillation. Expert Systems with Applications, 115, pp. 465–473.
17. Gehi, A.K., Sears, S., Goli, N., Walker, T.J., Chung, E., Schwartz, J., Wood, K.A., Guise, K. and Mounsey, J.P., 2012. Psychopathology and symptoms of atrial fibrillation: Implications for therapy. Journal of Cardiovascular Electrophysiology, 23(5), pp. 473–478.
18. Roberts-Thomson, K.C., Kistler, P.M. and Kalman, J.M., 2005. Atrial tachycardia: Mechanisms, diagnosis, and management. Current Problems in Cardiology, 30(10), pp. 529–573.
19. Fox, D.J., Tischenko, A., Krahn, A.D., Skanes, A.C., Gula, L.J., Yee, R.K. and Klein, G.J., 2008. Supraventricular tachycardia: Diagnosis and management., 83(12), 1400–1411.
20. Chung, K.Y., Walsh, T.J. and Massie, E., 1965. Wolff-parkinson-white syndrome. American Heart Journal, 69(1), pp. 116–133.
21. Al-Khatib, S.M. and Pritchett, E.L., 1999. Clinical features of Wolff-Parkinson-White syndrome. American Heart Journal, 138(3), pp. 403–413.
22. Surawicz, B., 1971. Ventricular fibrillation. The American Journal of Cardiology, 28(3), pp. 268–287.
23. Surawicz, B., 1985. Ventricular fibrillation. Journal of the American College of Cardiology, 5(6), pp. 43B–54B.
24. Wellens, H.J., 2001. Ventricular tachycardia: Diagnosis of broad QRS complex tachycardia. Heart, 86(5), pp. 579–585.
25. Gowda, R.M., Khan, I.A., Wilbur, S.L., Vasavada, B.C. and Sacchi, T.J., 2004. Torsade de pointes: The clinical considerations. International Journal of Cardiology, 96(1), pp. 1–6.
26. Antzelevitch, C., 2006. Brugada syndrome. Pacing and Clinical Electrophysiology, 29(10), pp. 1130–1159.
27. Semelka, M., Gera, J. and Usman, S., 2013. Sick sinus syndrome: A review. American Family Physician, 87(10), pp. 691–696.
28. Savalia, S. and Emamian, V., 2018. Cardiac arrhythmia classification by multi-layer perceptron and convolution neural networks. Bioengineering, 5(2), p. 35.
29. Isin, A. and Ozdalili, S., 2017. Cardiac arrhythmia detection using DL. Procedia Computer Science, 120, pp. 268–275.

30. Schwab, P., Scebba, G.C., Zhang, J., Delai, M. and Karlen, W., 2017, September. Beat by beat: Classifying cardiac arrhythmias with recurrent neural networks. In 2017 Computing in Cardiology (CinC) (pp. 1–4). IEEE.
31. Du, X., Cai, Y., Wang, S. and Zhang, L., 2016, November. Overview of DL. In 2016 31st Youth Academic Annual Conference of Chinese Association of Automation (YAC) (pp. 159–164). IEEE.
32. Wu, Z., Ding, X. and Zhang, G., 2016. A novel method for classification of ECG arrhythmias using deep belief networks. International Journal of Computational Intelligence and Applications, 15(04), p. 1650021.
33. Gowda, R.M., Khan, I.A., Wilbur, S.L., Vasavada, B.C. and Sacchi, T.J., 2004. Torsade de pointes: the clinical considerations. International Journal of Cardiology, 96(1), pp. 1–6.
34. Abdula, L. and Al-Ani, M. (2020). CNN-LSTM based model for ECG arrhythmias and myocardial infarction classification. Advances in Science Technology and Engineering Systems Journal, 5, pp. 601–606. 10.25046/aj050573.
35. Isin, A. and Ozdalili, S., 2017. Cardiac arrhythmia detection using deep learning. Procedia Computer Science, 120, pp. 268–275.

Chapter 2

Neural networks and LDA-based machine learning framework for the early detection of breast cancer

Saanjhi Saraogi[1], *Sakshi Saraogi*[1], *Asnath Victy Phamila Y*[1], *and Kalaivani Kathirvelu*[2]

[1]School of Computer Science and Engineering, Vellore Institute of Technology, Chennai, Tamil Nadu, India

[2]Department of Computer Science and Engineering, Vels Institute of Science, Technology and Advanced Studies, Chennai, Tamil Nadu, India

2.1 INTRODUCTION

A common and dangerous type of cancer that mostly affects women is breast cancer. It is one of the main causes of death for women, and early detection is essential for better survival rates and effective treatment. The prognosis is greatly impacted by the type and stage of cancer at diagnosis. Breast cancer can develop in various tissues, but it usually starts in the ducts or lobules of the breast. Moreover, there is a chance that cancer cells will spread to the lymph nodes under the arms, which presents more hazards. According to projections, approximately 13.4% of contemporary women will be diagnosed with cancer at some point in their lives, with breast cancer being the most prevalent and deadly type. Since the disease can be fatal if not caught in its early stages, early detection is essential. Every year, around 12% of women worldwide are affected by breast cancer, and this percentage is still rising [1]. An effective breast cancer treatment depends on early detection. Globally, the number of cases of breast cancer that are not discovered until they have progressed to an advanced stage is higher. It is difficult to create reliable prognostic models, which makes it harder for medical professionals to create therapeutic plans that will increase patient survival. Therefore, a great deal of work goes into creating methods that have as few faults as possible in order to improve accuracy. Researchers have used machine learning techniques to create computerized systems in response to the need for a quicker and more effective diagnosis system. The time-consuming nature of current breast cancer detection techniques including mammography, ultrasound, and biopsy is addressed by this strategy. Efficient tumor categorization and cell identification are made possible by the algorithms employed in these systems.

2.2 LITERATURE SURVEY

Numerous machine learning techniques have been investigated in earlier research studies on the diagnosis of breast cancer. Using the Wisconsin Breast Cancer dataset, one study [2] examined the effectiveness of Support Vector Machine (SVM), Random Forest, Decision Tree and K-Nearest Neighbor (KNN). The best classification results were obtained by KNN, which was followed by SVM, Random Forest, and Decision Tree. The effectiveness of SVM, Naive Bayes, and Artificial Neural Networks (ANN) in

DOI: 10.1201/9781003369059-3

conjunction with feature extraction/selection algorithms was examined in a different study [1]. The research dataset used for this study is the Wisconsin Diagnostic Breast Cancer (WDBC) dataset. SVM-LDA outperformed the other methods, according to the study, even though it took longer to compute. Researchers compared the performance of ANN and SVM with other classifiers like CNN, KNN, and Inception V3 in a study [3]. The outcomes of the experiment proved that ANN was a better option for diagnosing breast cancer than SVM and other classifiers. Researchers presented a novel approach for diagnosing breast cancer dubbed HA-BiRNN in a different study [4]. Among other machine learning methods, they used bidirectional recurrent neural networks, Naive Bayes classifiers, SVM classifiers, bi-clustering Ada Boost algorithms, and RCNN classifiers. The outcomes demonstrated that the DNN algorithm outperformed the other methods in terms of performance, efficiency, and image quality, better satisfying the needs of medical systems.

A new method for detecting breast cancer was presented in a recent study [5]. It combined deep learning techniques like artificial neural networks (ANN), convolutional neural networks (CNN), and recurrent neural networks (RNN) with machine learning techniques like logistic regression, support vector machine (SVM), K-nearest neighbor (KNN), Random Forest, Decision Tree, and Naive Bayes classifier. The outcomes demonstrated that the ANN and CNN models, respectively, had high accuracy rates of 97.3% and 99.3%. Researchers used picture categorization in another study [6] to create a novel approach to breast cancer diagnosis. They used the Random Forest (RF) algorithm, Convolutional Neural Network (CNN), Support Vector Machines (SVM), conventional Neural Networks (NN), and Bayesian approaches. The research showed that the CNN approach—which uses kernels to extract global features—performed better at detecting breast cancer than alternative methods. Additionally, using the Wisconsin Breast Cancer dataset, researchers compared the effectiveness of several machine learning techniques in a study [7]. Along with deep and convolutional neural networks, they also used ALEXNET for feature extraction and analysis of benign and malignant tumors. The Support Vector Machine outperformed all other models with a 94% accuracy rate and generated better results, according to the findings. The authors of a study publication [8] suggested a strategy for applying different machine learning algorithms to classify mammography images into benign, malignant, and normal categories. Random Forest, Convolutional Neural Networks (CNN), and Support Vector Machines were contrasted. Their simulations‘ outcomes demonstrated that CNN, the best classifier, classified digital mammograms with the highest accuracy by combining morphological and filtering techniques.

Researchers used a dataset from the University of Wisconsin Hospital's collection of Dr. William H. Walberg in another investigation [9]. In addition to using machine learning algorithms like logistic regression, SVM, K-NN, Decision Trees (DT), Naive Bayes, and Random Forests, they also used data visualization approaches. With all of the features at its disposal, the logistic regression model produced the best classification accuracy—98.1%. This suggests better performance a compared to the other studied approaches. In a different study [10], the authors used the Wisconsin Breast Cancer dataset to examine the effectiveness of logistic regression, Naive Bayes, Random Forest, and Support Vector Machine (SVM). The studies were carried out utilizing the ANACONDA Data Science Platform in a virtual setting. Out of all the studied approaches, Random Forest had the lowest error rate and the best accuracy, at 99.76%, according to the data. The effectiveness of several machine learning algorithms was examined in a research study [11], and the experimental findings revealed that Support Vector Machines (SVM) produced the best accuracy (97.13%) and the lowest error rate. The WEKA data mining tool was used in a simulated setting for the investigation. Three machine learning approaches—Bayesian networks, Random Forest (RF), and Support Vector Machine (SVM)—were contrasted in a different study [12]. The researchers found that the method employed had an impact on the classification results. SVMs demonstrated superior precision, specificity, and overall accuracy, whereas RFs demonstrated superior tumor classification accuracy.

Mirajkar and Lakshmi employed the Naive Bayes Classification algorithm in data mining to create a cancer prediction technique in a research study [13]. Their method's goal was to evaluate the risk of particular cancers, with a particular emphasis on ovarian and breast cancer. The study sought to categorize cancer symptoms and determine the probability of acquiring different types of cancer by utilizing the Naive Bayes algorithm. A different study [14] employed data mining for cancer diagnosis and prognosis using the Classification and Association framework technique. Using the FP method for Association Rule Mining, frequent patterns for detecting benign and aggressive forms of breast cancer were found. In the classification method, they also employed the Decision Tree algorithm to forecast the prognosis of breast cancer based on characteristics including age, gender, and symptom severity. According to the study, the diagnosis analysis was highly accurate, indicating that the approach could help doctors make decisions by facilitating early diagnosis and possibly preventing needless biopsies. Using a variety of classification data mining approaches, accurate prediction models for breast cancer were constructed in a study [15]. Using characteristics linked to regularity in cell size, the researchers classified tumor diagnoses as benign or malignant using the Wisconsin dataset. Prediction accuracy was used to gauge performance, and the Sequential Minimal Optimization algorithm outperformed other techniques like BF Tree and IBK, achieving the greatest prediction accuracy of 96.2%. Additionally, SMO showed a decreased mean absolute error (MAE) and a higher Kappa statistic (KS) of 0.92. Chi-square, Info Gain, and Gain Ratio tests revealed that all characteristics were significant for breast cancer survival. Using the WEKA toolset, researchers sought to determine the best method for forecasting cancer survival rates using a comparison analysis [16]. Using the SEER breast cancer dataset, they found that almost half of the patient records had missing data for specific features. Consequently, the dataset was cleared of those properties. Age, tumor size, and node size were among the critical clinical variables selected for examination. Three algorithms for categorization were assessed according to their accuracy, precision, and recall. As a result of the prognosis analysis's very acceptable accuracy, medical professionals may find it useful in making decisions regarding early diagnosis and maybe avoiding needless biopsies.

In a study [17], scientists examined the features of mammography pictures to create a model for predicting breast cancer. There were 250 patients in the sample, all of whom had benign or malignant tumors. For analysis, three classification algorithms (J48, CART, and ADTree) were employed; TP Rate, FP Rate, and precision were utilized to gauge performance. With an accuracy of 98.5%, the CART algorithm was the most accurate, closely followed by J48, which had a 98.1% accuracy. Using the same mammography pictures, the researchers suggested conducting additional testing with other categorization systems to examine how well they performed. A new method for predicting breast cancer was presented in a different study [18], which used a hybrid algorithm that included k-means with ELM (Extreme Learning Machine). Based on the features that were retrieved, the k-means method was utilized to cluster the tumors, whereas ELM classified the tumors more effectively and accurately. SVM was also included in the hybrid system to classify the images as normal, benign, or malignant. The system's effectiveness was assessed using a number of criteria, including accuracy, sensitivity, specificity, and Jaccard distance. The outcomes showed that the suggested hybrid system outperformed alternative approaches in correctly diagnosing cases of breast cancer. A review of the literature [19] focuses the data mining methods to diagnose and predict breast cancer. The results demonstrated the potential of data mining methods in revealing hidden patterns and supporting medical professionals in making decisions. It was stated that the diagnosis analysis accuracy when employing data mining classification techniques was quite respectable. Artificial Neural Networks (ANNs) showed better accuracy in prognosis than previous methods. The authors stressed the value of developing several models and experimenting with various algorithms in order to identify the model that performs the best in each unique situation. In order to increase accuracy, researchers adopted an ensemble technique in a study [20] that focused on neural network classification for breast cancer prediction. The 286 cases in the WBCD dataset that were categorized as benign or malignant were subjected to multiple classification approaches for analysis. Ninety-eight percent accuracy was achieved by the Tree Random classifier, which performed better. The researchers proposed utilizing an Ensemble classifier for additional analysis in an effort to potentially reach 100% accuracy.

A prototype for diagnosing and treating breast cancer patients based on clinical characteristics such as age, tumor size, and node size was created in study [21]. Thirteen classifiers, including Bayes-Net, Logistic, Multilayer Perceptron, J48, and others, were shown to accurately diagnose patients as healthy or ill after the study examined 37 classification rules. In study [22], data mining techniques were used to estimate the survival rate of patients with breast cancer. The attributes that had missing data were eliminated from the analysis of the SEER data by the researchers. Based on patient survival status, the dataset was split into two processes, and the C4.5 algorithm fared better in predicting survivability. Using the J48 Decision Tree algorithm, a prediction framework for the early diagnosis of breast cancer was developed in study [23]. With an accuracy of 94.56% on the Wisconsin Breast Cancer dataset, the J48 algorithm proved to be a useful diagnostic tool. A hybrid model for classifying breast cancer was constructed in study [24], incorporating methods from Decision Tree and Support Vector Machine. The model outperformed other categorization methods, with a 91% accuracy rate. A breast cancer prediction system based on a hybrid CART classifier approach with feature selection and bagging techniques was presented in study [25]. Increasing classification accuracy was the aim, and the researchers tried with different datasets related to breast cancer. Promising outcomes were observed in the accurate classification of breast cancer cases using the hybrid strategy that included feature selection with bagging.

From the extensive literature review, the following objectives were formulated:

- To develop an efficient neural network based machine learning model which is capable of distinguishing between benign and malignant breast cancer cells.
- To determine the most effective attributes for predicting whether a cancer is malignant or benign, and to assess the developed model's performance through calculations of metrics like F1 score, sensitivity, and accuracy.
- To identify the trends that can assist in selecting the appropriate model, hyper parameters to avoid producing suboptimal result and to minimize the loss function.

2.3 PROPOSED METHODOLOGY

Data preprocessing and pruning methods are pivotal in ensuring the integrity and dependability of datasets used to train machine learning models. The Wisconsin breast cancer dataset underwent various stages of preprocessing to ready it for model training. Prior to any analysis, a thorough check for missing attribute values was conducted on the dataset. As it turned out, the dataset was already complete without any missing values. This is not always the case in most datasets, where missing values are prevalent. In such instances, imputation techniques like filling in missing values with means, medians, or modes are employed to prevent the removal of samples containing incomplete data. To reduce dimensionality, PCA and LDA were employed. PCA reconfigures original features into a lower-dimensional space while preserving the most significant variance. On the contrary, LDA seeks optimal linear combinations of features that effectively differentiate between classes. Reducing feature count not only eases computational complexity but also aids in dimensionality reduction. By applying these data refinement techniques, the Wisconsin breast cancer dataset was refined in a dependable and top-quality manner. This enhancement strengthened the accuracy of machine learning models in identifying and categorizing instances of breast cancer. These preprocessing steps, when combined, played a pivotal role in establishing a robust and accurate machine learning framework for early breast cancer detection.

Prediction models have been created and tested by repeatedly training with the obtained dataset utilizing the relationships found. Using the testing dataset, the trained models were subjected to test, and several metrics were computed to assess the performance. Figures 2.1 and 2.2 show a diagram of the process' general design as well as the stages involved in each phase.

Logistic Regression, Random Forest, K-nearest neighbor, neural networks, Support Vector Machines, and Naive Bayes are some of the algorithms used for training.

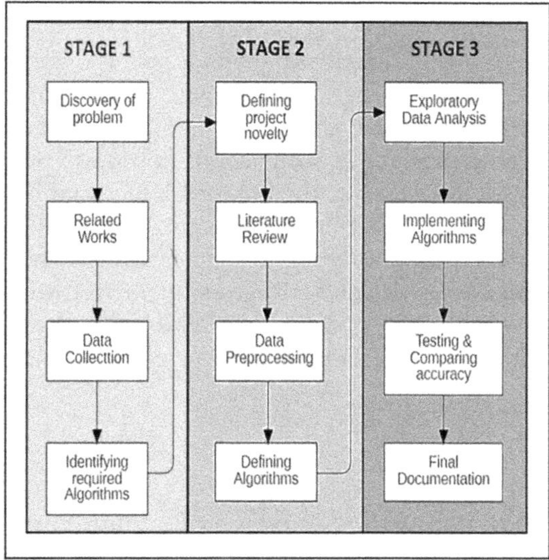

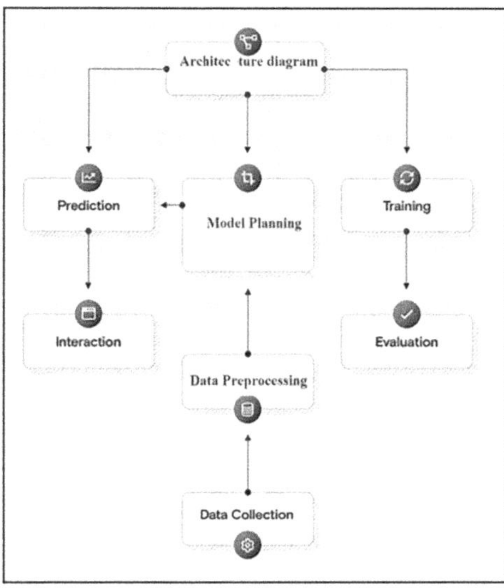

Figure 2.1 Stage wise phases involved in the process.

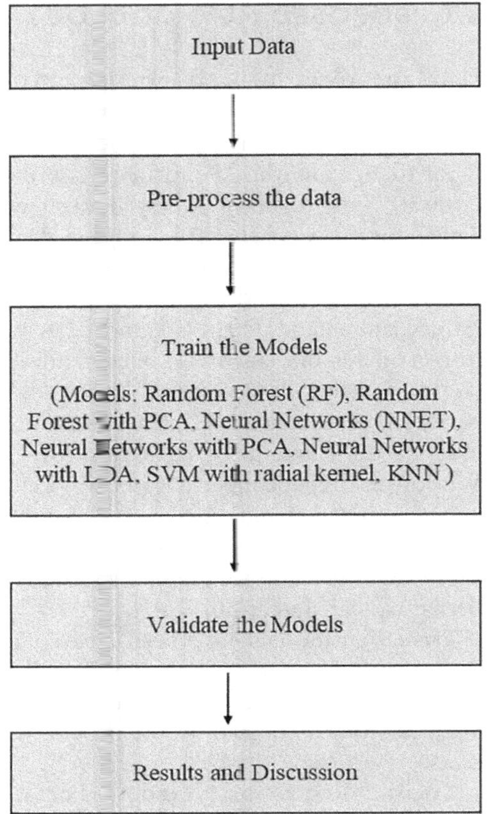

Figure 2.2 Overall architecture diagram.

2.3.1 Logistic Regression

In a linear regression, it is inappropriate to forecast the dependent variable using only the independent variable and the hyperplane that has been generated. Logistic Regression is therefore used when working with categorical data. Rather than forecasting continuous variables, Logistic Regression is used to make predictions about the truth or falsehood of an outcome. It serves as a classification tool. In Logistic Regression, the independent variable of the dependent variable is transformed using the sigmoid function, resulting in a probability expression ranging from 0 to 1. Because it offers probabilities and can categorize fresh samples using both continuous and discrete measures, Logistic Regression is frequently employed in machine learning. The assumption that the dependent and independent variables are linear, however, is a drawback of Logistic Regression. In some circumstances, this presumption may be problematic.

2.3.2 Random Forest

Multiple Decision Trees form the supervised learning method known as Random Forest. With a hierarchical structure, Decision Trees have nodes that indicate certain conditions on a collection of features and branches that segment the options and lead to leaf nodes. The leaf nodes are given their respective class labels. Both conditional inference tree methods and recursive partitioning can be used to build Decision Trees. Recursive partitioning involves deciding whether to divide or not split each node based on checks of attribute value, which results in the learning of the tree. The recursion stops when all members of a subset at a node have the same target variable value. Conditional Inference Tree, a statistical method, addresses multiple testing issues and utilizes non-parametric tests as splitting criteria to avoid overfitting. Since Random Forest can handle missing values, continuous, categorical, and binary data, it is appropriate for high-dimensional data modeling. However, it should be tuned carefully as it tends to overfit. It is worth noting that the size of the trees in Random Forest can consume significant memory, which can be a consideration for large datasets.

2.3.3 K-Nearest Neighbor

A straightforward and well-liked supervised learning technique in machine learning is K-Nearest Neighbor (KNN). Assuming that new and old examples are equivalent, it places the new instance in the category that is closest to the old ones. KNN categorizes new data points by assessing how similar they are to previously stored data points. The algorithm works by identifying the data points closest to the new point based on their distances. There are several ways to compute this distance, with specialists typically using the Euclidean distance. After that, a predetermined amount of points are divided into separate groups according to how close they are to one another. An odd number of points are selected in KNN, particularly when there are two classes. The majority vote among the nearest points determines the category assigned to the new data point. KNN is a straightforward technique and can handle large datasets. However, it has significant computational costs as the distance between each training sample and every data point must be calculated. Additionally, determining the value of K, the number of nearest neighbors, can impact the complexity of the algorithm.

2.3.4 Neural networks (NNET)

ANNisa biological neural network based mathematical model. In an ANN, nodes and edges are referred to as neurons and synapses, respectively. Neurons receive input data through weighted synapses, perform calculations, and either represent the results or pass them to subsequent neurons for further processing. The connections between neurons in neural networks are characterized by weights, which are adjusted through the learning process by iteratively processing data points. The neural network can be used to forecast classes or quantities for new input data points, including regression tasks, once all the weights have been learned. Neural networks have the capability to learn complex models, and they can act as "black boxes" without the need for extensive feature engineering prior to model training. Additionally, by employing a "deep" approach, more sophisticated models can be constructed and combined, enabling the discovery of new possibilities.

2.3.5 Support Vector Machine

The support vector machine (SVM) method looks for a hyperplane that may effectively split data points into several groups in an N-dimensional space, where N is the number of features. Any of the possible hyperplanes can be used to split the two classes of data points. Finding the hyperplane with the largest margin—which represents the biggest separation between data points from the two classes—is the aim. Hyperplanes, which are these decision boundaries, help categorize the data points. It is possible to designate distinct classes to each side of the hyperplane. The number of features also affects the hyperplane's size. Support vectors are the data points that are near the hyperplane and have an impact on its orientation and position. The classifier's margin can be raised by utilizing these support vectors. If we remove the support vectors, the hyperplane's position will change. Among the finest classifiers is SVM when dealing with high-dimensional data that has a clear separation margin. Due to its lengthier training requirements, it might not be appropriate for huge datasets, and noisy data tends to negatively impact its performance.

2.3.6 Naive Bayes

The Naive Bayes classifier, a probabilistic algorithm that applies the Bayes theorem and is predicated on the notion of strong (naive) independence, is among the best classification methods. It is assumed that the values of the features are independent of each other given the class variable. The classifier selects the class to which a given tuple belongs based on the highest likelihood. The Naive Bayes classifier is a supervised learning algorithm used in classification applications. Despite its simplicity, the Naive Bayes classifier is a very effective machine learning algorithm that is used in many diverse applications. Its application in practical settings is limited by the naive belief that each predictor or characteristic is independent. The "zero-frequency problem" is a flaw in the Naive Bayes method that results in the algorithm returning a category for a categorical variable that was absent from the training dataset but present with a zero probability in the test dataset. This difficulty can be resolved by applying a smoothing strategy. Another problem is that Naive Bayes requires large datasets to achieve optimal accuracy.

2.4 RESULTS AND DISCUSSION

This analysis makes use of the UC Irvine Machine Learning Repository's Breast Cancer Wisconsin (Diagnostic) Data Set. The data was collected by the University of Wisconsin in 1993 and comprises biopsy results from 569 patients at Wisconsin Hospital. The dataset consists of 569 instances, each containing 32 attributes. The objective is to forecast the presence or absence of cancer based on the provided features, and the qualities contain information about both cancerous and non-cancerous cells. The value of each attribute is displayed numerically. The "Target" variable indicates whether a patient has been diagnosed with "Benign" or "Malignant" cancer. A value of "Malignant" signifies the presence of cancer, while "Benign" indicates the absence of cancer. The key particulars about the dataset are:

- Class distribution: 357 instances classified as benign; 212 instances classified as malignant
- Number of instances: 569
- Number of attributes: 32, including an ID number and the diagnosis

Numerous real-valued properties including radius, texture, area, perimeter, compactness, smoothness, concave spots, concavity, symmetry, and fractal dimension are present in the dataset. Figures 2.3 to 2.14 and Table 2.1 illustrate the findings and conclusions.

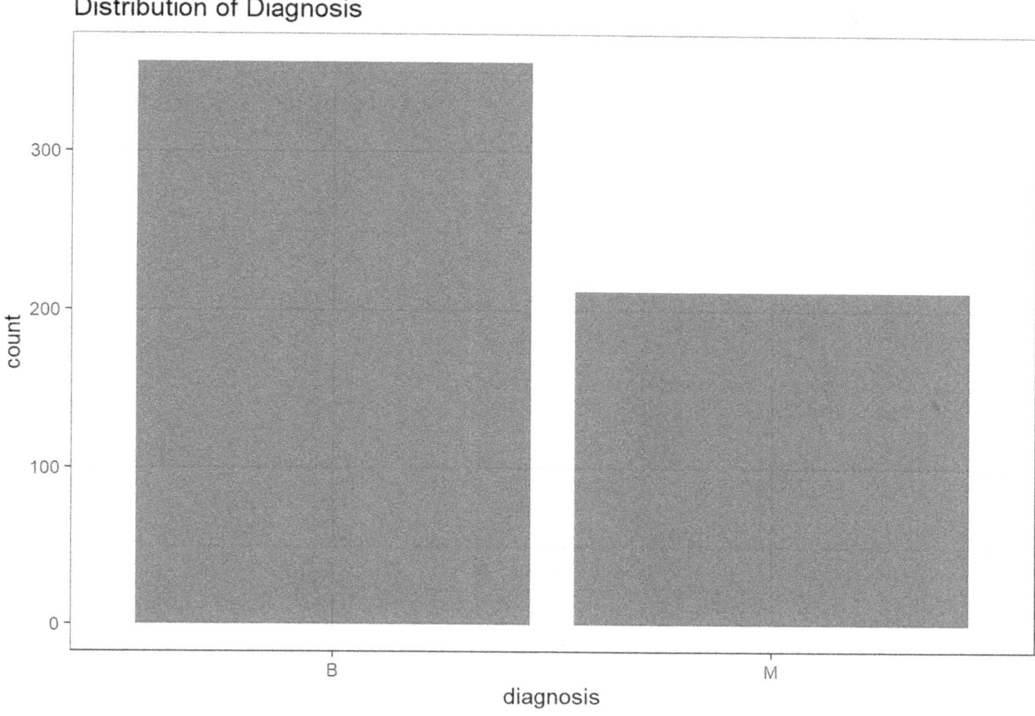

Figure 2.3 Distribution of diagnosis (target variable).

INFERENCE: Diagnosis is the target variable, which is slightly unbalanced.

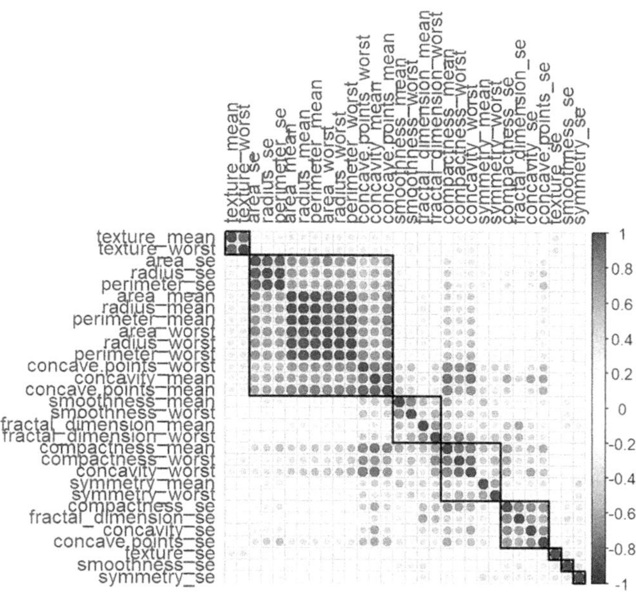

Figure 2.4 Correlation among multiple factors.

INFERENCE: The graph illustrates the presence of strong correlations among multiple factors. The performance of different methods is enhanced when strongly correlated features are eliminated from the dataset. The models can concentrate on the most insightful and independent factors by removing duplicate or strongly correlated characteristics, which improves performance and accuracy.

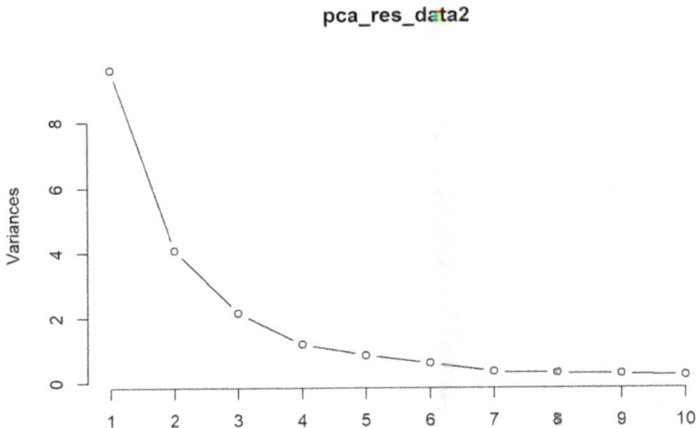

Figure 2.5 Variance.

INFERENCE: Principal Component Analysis (PCA)'s main objective is to keep as much variance as feasible while reducing the dimensionality of a dataset with many variables that are weakly or strongly connected. Principal components (PCs), a new collection of orthogonal variables created by altering the original variables, are used to achieve this. As we move down the order of principal components, the amount of variance retained from the original variables decreases. PCA allows for a more concise representation of the data while preserving the most important information.

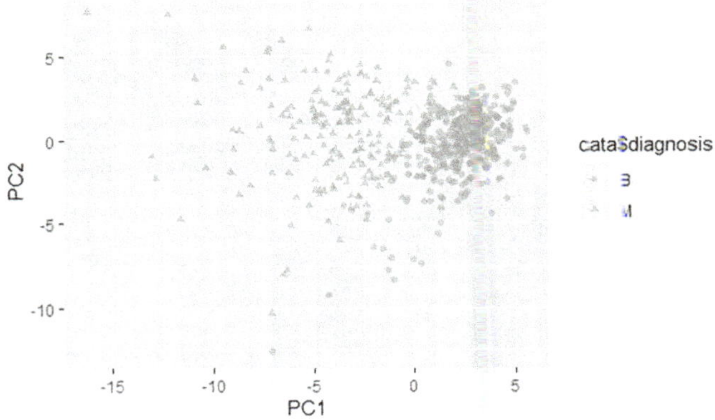

Figure 2.6 Principal components.

INFERENCE: The data of the first two components exhibit clear separation into two distinct classes. This separation is attributed to the relatively low variance explained by these components. Due to the limited overlap between the classes, the data can be easily distinguished and classified accurately.

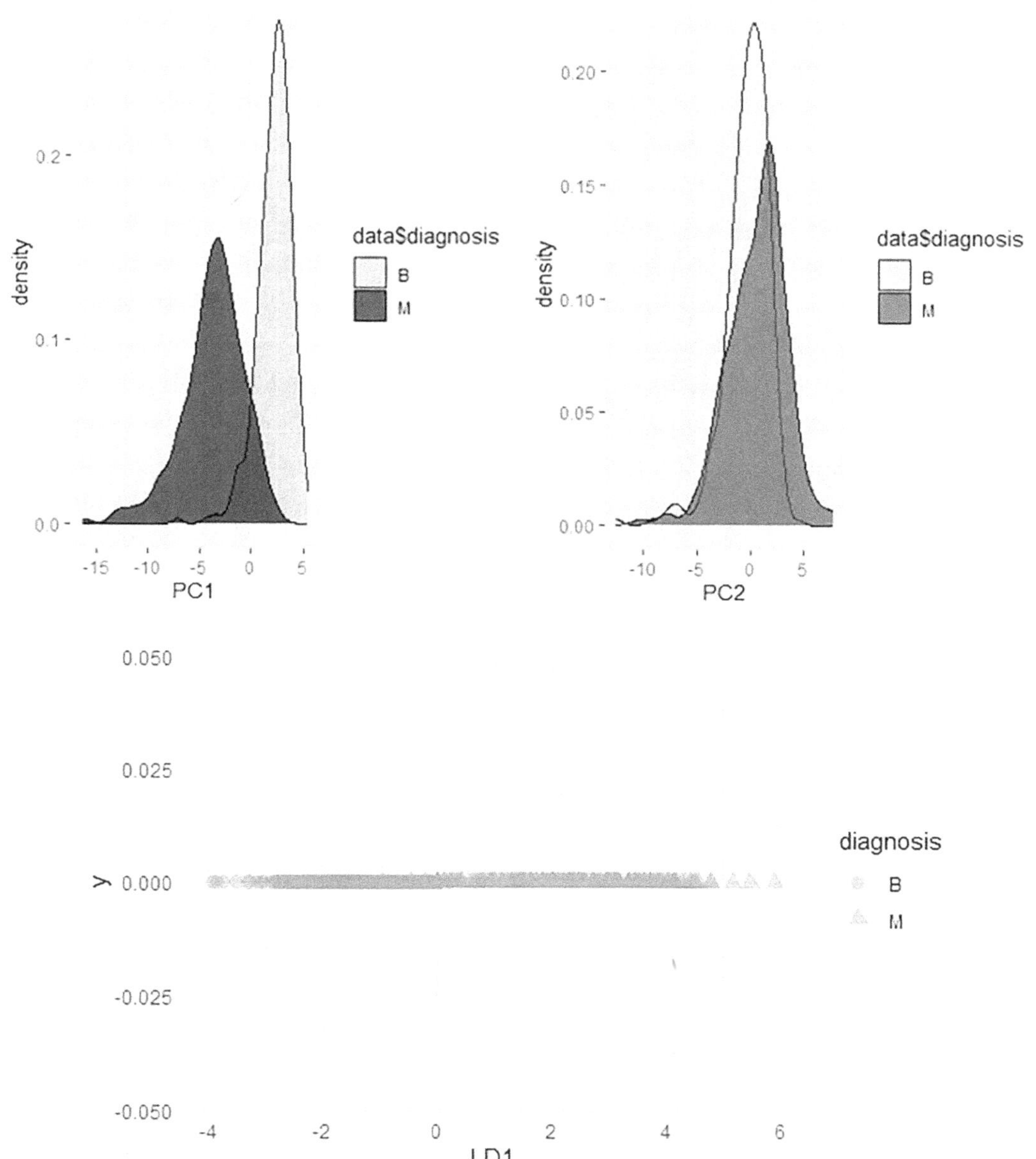

Figure 2.7 Linear discriminant analysis.

INFERENCE: A statistical technique called linear discriminant analysis (LDA) analyzes the distribution of predictors separately within each answer class. The Bayes theorem is then used to calculate the likelihood of class membership. It is crucial to remember that LDA considers each class to have a normal distribution with a unique mean and shared variance. LDA aims to find the linear combination of predictors that best distinguishes between various response classes by examining the distribution of predictors.

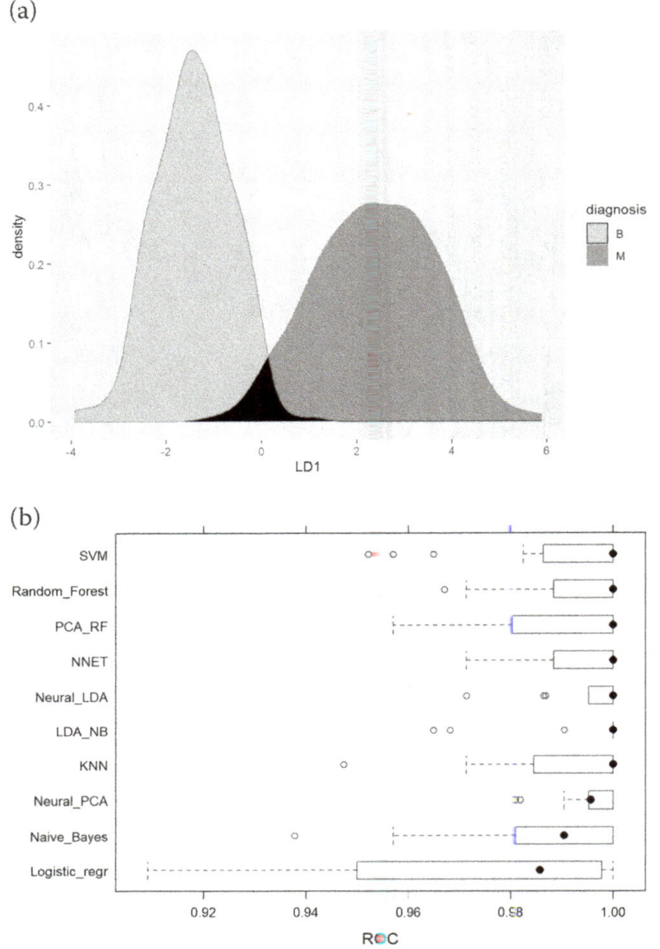

Figure 2.8 (a) and (b) ROC (receiver operating characteristic).

INFERENCE: The Receiver Operating Characteristic (ROC) shows how well a classification model performs at different categorization criteria. For various threshold values, it displays the relationship between the Sensitivity and Specificity. One popular statistic for evaluating the effectiveness of the model is the area under the ROC curve (AUC). Regardless of the set threshold, the AUC shows the model's overall capacity to distinguish between the positive and negative classes. It offers a single value that sums up the predictive ability of the model, making it a reliable evaluation metric.

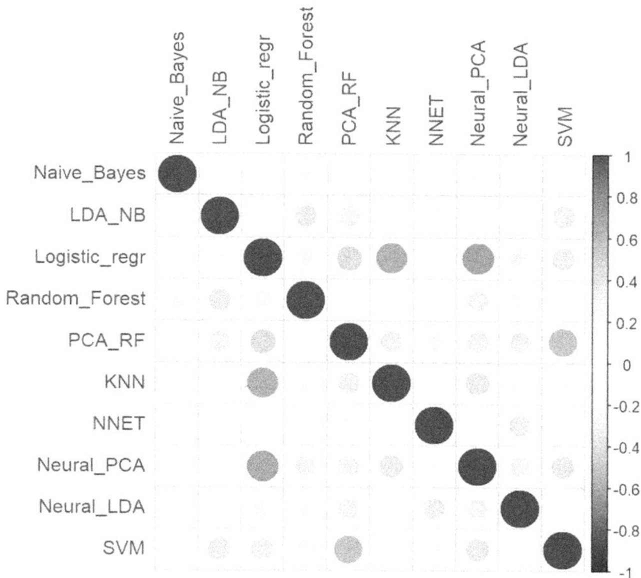

Figure 2.9 Correlation plot.

INFERENCE: Correlation Plot

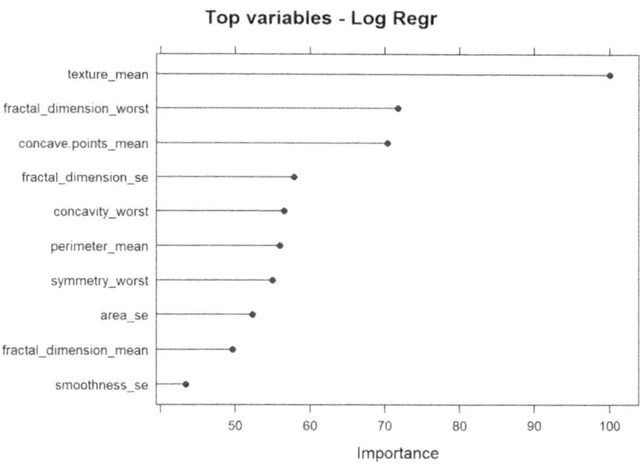

Figure 2.10 Logistic regression.

INFERENCE: The plot earlier showcases the essential variables that contribute significantly to the model and enable accurate predictions in Logistic Regression. These variables have been identified as the most influential factors for achieving the best prediction performance.

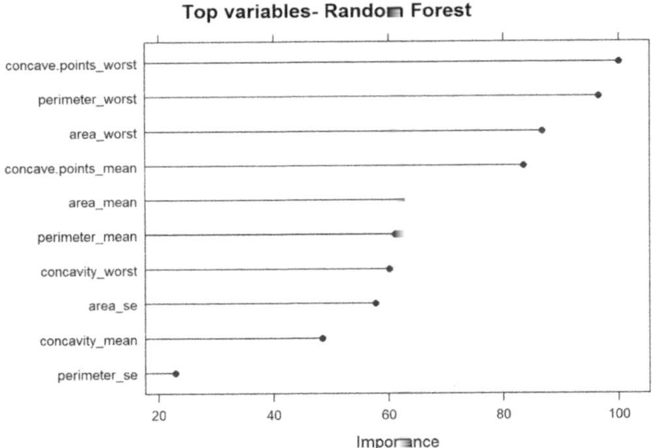

Figure 2.11 Random Forest.

INFERENCE: The plot earlier displays the most critical variables that enable accurate predictions and have the highest contribution to the Random Forest model. These variables have been identified as the key factors for achieving optimal prediction performance.

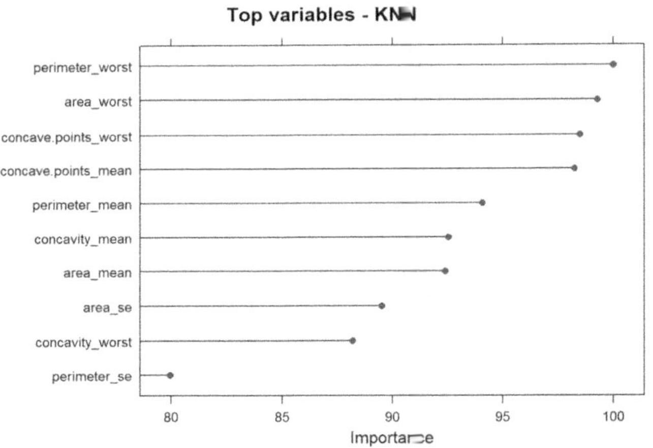

Figure 2.12 KNN.

INFERENCE: The plot earlier showcases the essential variables that enable optimal prediction and have the greatest impact on the KNN model. These variables have been identified as the most influential factors for achieving accurate predictions.

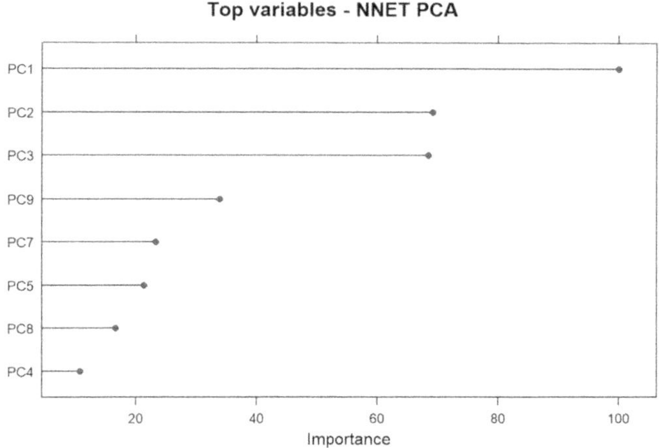

Figure 2.13 Neural networks PCA.

INFERENCE: The figure earlier highlights the critical elements that are essential to making the best prediction and that significantly contribute to the NNET model. These variables have been identified as the most influential factors for accurate predictions.

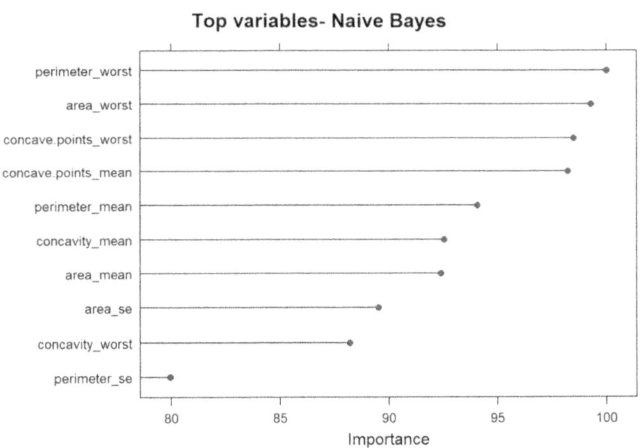

Figure 2.14 Naive Bayes.

INFERENCE: The plot earlier displays the crucial variables that contribute significantly to the prediction and have the highest impact on the Naive Bayes model. These variables have been identified as the most important for accurate predictions (Table 2.1).

Accuracy serves as the baseline for evaluating a model's performance in classification tasks. It determines what proportion of all of the model's forecasts were correct. A higher accuracy number indicates a more accurate model.

Precision, which is also known as the Positive Predictive Value (PPV), focuses on how reliable positive predictions are. It determines the percentage of true positive predictions out of all the anticipated positive events. A model with a higher accuracy value and fewer false positives is considered more accurate.

Table 2.1 (a) and (b) Performance metrics of all the models

(a)

Metric	***Naive Bayes***	***LDA_NB***	***Logistic_regr***	***Random Forest***	***PCA_RF***	***KNN***	***NNET***	***Neural PCA***	***Neural_LDA***	***SVM***
Sensitivity	0.9047619	0.9285714	1.0000000	0.9761905	0.9523810	0.9285714	0.9523810	1.0000000	0.9761905	0.9523810
Specificity	0.9577465	0.9859155	0.9436620	0.9859155	0.9718310	1.0000000	0.9859155	0.9718310	0.9859155	0.9718310
PosPred Value	0.9268293	0.9750000	0.9130435	0.9761905	0.9523810	1.0000000	0.9756098	0.9545455	0.9761905	0.9523810
NegPred Value	0.9444444	0.9589041	1.0000000	0.9859155	0.9718310	0.9594595	0.9722222	1.0000000	0.9859155	0.9718310
Precision	0.9268293	0.9750000	0.9130435	0.9761905	0.9523810	1.0000000	0.9756098	0.9545455	0.9761905	0.9523810
Recall	0.9047619	0.9285714	1.0000000	0.9761905	0.9523810	0.9285714	0.9523810	1.0000000	0.9761905	0.9523810
F1	0.9156627	0.9512195	0.9545455	0.9761905	0.9523810	0.9629630	0.9638554	0.9767442	0.9761905	0.9523810
Prevalence	0.3716814	0.3716814	0.3716814	0.3716814	0.3716814	0.3716814	0.3716814	0.3716814	0.3716814	0.3716814
Detection Rate	0.3362832	0.3451327	0.3716814	0.3628319	0.3539823	0.3451327	0.3539823	0.3716814	0.3628319	0.3539823
Detection Prevalence	0.3628319	0.3539823	0.4070796	0.3716814	0.3716814	0.3451327	0.3628319	0.3893805	0.3716814	0.3716814
Balanced Accuracy	0.9312542	0.9572435	0.9718310	0.9810530	0.9621060	0.9642857	0.9691482	0.9859155	0.9810530	0.9621060

(b)

Sl. No.	***Metric***	***Best_model***	***Value***
1	Sensitivity	Logistic_regr	1.0000000
2	Specificity	KNN	1.0000000
3	PosPred Value	KNN	1.0000000
4	NegPred Value	Neural_PCA	1.0000000
5	Precision	KNN	1.0000000
6	Recall	Neural_PCA	1.0000000
7	F1	Neural_PCA	0.9767442
8	Prevalence	Random_Forest	0.3716814
9	Detection Rate	Logistic_regr	0.3716814
10	Detection Prevalence	Logistic_regr	0.4070796
11	Balanced Accuracy	Neural_PCA	0.9859155

Remember, also known as Sensitivity or True Positive Rate, is the model's ability to accurately classify positive events. It determines the proportion of real positive projections among the actual positive examples. Recall is calculated by dividing the total number of true positives by the sum of true positives and false negatives. A greater recall score indicates fewer false negatives, which is a measure of the model's effectiveness in recognizing positive cases. The precision and recall products are multiplied by two to get the F1 Score, which is then divided by both precision and recall. The F1 score comes in handy when the dataset is imbalanced and the percentage of positive and negative examples changes considerably.

The Neural Network with LDA model has an outstanding F1 score in the diagnosis of breast cancer, indicating that it can accurately and reliably identify cases of malignant breast cancer. This model's high sensitivity in identifying events that have a favorable influence makes it a valuable tool for the early identification and detection of breast cancer.

2.5 CONCLUSION

The second most prevalent cause of cancer-related fatalities in women is breast cancer, which affects more women than any other type of cancer. There is a dearth of research on data cleaning and pruning strategies to prepare datasets for mining, despite the fact that numerous studies have examined classification algorithms for breast cancer prediction. A high-quality dataset has been found to increase accuracy, and choosing the right algorithms based on such datasets can result in the development of prediction systems. These tools can be used to determine the best course of action for breast cancer patients. Treatment choices depending on breast cancer stage can be informed by knowledge extracted from pertinent databases using data mining and machine learning approaches.

The Wisconsin Madison Breast Cancer Diagnosis Problem was employed in this work as a job for pattern categorization. Naive Bayes, Support Vector Machine (SVM), Neural Networks (NNET), Random Forest (RF), K Nearest Neighbors (KNN), and Logistic Regression were among the machine learning models that were assessed. To identify the linear combination of features that distinguishes between two or more classes, linear discriminant analysis was used. The model with the highest accuracy and most sensitivity (low false-negative rate) was found. When the models were compared in terms of precision, accuracy, and dataset size, it was discovered that neural networks employing Linear Discriminant Analysis (LDA) performed better than the methods currently in use. In terms of F1 score, sensitivity, and balanced accuracy, the Neural Network with LDA model showed the best results, attaining values.

Hypothesis testing was done to compare the performance metrics of the Neural Network with the LDA model to other models in order to further support the claim that the Neural Network with LDA model greatly outperformed other methodologies. The alternative hypothesis is that the Neural Network with the LDA model performs much better than the other models, rejecting the null hypothesis that there is no discernible difference in performance amongst the models. The observed performance differences were found to be statistically significant after applying the proper statistical tests and computing p-values.

Confidence intervals were also calculated in order to determine the range of values that the genuine performance metrics of the models are likely to fall within. The confidence intervals of the Neural Network with the LDA model do not overlap with those of other models, which provide further evidence of its superiority.

The study can be further extended by exploring the use of imbalanced approaches before analysis, computation of ROC (AUC), and the consideration of various stacking models.

2.6 FUTURE RESEARCH AND FUTURE SCOPE

Imbalanced datasets are common in medical applications and the class imbalance occurs when one class (e.g., malignant cases) is significantly outnumbered by the other class (e.g., benign cases). This presents a number of difficulties that may affect how well machine learning models work. Because it is more prevalent in the dataset, machine learning models frequently favor the majority class. Consequently, the minority class may be overlooked, leading to lower sensitivity and accuracy for detecting the critical class (e.g., malignant cases). Since a classifier that consistently predicts the majority class could nonetheless achieve high accuracy, traditional accuracy may not be an effective evaluation metric for imbalanced datasets. AUC-ROC, F1 score, and the precision-recall curve are superior measures for evaluating the performance of the model. Undersampling, which involves removing samples from the majority class to balance the dataset, can result in the loss of pertinent data and hinder the model's capacity to recognize significant patterns. The true distribution of the minority class may not be captured by oversampling approaches (like SMOTE) that replicate or create synthetic samples of the minority class.

To mitigate the challenges posed by imbalanced datasets, appropriate sampling or data augmentation techniques can be employed. To create a balanced dataset, samples from the majority class can be eliminated. This can help minimize bias. However, as previously mentioned, it might result in the loss of important data. Generating synthetic samples or duplicating existing ones for the minority class can help balance the dataset. By extrapolating characteristics from existing minority class samples, methods like the Synthetic Minority Over-sampling Technique (SMOTE) produce synthetic samples. Many machine learning algorithms allow assigning different weights to classes. By assigning higher weights to the minority class, the model pays more attention to correctly classifying the minority samples. Ensemble models like Random Forest and Boosting algorithms (e.g., AdaBoost) can be used, as they are naturally less affected by class imbalance and can provide more robust predictions. The potential consequences and impact of developing a trustworthy machine learning and data mining-based breast cancer prediction system are substantial. A robust prediction system can aid in early breast cancer detection, allowing for timely interventions and potentially improving patient survival rates. Machine learning models can analyze patient-specific data to recommend tailored treatment plans based on the individual's characteristics and cancer stage. By lowering the need for expensive treatments in advanced stages, early detection and individualized treatment programs may result in cost savings for patients and healthcare providers. Integrating the system into clinical practice can serve as an additional tool for healthcare professionals, providing them with valuable insights to make well-informed decisions. The predictive system can contribute to ongoing research by providing a vast amount of data that can be anonymized and used for further analysis and advancement of medical knowledge. With advancements in telemedicine and digital health, a reliable breast cancer prediction system can be made accessible to patients and healthcare providers worldwide, thereby bridging the gap in healthcare disparities.

However, it is essential to ensure ethical considerations, data privacy, and transparent communication with patients regarding the use of their medical data. The integration of such systems into clinical practice should always be done in collaboration with medical experts to ensure safe and effective implementation. Continuous monitoring and updating of the system based on new data and research are crucial to maintain its accuracy and relevance in clinical settings.

REFERENCES

1. Omondiagbe D.A., Veeramani S. and Sidhu A.S., "Machine Learning Classification Techniques for Breast CancerDiagnosis", IOP Conference Series: Materials Science and Engineering. Vol. 495, pp. 1–16. IOP Publishing (2019).
2. Ak, M.F. "A Comparative Analysis of Breast Cancer Detection and Diagnosis Using Data Visualization and Machine Learning Applications", Healthcare 2020, 8, 111, pp. 1–23.
3. Wadkar K., Pathak P. and Wagh N., "Breast Cancer Detection Using ANN Network and Performance Analysis with SVM", International Journal of Computer Engineering and Technology (2019), 10, 75–86.
4. Reddy Vaka A., Soni B. and Reddy S., "Breast Cancer Detection by Leveraging Machine Learning", Ict Express (2020), 6(4), pp. 320–324.
5. Tiwari M., Bharuka R., Shah P. and Lokare R., "Breast Cancer Prediction Using Deep Learning and Machine Learning Techniques", (March 22, 2020). Available at SSRN: https://ssrn.com/abstract=3558786
6. Nahid A.-A. and Kong Y., "Involvement of Machine Learning for Breast Cancer Image Classification: A Survey", Computational and Mathematical Methods in Medicine (2017), 2017, 1–29.
7. Kashif M., et al. "Breast Cancer Detection and Diagnostic with Convolutional Neural Networks." Artificial Intelligence and Internet of Things. CRC Press (2021), 65–84.
8. Vasundhara S.., Kiranmayee B.V. and Chalumuru S., "Machine Learning Approach for Breast Cancer Prediction", International Journal of Recent Technology and Engineering (IJRTE) (2019), 10, 98–103.
9. Ak M.F., "A Comparative Analysis of Breast Cancer Detection and Diagnosis Using Data Visualization and Machine Learning Applications", Healthcare, MDPI (2020), 8, 1–23.
10. Sivapriya J., Aravind Kumar V., SiddarthSai S. and Sriram S., "Breast Cancer Prediction Using Machine Learning", International Journal of Recent Technology and Engineering (IJRTE) (2019), 8, 4879–4881.
11. Asri H., Mousannifb H., Al Moatassime H. and Noeld T., "Using Machine Learning Algorithms for Breast Cancer Risk Prediction and Diagnosis", Procedia Computer Science (2016), 83, 1064–1069.
12. Bazazeh D. and Shubair R., "Comparative Study of Machine Learning Algorithms for Breast Cancer Detection and Diagnosis", IEEE International Conference on Electronic Devices, Systems and Applications (ICEDSA) (2016).
13. Mirajkar P. and Lakshmi P., "Prediction of Cancer Risk in Perspective of Symptoms using Naive Bayes Classifier", International Journal of Engineering Research in Computer Science and Engineering (2017), 4(9), 145–149.
14. Majali J., Niranjan R., Phatak V. and Tadakhe O., "Data Mining Techniques for Diagnosis and Prognosis of Cancer", International Journal of Advanced Research in Computer and Communication Engineering (2015), 4(3), 613–616.
15. Chaurasia V. and Pal S., "A Novel Approach for Breast Cancer Detection Using Data Mining Techniques", International Journal of Innovative Research in Computer and Communication Engineering (2014), 2, 2456–2465.
16. Zand H.K., "A Comparative Survey on Data Mining Techniques for Breast Cancer Diagnosis and Prediction", Indian Journal of Fundamental and Applied Life Sciences (2015), 5, 4330–4339.
17. Padmapriya B. and Velmurugan T., "Classification Algorithm Based Analysis of Breast Cancer Data", International Journal of Data Mining Techniques and Applications (2016), 5, 43–49.
18. Chidambaranathan S., "Breast Cancer Diagnosis Based on Feature Extraction by Hybrid of k-Means and Extreme Learning Machine Algorithms", ARPN Journal of Engineering and Applied Sciences (2016), 11, 4581–4586.
19. Gupta S., Kumar D. and Sharma A., "Data Mining Classification Techniques Applied for Breast Cancer Diagnosis and Prognosis", Indian Journal of Computer Science and Engineering (2011), 2, 188–195.

20. Chandrasekar R.M., Palaniammal V. and Phil M., "Performance and Evaluation of Data Mining Techniques in Cancer Diagnosis", IOSR Journal of Computer Engineering (2013), 15, 39–44.
21. Joshi J., Doshi R. and Patel J., "Diagnosis and Prognosis Breast Cancer Using Classification Rules", International Journal of Engineering Research and General Science (2014), 2, 315–323.
22. Bellaachia A. and Guven E., "Predicting Breast Cancer Survivability Using Data Mining Techniques" IOSR Journal of Dental and Medical Sciences (2006), 1–4.
23. Sumbaly R., Vishnusri N. and Jeyalatha S., "Diagnosis of Breast Cancer Using Decision Tree Data Mining Technique", International Journal of Computer Applications (2014), 98, 16–24.
24. Sivakami K., "Mining Big Data: Breast Cancer Prediction Using DT-SVM Hybrid Model", International Journal of Scientific Engineering and Applied Science (2015), 1, 418–429.
25. Lavanya D. and Rani K.U., "Ensemble Decision Tree Classifier for Breast Cancer Data", International Journal of Information Technology Convergence and Services (2016), 2(1), 17–24.

Chapter 3

Advanced deep learning algorithms for early ocular disease detection using fundus images

Shubhashree A[1], *Divya B S*[1], *and Thompson Stephan*[2]

[1]Department of Computer Science and Engineering, M S Ramaiah University of Applied Sciences, Bengaluru, Karnataka, India

[2]Department of Computer Science and Engineering, Graphic Era Deemed to be University, Dehradun, Uttarakhand, India

3.1 INTRODUCTION

Ocular diseases (ODs) that can result in blindness have become incredibly common during the past twenty years. Examples include trachoma, cataracts, untreated refractive errors, diabetic retinopathy, age-related macular degeneration, and DR. According to a recent World Health Organization (WHO) assessment on vision, more than 2.2 billion individuals worldwide are visually impaired. At least 45% of these incidents might have been avoided or still need to be resolved [1]. Any ailment or disorder that impairs the eye's ability to function normally or negatively affects the eye's visual acuity is referred to as an ocular disease. Almost everyone experiences visual issues at some point in their lives. Others require the care of a specialist, while others are amateurs that do not appear on reports or may be handled at home [2]. Globally, fundus problems are the main reason why people go blind. The most prevalent eye diseases are age-related macular degeneration, cataract, glaucoma, and diabetic retinopathy (DR) (AMD). By 2030, there will be over 400 million people with DR, per related research [3]. These eye conditions are becoming a significant worldwide health issue. Most importantly, the ophthalmic condition is fatal and may leave patients permanently blind. In clinical settings, early detection of these illnesses can prevent visual damage. The number of ophthalmologists and the number of patients, however, is significantly out of proportion. Additionally, manually evaluating the fundus takes a lot of time and is highly dependent on the expertise of ophthalmologists. This makes thorough fundus screening more challenging. Therefore, automated computer-aided diagnostic methods are essential for identifying eye problems. This is a typical misconception [3]. Globally, there is a vast range in the prevalence of eye disorders based on characteristics including age, gender, employment, lifestyle, economic status, cleanliness, habits, and conventions. According to research that studied individuals in tropical and temperate countries, irresistible eye infections are more common in tropical populations because of variables including dust, humidity, sunshine, and other natural elements [4]. Additionally, eye disorders present themselves in communities differently in developing and industrialized nations. There are substantial rates of ocular morbidity in many developing nations, notably in Asia, which are underdiagnosed and neglected [5]. Globally, 285 million individuals are estimated to have visual impairments, of which 246 million are estimated to have poor eyesight and 39 million to be blind [6]. The World Health Organization (WHO) estimates that 2.2 billion individuals worldwide have a close-up or distant vision issue [7]. Estimates suggest that half of these situations might have been avoided or resolved. In addition to those who have near vision impairment due to uncorrected presbyopia (826 million), there are 1 billion people who have moderate-to-severe distance vision impairment or blindness because

DOI: 10.1201/9781003369059-4

of untreated cataract (94 million), glaucoma (7.7 million), corneal opacities (4.2 million), diabetic retinopathy (3.9 million), and trachoma (2 million) [8]. The primary causes of visual impairment include uncorrected refractive errors, cataracts, age-related macular degeneration, glaucoma, diabetic retinopathy, corneal opacity, trachoma, hypertension, and other conditions [9]. Extraordinarily little study has been done on the prevalence of blindness and visual impairment in Bangladesh. Most of the population of the nation lives in rural areas. Over 80% of people who live in cities nowadays need medical attention, yet there aren't many ophthalmology services available. Although there are more businesses providing services for blindness, the incidence is still low [10]. Figure 3.1 shows the different retinal color fundus images with different ODs.

Ocular illness identification is time-consuming and expensive since it is entirely thorough and necessitates several sessions for a patient to go through. A map of high-risk groups and the quick diagnosis of ocular illness may both be possible with an automated diagnostic technique. Our motivation is to lower the risk to doctors by using this automated tool, which is quick to interpret the results and a patient may not experience continuous trauma by attending many sessions scheduled by the eye care professionals. This method may also be cost-effective because it lowers the risk that patients with cataracts or other eye-related diseases will harm themselves. The proposed work in this chapter attempts to develop an automated digital system for the diagnosis process that distinguishes between subjects with normal vision and those with ocular illness. It offers a desktop program with a graphical user interface (GUI) where the user may submit a test image of the eye and get findings with predictions on the GUI. The prognosis, the planning of the treatment, and correct second opinions to clinicians regarding the biological origin of the eye ailment all depend on accurate screening of ocular disease/normal patients. The entire process would be automated using DL, which is quick and efficient. The low socioeconomic group would have fewer visits and less treatment burden as a result.

The goal of the study is to simultaneously diagnose interleaved ODs from color fundus images using an ML-CAD framework based on DL. Utilizing a current, widely accessible ML dataset (RFMiD), which comprises a wide range of difficult ocular disorders, the

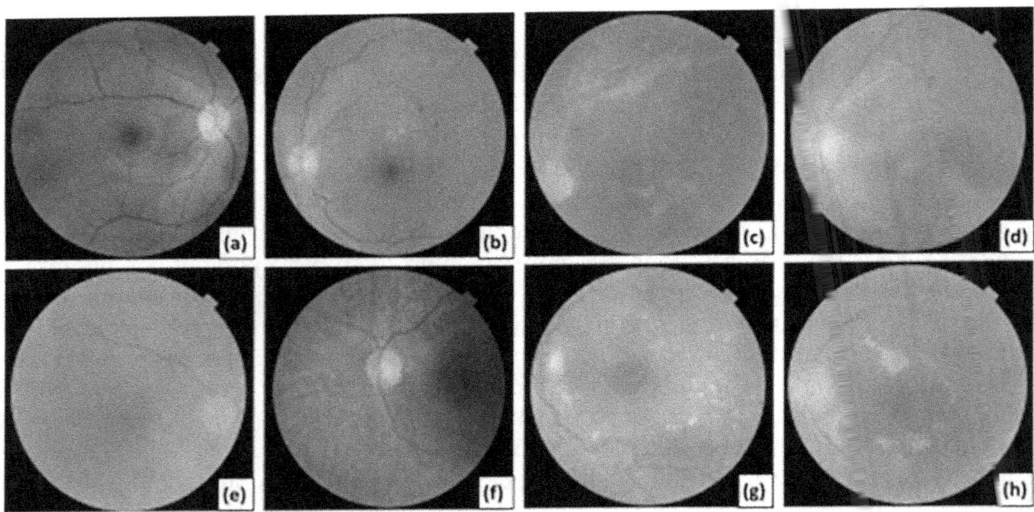

Figure 3.1 Different retinal color fundus images with different ODs. (a) Normal, (b) DR, (c) RT, (d) MH and MS, (e) MH and DN, (f) MH, MYA, and ODC, (g) DR, LS, and TV, and (h) EDN, ODP, and TSLN.

usefulness of the proposed framework is confirmed. Using five different indicators, we evaluate the performance of the suggested framework in comparison to that of other frameworks and built-in models. The experimental findings show how useful and better the suggested framework is. The suggested framework can identify more than 29 ODs, in contrast to existing numerous ocular disorders frameworks that can only identify ten ODs.

3.1.1 Application requirements and constraints

1. High-level requirements for the proposed work:
   - An application with an intuitive user interface that automates the diagnosis of Ocular disease and Cognitive Normal subjects.
   - Provides an option to save the predictions for future references.
   - Privileges the user to view the uploaded image, which helps in cross-verification of the uploaded image.
2. Constraints for the proposed work:
   - Data is not stored in a database, and hence the data is not centralized.
   - The application is a stand-alone desktop application.
   - The application is supported by the Windows operating system.

3.2 METHODOLOGY

The proposed work aims to enhance performance and automate the classification of subjects with multiple ocular diseases, utilizing the Transfer learning method in conjunction with various deep learning architectures, learning rates, and optimizers, all applied to the Ocular Disease Intelligent Recognition (ODIR) dataset. The objectives encompasses initial data pre-processing, which included image tagging and flipping for dataset diversification, as well as the enhancement of image visibility through contrast-limited adaptive histogram equalization (CLAHE). Four distinct deep learning models (VGG-19, MobileNet-v2, EfficientNetB3, and ResNet-34) were reconstructed using transfer learning with a focus on decreasing learning rates and using different optimizers. Additionally, the trained model is deployed on the Gradio App for prediction purposes. The research process involves a literature survey, comprehensive data pre-processing, deep learning model selection and evaluation, UI finalization, and the subsequent development and integration of the chosen UI with the classification model to create an executable file. This chapter soughts to contribute to the field of multi-label classification of ocular diseases by harnessing advanced deep learning techniques and transfer learning, ultimately delivering an efficient, user-friendly solution for disease diagnosis and classification. The organized ophthalmic database, known as Ocular Disease Intelligent Recognition (ODIR), comprises data from 5,000 individuals. This dataset encompasses age information, color fundus images of both the left and right eyes, and diagnostic keywords provided by medical professionals. ODIR‘s primary objective is to offer a comprehensive representation of real-life patient data collected from various hospitals and healthcare institutions throughout China. Shanggong Medical Technology Co., Ltd. has meticulously compiled this dataset. These healthcare organizations utilize a variety of commercially available cameras, such as Canon, Zeiss, and Kowa, to capture fundus images, resulting in varying image resolutions. To ensure data quality, trained human assessors meticulously assigned labels to the annotations. Patients were categorized into one of eight groups, including "normal," "diabetes," "glaucoma," "cataract," "AMD," "hypertension," "myopia," and "other diseases/abnormalities." The architectural design of the proposed system is visually represented in Figure 3.2. The flow of data within this architecture is

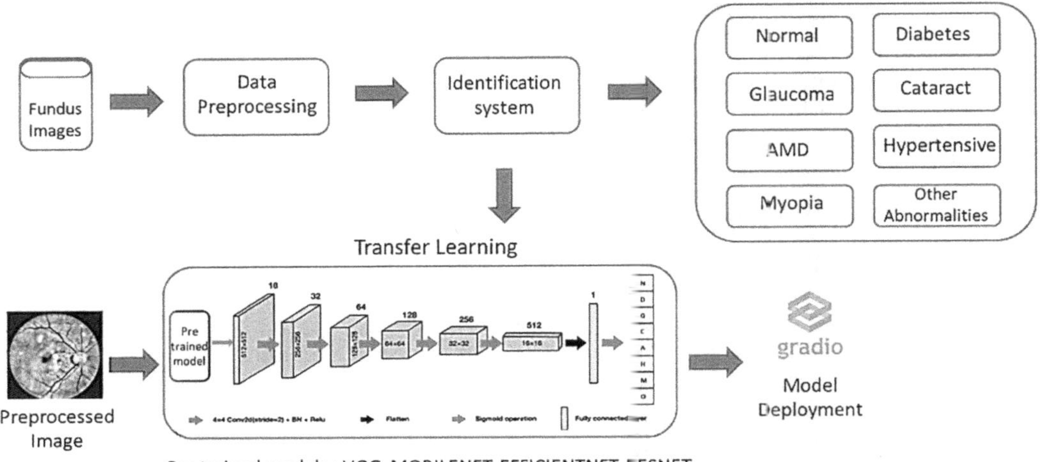

Figure 3.2 Architectural design of the proposed system.

comprehensively depicted in Figure 3.3. Additionally, Figure 3.4 provides an illustrative sample data frame, allowing for a detailed understanding of the data structure. Furthermore, the graphical representations in Figure 3.5 vividly showcase the diagnostic distributions, providing valuable insights into the distribution patterns of the diagnostic categories.

3.3 LEVERAGING TRANSFER LEARNING IN MACHINE LEARNING

Transfer learning represents a valuable approach in machine learning, where instead of initiating the development of a deep neural network from scratch for a particular task, the utilization of pre-existing knowledge from a model trained in a different domain or source task is preferred. This approach enables the application of previous learning to address fresh and related challenges. Essentially, within transfer learning, the computer relies on the insights and understanding acquired from previous experiences to enhance predictions for a new task. The benefits of transfer learning encompass notable reductions in training time and potential enhancements in neural network performance. This technique proves particularly advantageous in scenarios where data may be limited, as it allows the exploitation of the wealth of information encoded in models trained on larger and more diverse datasets, ultimately amplifying the efficiency and effectiveness of machine learning solutions. The diagram presented in Figure 3.6 illustrates the architectural framework and concept of transfer learning.

3.3.1 Classification using VGG-19 model

The VGG-19 model, created by researchers at the University of Oxford, saw its introduction in 2015. Renowned for its exceptional image classification capabilities, the model achieved an impressive accuracy rate of 92.7% on the ImageNet dataset. Its architectural foundation relies on an extensive assembly of small convolutional filters, enabling it to effectively comprehend intricate pixel relational data. In preparation for deploying the VGG-19 classification model, the initial step involves downloading the essential libraries and dependencies to ensure compatibility with the model's environment. The VGG-19 model

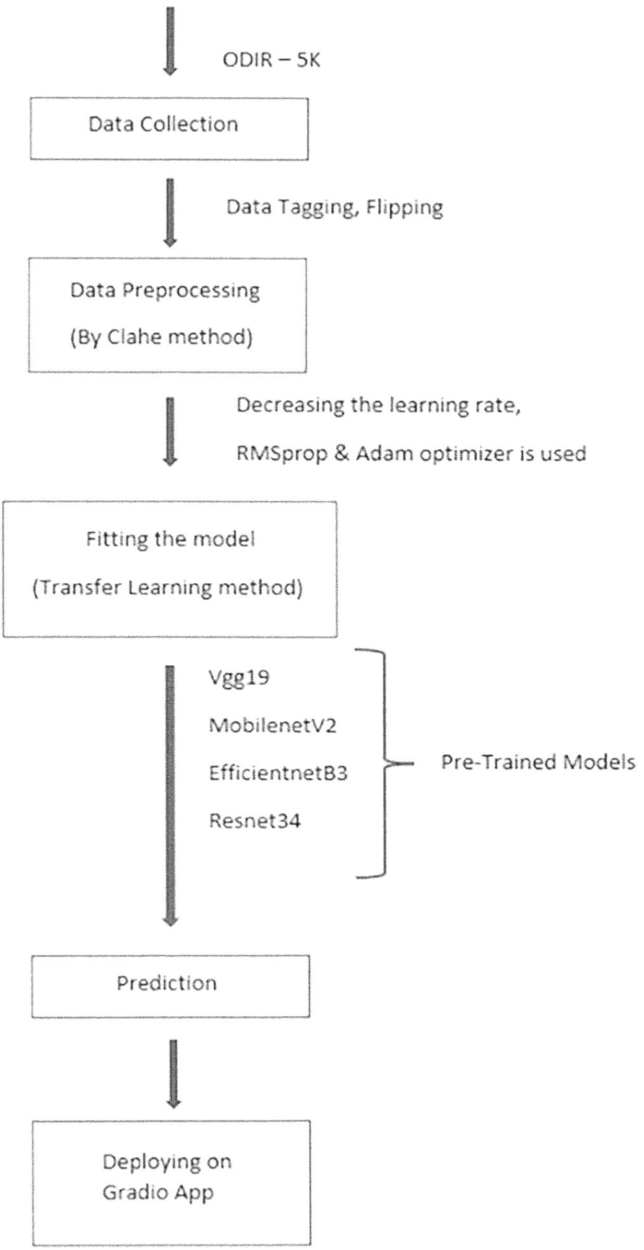

Figure 3.3 Data flow.

necessitates a specific data input size of 224 Ã—224, prompting adjustments to the dimensions of our training images accordingly. Subsequently, the acquired images underwent preprocessing to align them with the VGG-19 model's requirements. The ImageDataGenerator module from the Keras library was instrumental in this task. During this preprocessing stage, specific configurations were established: the re-scale value was set at 1/255, the shear range at 0.2, the zoom range at 0.2, and horizontal flipping was enabled.

	ID	Patient Age	Patient Sex	Left-Fundus	Right-Fundus	Left-Diagnostic Keywords	Right-Diagnostic Keywords	N	D	G	C	A	H	M	O	filepath	labels	target	filename
0	0	69	Female	0_left.jpg	0_right.jpg	cataract	normal fundus	0	0	0	1	0	0	0	0	../input/ocular-disease-recognition-odir5k/ODI...	['N']	[1, 0, 0, 0, 0, 0, 0, 0]	0_right.jpg
1	1	57	Male	1_left.jpg	1_right.jpg	normal fundus	normal fundus	1	0	0	0	0	0	0	0	../input/ocular-disease-recognition-odir5k/ODI...	['N']	[1, 0, 0, 0, 0, 0, 0, 0]	1_right.jpg
2	2	42	Male	2_left.jpg	2_right.jpg	laser spot, moderate non proliferative retinopathy	moderate non proliferative retinopathy	0	1	0	0	0	0	0	1	../input/ocular-disease-recognition-odir5k/ODI...	['D']	[0, 1, 0, 0, 0, 0, 0, 0]	2_right.jpg
3	4	53	Male	4_left.jpg	4_right.jpg	macular epiretinal membrane	mild nonproliferative retinopathy	0	1	0	0	0	0	0	1	../input/ocular-disease-recognition-odir5k/ODI...	['D']	[0, 1, 0, 0, 0, 0, 0, 0]	4_right.jpg
4	5	50	Female	5_left.jpg	5_right.jpg	moderate non proliferative retinopathy	moderate non proliferative retinopathy	0	1	0	0	0	0	0	0	../input/ocular-disease-recognition-odir5k/ODI...	['D']	[0, 1, 0, 0, 0, 0, 0, 0]	5_right.jpg

Figure 3.4 Sample data frame.

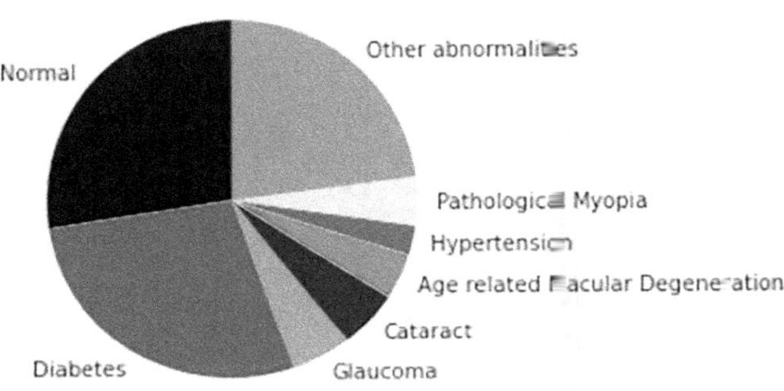

Figure 3.5 Diagnostic distributions.

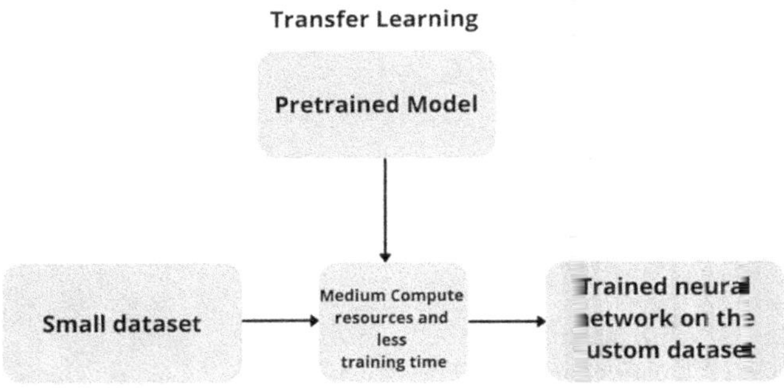

Figure 3.6 Architectural framework of transfer learning.

The responsibility of the ImageDataGenerator function lies in generating the preprocessed images, adhering to the parameters we've defined, to facilitate their utilization by the VGG-19 model. To empower the VGG-19 model to effectively train and predict eight distinct categories of eye diseases, two additional Dense layers were integrated into the existing VGG-19 architecture. For model training and prediction, we employ the categorical cross-entropy loss function and the RMSprop optimizer, along with the application of the sigmoid activation function. Following the parameter configuration , the model undergoes training over 50 iterations on the training dataset. Evaluation of the training's performance occurs upon its completion, specifically concerning its performance on the validation dataset.

3.3.2 Classification using MobileNet-v2

Google's MobileNet-v2 image classification model is designed with the primary objective of achieving efficient real-time classification, even within resource-constrained computing environments such as mobile devices. Similar to the initial two models discussed, this model also employs transfer learning, having been pretrained using the extensive ImageNet dataset. In the architecture of this image classification framework, the residual blocks follow an inverted residual structure, characterized by input and output layers comprised of slender bottleneck layers. Furthermore, this model employs lightweight convolutions, and its thin layers are devoid of non-linearities. For the utilization of the MobileNet-v2 model on the ODIR dataset, the initial step involved the conversion of the dataset images into a TensorFlow dataset format within the Colab notebook environment. The creation of the TensorFlow dataset was facilitated through the utilization of the TensorFlow framework's ImageFolder API. Subsequently, the MobileNet-v2 classification model was instantiated, with the classification layers being contingent on the preceding layer prior to the application of the flatten operation. The model's configuration featured categorical cross-entropy as the designated loss function and accuracy as the evaluation metric. Finally, to assess the model's performance, graphical representations were generated, depicting the relationship between Accuracy and Epoch as well as Cross Entropy and Epoch.

3.3.3 Classification using EfficientNetB3

EfficientNetB3 stands out as an advanced model renowned for its proficiency in categorizing custom images. Crafted by Google Brain, this state-of-the-art, CNN-based model represents an open-source innovation. The model's inception took place within the framework of the Jupyter Notebook platform and harnessed the capabilities of the Keras deep learning framework. Employing a supervised learning approach, we undertook the task of training the EfficientNetB3 model on the ODIR dataset. The model's training process involved supplying the deep neural network with the distinctive attributes of the training images. Its core function revolves around the prediction of the likelihood that the test images belong to specific classes. In this context, the model's prediction is synonymous with the class exhibiting the highest probability, as determined by the model's computations.

3.3.4 Classification using Resnet-34

The convolutional neural network architecture recognized as Resnet is frequently employed in the capacity of a classification model. To prepare for our study, we engaged in the pretraining of the Resnet-34 model, utilizing the extensive Imagenet dataset, an expansive collection encompassing 14 million images classified into 1000 distinct categories. Subsequently, we harnessed the ODIR dataset to further refine and adapt this model, aligning it for the precise task of ocular illness classification. The methodology applied here aligns with the concept of transfer learning, a practice that entails the retraining of an image classification model originally trained on dissimilar images. While the construction of the Resnet-34 model may appear intricate, the process commenced with the incorporation of the dataset within a Jupyter Notebook, facilitating the subsequent training of the Resnet-34 model. Following this, a customized pretrained Resnet image classification model was procured for use in our study.

3.4 EVALUATION METRICS

Assessment metrics, such as accuracy, precision, recall, F1 score, and others from reference [18], have been employed for the analysis of the data generated by the classification models, ensuring clarity and comprehensibility in our evaluation.

Loss Function: Each classifier model employs Binary Cross-Entropy (BCE) as the loss function. For each instance and label, the problem is treated as a binary classification task, predicting the presence (1) or absence (0) of the label.

1. Application of a sigmoid activation function to the model's output for each label is essential. The sigmoid function transforms the model's raw output into a probability value within the range of 0 to 1, indicating the likelihood of the label's presence.
2. BCE loss is independently calculated for each label, following this formula:

$$BCE(y_i, \hat{y}_i) = -[y_i \cdot log(\hat{y}_i) + (1 - y_i) \cdot log(1 - \hat{y}_i)]$$

- The true label (0 or 1) is represented as y_i.
- The predicted probability of the label being 1 is denoted as $\hat{y}_i$.

3. Subsequently, an averaging process is performed on the BCE losses across all labels to compute the overall loss for the multi-label classification problem.

This loss function demonstrates its suitability for multi-label classification by enabling independent predictions for each label and accommodating scenarios where an instance may belong to multiple classes concurrently.

3.5 EXPERIMENTAL RESULTS

To assess the effectiveness of the four classification models, a total of four distinct experiments were conducted, specifically involving VGG-19, MobileNet-v2, EfficientNetB3, and Resnet-34.

3.5.1 VGG-19 model

Figure 3.7a depicts an accuracy plot detailing the training and validation data, illustrating that despite fluctuations throughout the training process, the validation accuracy eventually stabilizes. Some slight overfitting is noticeable in the validation data, observed within the space between the two plotted lines. Additionally, Figure 3.7b illustrates the loss plot for both the training and validation data. According to this graph, as the number of epochs increases, the training loss decreases until the two lines nearly converge. Similar to the training loss, the validation loss displays relatively consistent variability. Notably, the classifier achieves an AUC of 96.80%. Figure 3.7c presents the Confusion Matrix for VGG-19, while Figure 3.7d provides insights into the accuracy, precision, and recall results for VGG-19.

3.5.2 MobileNet-v2 model

When examining the outcomes derived from diverse hyperparameter configurations, this particular model achieved its peak accuracy after 50 epochs, with a batch size set to 32. The

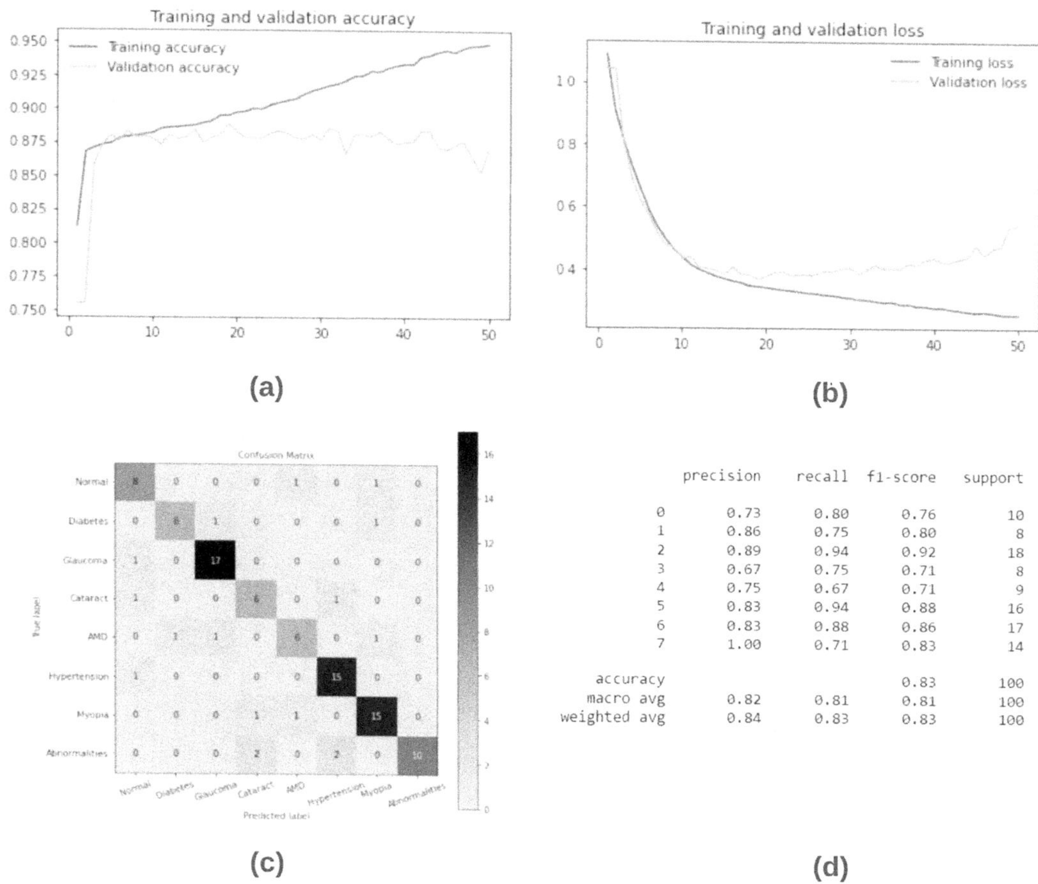

	precision	recall	f1-score	support
0	0.73	0.80	0.76	10
1	0.86	0.75	0.80	8
2	0.89	0.94	0.92	18
3	0.67	0.75	0.71	8
4	0.75	0.67	0.71	9
5	0.83	0.94	0.88	16
6	0.83	0.88	0.86	17
7	1.00	0.71	0.83	14
accuracy			0.83	100
macro avg	0.82	0.81	0.81	100
weighted avg	0.84	0.83	0.83	100

Figure 3.7 Performance analysis of VGG-19 model.

accuracy achieved was 83%, while the model's AUC stood at an impressive 96.83%. In Figure 3.8a, the accuracy plot reveals noteworthy patterns when using both training and validation data. Notably, the lines exhibit considerable separation during the training phase, with sporadic convergence points characterized by relatively low accuracy for the testing data but an increase in accuracy for the training data. Figure 3.8b illustrates the loss plot across both training and validation datasets, demonstrating dynamic fluctuations throughout the training process. Notably, as the number of epochs increases, the testing loss declines while the training loss ascends. Figure 3.8c visually represents the Confusion Matrix for MobileNet-v2, while Figure 3.8d presents detailed insights into accuracy, precision, and recall results for MobileNet-v2.

3.5.3 EfficientNetB3

An accuracy plot that includes both training and validation data is shown in Figure 3.9a. This graph shows how the validation accuracy fluctuates throughout training before settling. A gap between the two lines shows that the validation data were overfit. Notably, accuracy shows a rising trend as the number of epochs rises. The loss curve for the training and

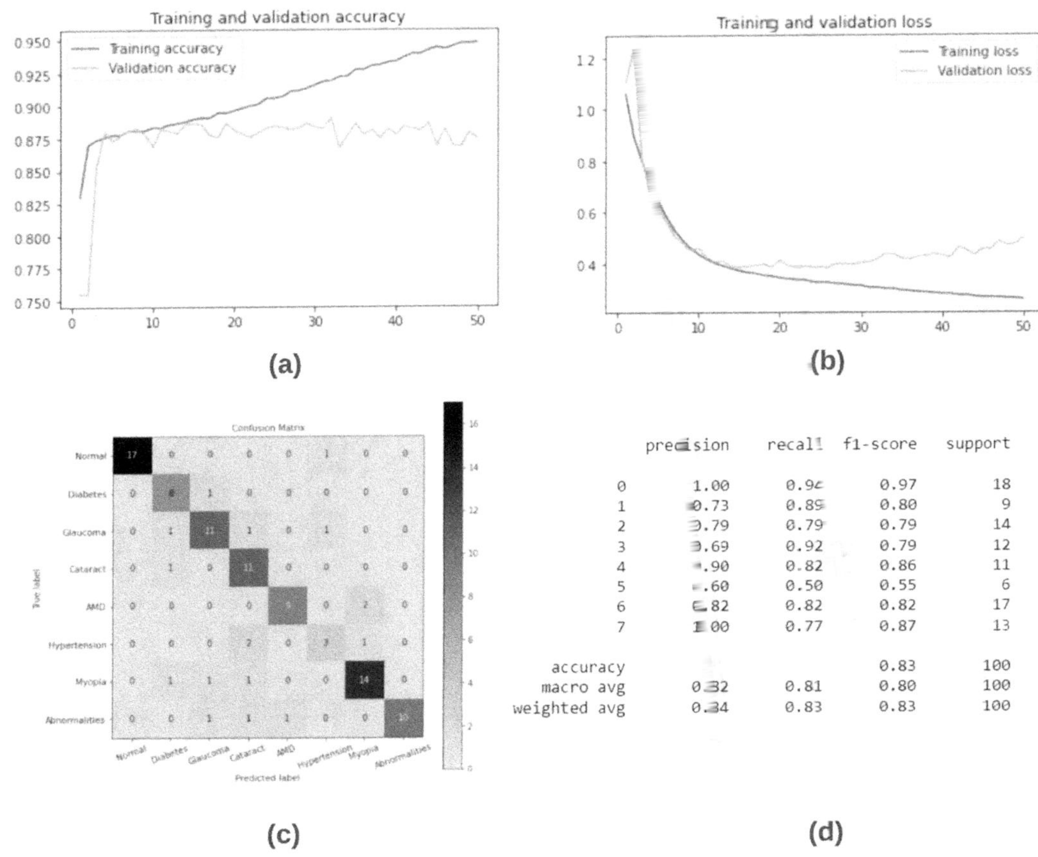

	precision	recall	f1-score	support
0	1.00	0.94	0.97	18
1	0.73	0.89	0.80	9
2	0.79	0.79	0.79	14
3	0.69	0.92	0.79	12
4	0.90	0.82	0.86	11
5	0.60	0.50	0.55	6
6	0.82	0.82	0.82	17
7	1.00	0.77	0.87	13
accuracy			0.83	100
macro avg	0.82	0.81	0.80	100
weighted avg	0.84	0.83	0.83	100

Figure 3.8 Performance analysis of MobileNet-v2 model.

validation datasets is shown in Figure 3.9b. The training loss decreases as the number of epochs increases, as shown in this graph, with the two lines almost converging. The validation loss maintains a rather constant variation pattern, much like the training loss does. The classifier's AUC attains a commendable score of 96.73%. Figure 3.9c provides a visual representation of the Confusion Matrix for EfficientNetB3, while Figure 3.9d furnishes detailed insights into the accuracy, precision, and recall outcomes for EfficientNetB3.

3.5.4 Resnet-34

Figure 3.10a portrays the accuracy plot encompassing both training and validation data. This graph illustrates the fluctuation in validation accuracy during the training process, eventually stabilizing. Notably, the presence of a gap between the two lines suggests overfitting in the validation data. Furthermore, the accuracy metric exhibits an upward trend with an increasing number of epochs. Meanwhile, Figure 3.10b visualizes the loss plot for both the training and validation datasets. As indicated by this graph, the training loss diminishes with the rising number of epochs, with the two lines approaching convergence.

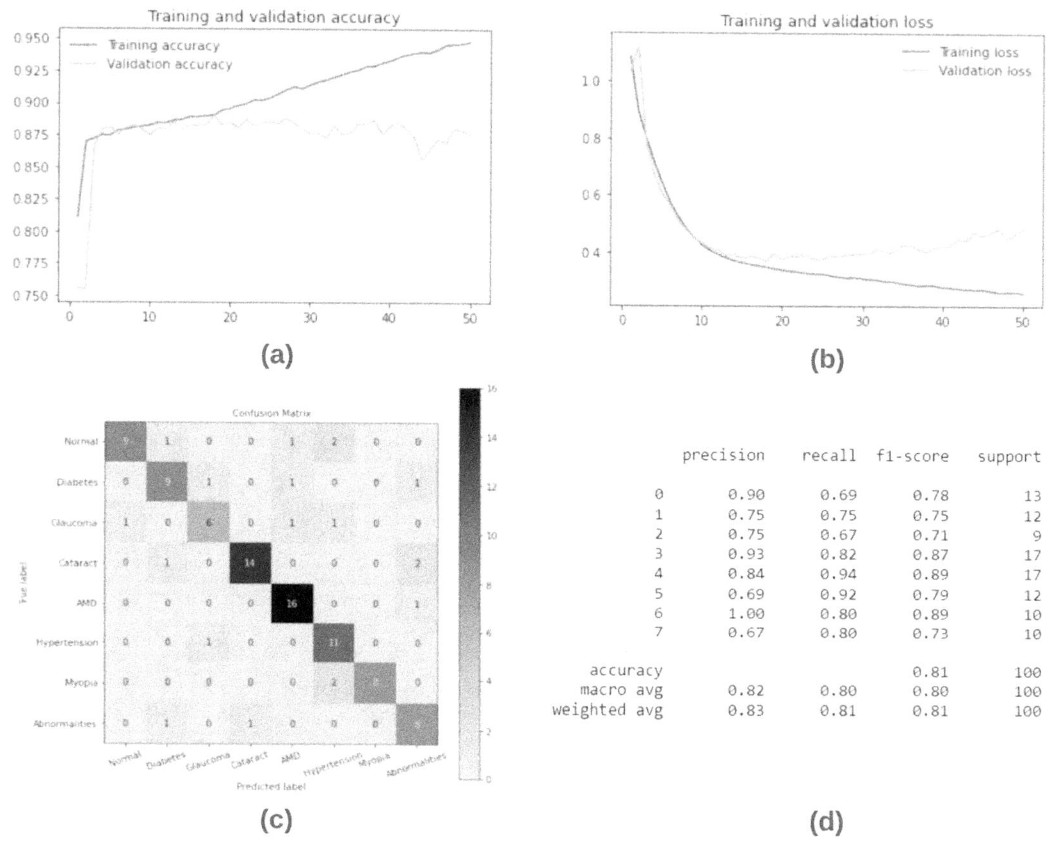

	precision	recall	f1-score	support
0	0.90	0.69	0.78	13
1	0.75	0.75	0.75	12
2	0.75	0.67	0.71	9
3	0.93	0.82	0.87	17
4	0.84	0.94	0.89	17
5	0.69	0.92	0.79	12
6	1.00	0.80	0.89	10
7	0.67	0.80	0.73	10
accuracy			0.81	100
macro avg	0.82	0.80	0.80	100
weighted avg	0.83	0.81	0.81	100

Figure 3.9 Performance analysis of EfficientNetB3 model

Similar to the training loss, the validation loss demonstrates a relatively consistent variance pattern. Figure 3.10c visually presents the Confusion Matrix for EfficientNetB3, while Figure 3.10d provides in-depth insights into the accuracy, precision, and recall results for EfficientNetB3.

Among the various machine learning models trained, it was observed that the MobileNet-v2 Model consistently delivered the most accurate predictions when subjected to testing and comparison. The outcomes reveal an AUC score of 96.83%. The comprehensive results from all four models, along with their comparative analysis, are presented in Table 3.1.

3.5.5 Graphical user interface and functionality

An intuitive graphical user interface (GUI) has been meticulously developed utilizing Gradio for seamless interaction with the Python algorithm. This GUI, tailored for Windows-based devices, empowers users to effortlessly upload images and obtain corresponding results. Notably, this GUI offers a convenient option to preserve the results for future reference, enhancing the utility of the system. The model diagram that intricately merges the GUI with the deep learning model is thoughtfully illustrated in Figure 3.11, providing a comprehensive overview of the system's architecture. The functionalities encapsulated within the GUI encompass the following:

1. **Image Upload:** Users are afforded the flexibility to select and upload their desired images, facilitating predictions for the specified image. Upon selection from the local drive, the input image undergoes necessary pre-processing, enabling the algorithm to generate predictions for the image's class.

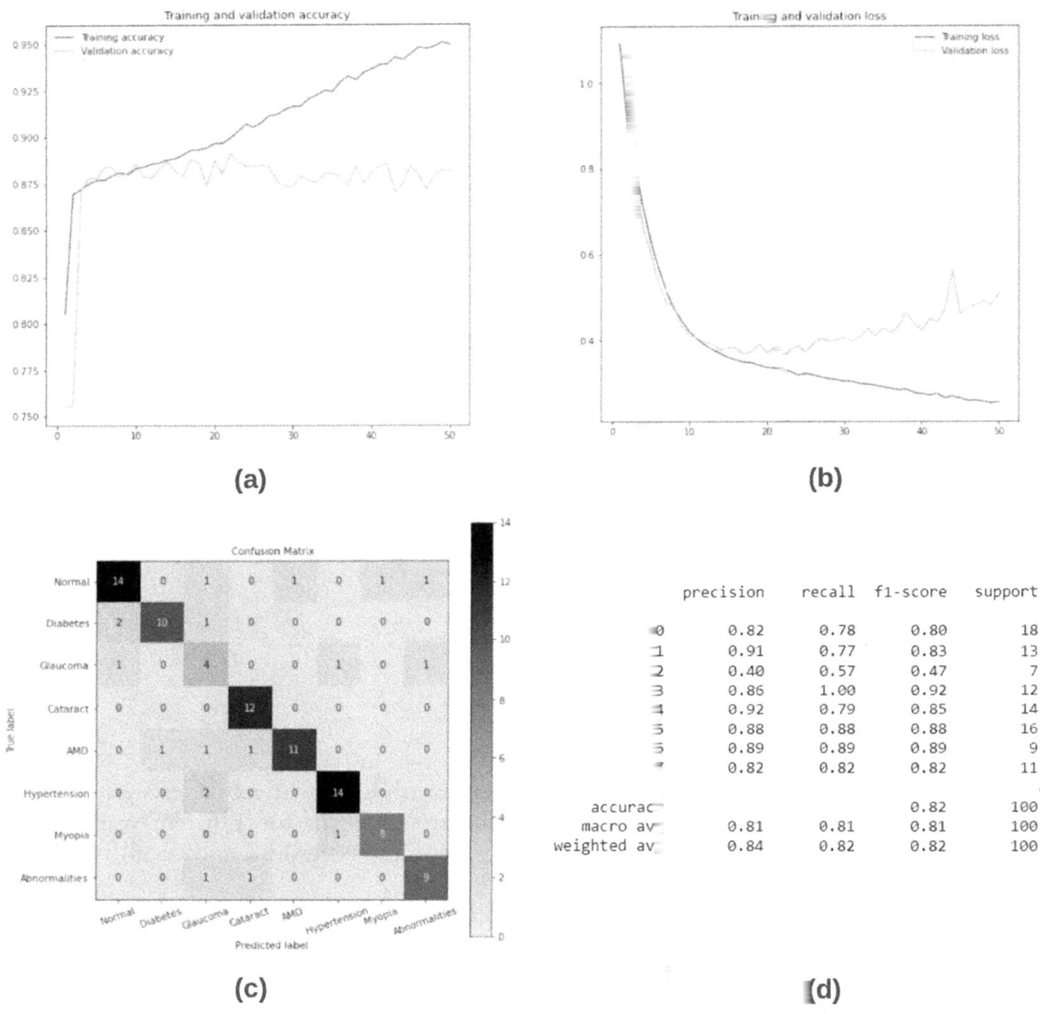

Figure 3.10 Performance analysis of Resnet-34 model.

Table 3.1 Performance metrics and hyperparameter settings for various models

Methods	*Accuracy (%)*	*AUC (%)*	*Learning rate*	*Optimizer*
VGG-19	83	96.8	0.001	RMSPROP
MobileNet-v2	83	96.83	0.0001	ADAM
EfficientNetB3	81	96.73	0.01	RMSPROP
ResNet-34	82	96.87	0.0001	ADAM

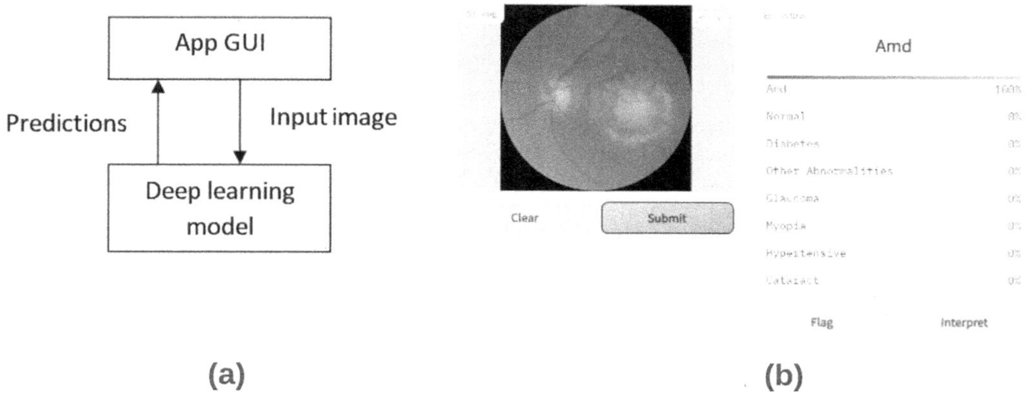

Figure 3.11 Integration of GUI and deep learning model.

2. **Link Sharing:** The system generates a shareable link through Gradio, which users, including neurologists and end-users, can readily access via any standard web browser. This link empowers them to effortlessly upload MRI images and receive predictions. The ensuing dialog box furnishes valuable prediction details, including the predicted class. A visual representation of the application is encapsulated in Figure 3.11b, showcasing an instance where an originally uploaded AMD image yields an "AMD" prediction within the GUI interface.

3.6 CONCLUSION

In this study, a desktop application with an intuitive GUI was developed for Ocular Disease classification. The dataset used, known as the ODIR dataset, was sourced from Kaggle. Four distinct deep learning models underwent training on this dataset, with each model's performance evaluated based on accuracy. MobileNet-v2 Model demonstrated the best balance of training time and accuracy, achieving an accuracy rate of 83%. Resnet-34, despite longer training times, achieved an accuracy rate of 82%. EfficientNetB3 lagged behind in terms of accuracy. Notably, MobileNet-v2 also outperformed the other architectures when considering AUC and accuracy metrics. The GUI, designed using the Gradio designer tool, enables users to upload images for predictions through shareable links. Future work could involve exploring custom CNN models specific to this dataset and enhancing the GUI with additional user options. Additionally, model performance can be optimized through hyperparameter adjustments and the incorporation of data augmentation techniques to improve accuracy. To enhance user convenience, the system could be designed to allow users to download and save predictions in spreadsheet format.

REFERENCES

1. Elloumi, Y., Akil, M., Boudegga, H.: Ocular diseases diagnosis in fundus images using a deep learning: approaches, tools and performance evaluation. In: Real-Time Image Processing and Deep Learning 2019, vol. 10996, pp. 221–228 (2019).
2. Li, T., Bo, W., Hu, C., Kang, H., Liu, H., Wang, K., Fu, H.: Applications of deep learning in fundus images: a review. Medical Image Analysis **69**, 101971 (2021).

3. Adio, A., Alikor, A., Awoyesuku, E.: Survey of pediatric ophthalmic diagnoses in a teaching hospital in Nigeria. Nigerian Journal of Medicine: Journal of the National Association of Resident Doctors of Nigeria **20**(1), 105–108 (2011).
4. Paudel, P., Ramson, P., Naduvilath, T., Wilson, D., Phuong, H.T., Ho, S.M., Giap, N.V.: Prevalence of vision impairment and refractive error in school children in Ba Ria – Vung Tau province, Vietnam. Clinical & Experimental Ophthalmology **42**(3), 217–226 (2014).
5. Edussuriya, K., Sennanayake, S., Senaratne, T., Marshall, D., Sullivan, T., Selva, D., Casson, R.J.: The prevalence and causes of visual impairment in central Sri Lanka: the Kandy eye study. Ophthalmology **116**(1), 52–56 (2009).
6. Katibeh, M., Pakravan, M., Yaseri, M., Pakbin, M., Soleimanizad, R.: Prevalence and causes of visual impairment and blindness in central Iran; the Yazd eye study. Journal of Ophthalmic & Vision Research **10**(3), 279 (2015).
7. Steinmetz, J.D., Bourne, R.R., Briant, P.S., Flaxman, S.R., Taylor, H.R., Jonas, J.B., Abdoli, A.A., Abrha, W.A., Abualhasan, A., Abu-Gharbieh, E.G., *et al.*: Causes of blindness and vision impairment in 2020 and trends over 30 years, and prevalence of avoidable blindness in relation to vision 2020: the right to sight: an analysis for the global burden of disease study. The Lancet Global Health **9**(2), 144–160 (2021).
8. Bourne, R.R., Dineen, B.P., Ali, S.M., Huq, D.M.N., Johnson, G.J.: Prevalence of refractive error in Bangladeshi adults: results of the national blindness and low vision survey of Bangladesh. Ophthalmology **111**(6), 1150–1160 (2004).
9. Hossain, M.F., Nandi, D.C., Ahsan, N.: Knowledge, attitude and practices regarding common eye disease in Bangladesh: a study of Cumilla zone. Knowledge, Attitude and Practices Regarding Common Eye Disease in Bangladesh: A Study of Cumilla Zone **25**(4), 2279–0845 (2020).
10. AndrewMvd: Ocular Disease Recognition (ODIR5K) https://www.kaggle.com/datasets/andrewmvd/ocular-disease-recognition-odir5k. Accessed: [Insert Date] (2023).

Part 2

Disease detection and diagnosis

Chapter 4

A vision transformer-based approach for brain tumor detection

Piyush Kumar[1], *Radhika Goyal*[2], *Shubham Garg*[2], *Shuchi Mala*[2], *Ronit Bali*[2], *and Anukansha Sharma*[2]

[1]Department of General Management, Amity Business School, Amity University, Noida, Uttar Pradesh, India

[2]Department of Computer Science and Engineering, Amity School of Engineering and Technology, Amity University, Noida, Uttar Pradesh, India

4.1 INTRODUCTION

The brain itself is the most complex part of the human body which controls everything in the body from thoughts to storing memories, containing emotions, consisting of sensory skills like touch, breathe, and temperature regulation, motor skills, and many other activities. The normal adult brain weighs about 1.3 kilograms and is around 60% fat while the other 40% contains water, proteins, carbohydrates, and much more. The brain receives signals from all parts of the body via neural signals through the central nervous system. The central nervous system contains trillions of neurons called nerve cells which pass information. The brain is divided into three parts, which include cerebrum, brainstem, and cerebellum [1].

The cerebrum is the front part of the brain containing the cerebral cortex at the center of the brain. The cerebrum is the largest portion among all three parts of the brain, which initiates and coordinates movements and regulates temperature. It enables the human body to perform sense activities that include speaking, hearing, smelling, touching, tasting, and watching. Further, it supports in reasoning, problem-solving, learning, and understanding, expressing emotions, etc. The cerebral cortex divides the brain into two parts. The right side of the brain controls the left part of the brain and vice versa. Corpus callosum is the path through which both parts of the brain communicate with each other. It is a C-shaped structure of white matter which is present in the center of the brain [1].

The brainstem connects the cerebrum with the spinal cord. It is further sub-divided into midbrain, pons, and medulla. The midbrain is one of the most complex structures in the brain, containing different neuron clusters, neural pathways, and many others. The midbrain facilitates various functions such as listening and movement to computing responses and ecological changes. The pons is the source of four of 12 cranial nerves enabling activities like chewing, focus, blinking, and facial expressions. It is the linkage between midbrain and medulla. The medulla is at the bottom of the brainstem where the brain meets the spinal cord. The medulla is responsible for inhalation, blood flow, CO_2, as well as oxygen. It also supports reflexive activities like vomiting, swallowing, coughing, etc. [1].

The cerebellum is a fist-size portion of the brain situated behind the head. It is located directly above the brainstem and below the temporal and occipital lobes. It also contains two hemispheres; the external portion contains neurons and the internal portion interconnects with the cerebral cortex. The major function of the cerebellum is to maintain posture, balance, and equilibrium and synchronize voluntary muscle movements.

The brain is covered with three layers of protective covering known as meninges to cover the brain and spinal cord. The outer most layer is called "Dura matter" and has two layers,

DOI: 10.1201/9781003369059-6

one is the periosteal layer and the meningeal layer is below it. The second layer is an arachnoid layer, which is a thin, web-like layer of connective tissues without any blood vessels or nerves. Cerebrospinal fluid is a fluid present below the arachnoid which provides cushion to the entire central nervous system. Below the arachnoid is pia matter, which contains arteries and veins.

Apart from the bodily activities, the brain contains various glands which are necessary for the well-being of a human. Glands like the pituitary gland, hypothalamus, amygdala, hippocampus, pineal gland, ventricles, and cerebrospinal fluids have a different role to play in the body. The pituitary gland is also known as the "master gland," which is found deep in the brain and in the forehead. It further governs other glands and regulates the flow of hormones from the thyroid, testicles, ovaries, adrenals, etc. The hypothalamus is located above the pituitary gland and sends chemical signal that controls its function. It helps with sleep patterns, regulates body temperature, controls hunger and thrust. The amygdala is in each half of the brain that controls and regulates emotions and memories [1].

A brain tumor is a severe disease caused when abnormal cells or masses start growing inside of the brain. Brain tumors are mostly of two types: one is cancerous, also known as malignant, and the other one is non-cancerous, known as benign. A malignant brain tumor is more dangerous than a benign tumor, as it can be spread in other parts of the brain and CNS. Major symptoms of brain tumors are headaches, which are severe while waking up in the morning, while sneezing or coughing, and it can occur while one is asleep. Vomiting, seizures, blurred vision, and weakness in the limbs can be other symptoms too. Other than this, memory loss, confusion, loss of balance, dizziness, and difficulty swallowing food are a few common symptoms that are signs of having brain tumor. Pituitary brain tumor causes lack of menstruation in women, sensitivity to heat and cold, low blood pressure, obesity, enlargement of hands and feet, etc. [2].

Benign and malignant have different types of brain tumors. As discussed earlier, benign tumors are not dangerous, thus its types include Chordomas, which grow at the base of the skull. Gangliocytomas are rare tumors found in nerve cells. Meningiomas are the most common type of tumor which form meninges. Pituitary adenomas are benign tumors found in the pituitary gland. Last, Schwannomas are again one of the most common types of brain tumor found in adults. This tumor develops Schwann cells in the peripheral nervous system.

Further, about 78% of malignant tumors are gliomas. These develop glial cells. Thus, types of gliomas include Astrocytoma, Glioblastoma, and Oligodendroglioma. The Astrocytoma forms star-shaped glial cells known as astrocytes. These are mostly found in the cerebrum and are a very common type of brain tumor. Glioblastomas are fast-growing astrocytes. Oligodendroglioma is a very uncommon tumor which begins in the cells that create myelin. Last, medulloblastoma is another type of malignant brain cancer which grows faster and is formed in the base of the skull commonly found in children [3].

In the United States, it is estimated that around 7,00,000 people have primary brain tumors, while around 88,970 people are going to get diagnosed in the year 2022. Of all the 7,00,000 people with brain tumors, 71% of them have benign tumors, while the remaining 29% are malignant. On the other hand, 58% of tumors occur in females, while 42% occur in males. Also, the median age of the diagnosis of a brain tumor was found to be 61 years. Furthermore, 18,200 people have lost their lives due to brain cancer in the year 2022, whereas the average survival rate of patients with a primary tumor is 75.7%. Brain tumors are also found in children in early childhood [4].

Around 13,000 children are found to have benign tumors in the US. It is also the leading cause of cancer-related death among children between 0 and 14 years. Around 31,000 adolescents and young adults are estimated to have benign tumors in the United States.

Around 12,000 adolescents and young adults were diagnosed in the year 2022. There has never been any medicine developed specifically for malignant brain tumors. Further, it represents the highest pre-patient initial cost of care for any cancer group. Its annualized mean net cost of care approached $150,000 [4].

In India, the prevalence of brain tumors is around 5–10% per 100,000 people. Further, according to the International Association of Cancer Registries (IARC), more than 28,000 cases of brain tumors are recorded in India each year, while more than 24,000 people die to due to brain cancer in India [5].

As it is known that the brain is a complex organ of the body, diagnosis of brain tumors is also a complex process. If one is experiencing symptoms of a brain tumor, the doctors must examine the physical and neurological aspects of the body such as symptoms, past health conditions, mental status, hearing, vision, etc. Based on the examinations, the doctors or the specialists recommend tests that include MRIs or magnetic resonance imaging tests, biopsy tests, spinal tap tests, etc. [3].

The MRI test is one of the best methods to detect brain tumors. This test enables the doctors to detect the exact size, position, and other details of the tumor. A biopsy is done to remove a small part of the tumor for study by a neurosurgeon. Further, if the tumor is difficult to remove, the surgeons perform a stereotactic biopsy, where they insert a needle in the skull to take a sample of the tumor. For a spinal tap, the surgeon removes the cerebrospinal fluid around the spine.

For treating brain tumors, neurosurgeons use methods like brain surgery, radiation therapy, brachytherapy, chemotherapy, and immunotherapy. Brachytherapy is a type of radiation therapy where the doctors place radioactive seeds in or near the cancer. Ration therapy is the therapy where high doses of X-rays destroy the brain tumor cells. Chemotherapy is a type of treatment where anti-cancer medicines are given to the patients whether in the form of pill or in the form of injection. Last, immunotherapy is a kind of treatment where the body's immune system helps to do its job in fighting cancer [3].

A Magnetic Resonance and Imaging (MRI) or CT scan is one of the most common ways to detect brain tumors. The detection of a tumor is itself a complex task, and to make these complex tasks easier, there is a need for image recognition and computer vision. Artificial Intelligence and machine learning are paving their way to make these complex detections easier every single day. To classify tumors from complex MRI images, different algorithms, neural networks, and transfer learning algorithms such as VGG16, VGG19, ResNet50, AlexNet, CoatNet, GoogleNet, etc. are applied. These help in not only detecting the tumor but also helping in detecting the type of tumor in the brain. Thus, based on the dataset provided to these algorithms, it detects whether the tumor is glioma, benign, or malignant.

In this chapter, the objective is to detect whether the image of the brain is tumorous or not using transfer learning and state-of-the-art algorithms, comparing the accuracies, precision, recall, and F1 score of the models.

4.2 LITERATURE REVIEW

In this article [6], the objective is to detect the early growth of brain tumors among children and the elderly, who are the most vulnerable to brain tumors. It is a severe kind of cancer characterized by unregulated brain cell proliferation within the skull. Because of their variety, tumor cells are notably difficult to categorize. CNN is the most used machine learning method for visual learning and detection of brain tumors. This paper suggests applying min-max normalization on a CNN-based dense Efficient Net to categorize 3260

T1-weighted contrast-enhanced brain MRI images into 4 groups i.e., glioma, meningioma, pituitary, and no tumor. The designed network is an Efficient Net variation with inclusion of dense and drop-out layers. Likewise, the researchers applied data augmentation in conjunction with min-max normalization to boost the contrast of tumor cells. The dense layer has the edge of properly categorizing a limited library of images. Therefore, the suggested technique outperforms the competition in terms of total performance. According to the experimental data, the suggested model was 99.97% correct during training and 98.78% correct during testing. The newly constructed Efficient Net CNN architecture, with excellent accuracy and a positive F1 score, could be a beneficial decision-making tool in the research of brain tumor diagnostic tests.

In this article [7], the authors discovered the essentials of brain cancer using deep learning methods for better foundation in the domain of computer vision. The authors used attributes of image processing methods such as scaling, contrast enhancement, and threshold is based on DNN (deep neural networks). The CT scan data was taken from Kaggle website which contained 300 training images and 253 testing images. Further each training data contained 95 normal images and 155 brain tumor images. For pre-processing the researchers have used midpoint filtering and grayscale. The precision of the model was 88% with accuracy of 85%.

In this article [8], the objective was to analyze the tumor localization in brain. There are various developing image processing techniques to analyze every body part like hyperspectral imaging. Hyperspectral imaging is the many colors depiction of tissue. It compares the tissue with former image models. The proposed model was performed on dataset taken from Kaggle website. The dataset contained 250 sample images. Further, the dataset was divided in 80:20 proportion in which 80% of the data was applied for training purposes whereas 20% was applied for testing purposes. In this article, hyperspectral imaging is used. Combining k-based clustering algorithms such as k-nearest neighbor and k-means clustering to locate tumors. In both algorithms, the value of 'k' is predicted using an optimization method known as the firefly algorithm. In comparison to existing strategies, the proposed model got better results with 96.47% accuracy, 96.32% sensitivity, and 98.24% specificity.

In this article [9], images can be blended using repetition region tactics or in spatial space. Given that these techniques can handle the concept of edges in an image, repeat region processes will be chosen. In a picture combination, the resulting combined photographs will be more illuminating than the component data pictures, making them better suited for depiction concerns. Counterfeit information (manufactured reasoning) calculations are expected to play a significant role in managing grasping therapy in the therapeutic benefits sector and managing rewritten prescription. This evaluation work looks at the role of image blending in a model of superior frontal brain development, and this intelligent blend-based sickness representation model can be employed for altered prescription more generally. The incredible blended images will deliver better request outcomes than employing individual data photographs. The difference limited the preprocessing of input images, like X-beam and SPECT images, using a flexible histogram evening out approach from the beginning.

The discrete cosine change-based mix approach is used to combine photos of benign and dangerous class-mind malignant growths. Support vector machine classifiers, KNN classifiers, and decision tree classifiers are attempted using details procured from combined and separated photos, and the outcome obtained from individual information pictures. Surveys of classifier shows are conducted using the cutoff values for accuracy, precision, review, expresses, and F1 score. When using detached highlights from combined images, SVM classifier performed finer than KNN and decision tree classifiers, yielding the best accuracy of 96.8%, precision of 95%, review of 94%, expresses of 93%, and F1 score of 91%. The proposed framework's results are distinct from those of already-in-use frameworks and provide pleasing results.

The authors [10] have used ResNet101 pre-trained model for transfer learning on normalized data. However, this method generates inessential features, which reduce accuracy. To overcome this, particle swarm optimization and differential evaluation algorithms have been utilized. This outputs desirable feature vectors which are fused into one single vector to which PCA is applied for further optimization. Then it is fed to classifiers for identifying brain tumors. The dataset used for this system is BRATS 2018 dataset consisting of 130,200 images with four classes of tumors. The proposed model had an accuracy of 94.4%. It also had an execution time speed-up of 25.5x. However, the fusion process increased the computational time throughout the testing period.

In this article [11], the authors developed a 3D CNN architecture which was then passed to pre-trained CNN model for feature extraction which included VGG19 was used. The dataset used in this article was 3 BRATS datasets of 2015, 2017, and 2018, which resulted in 98.32%, 96.97%, and 92.67% accuracy. Each dataset contained four distinct categories: Flair, T1CE, T1, and T2, along with ground truth images. These databases consist of HGG and LGG pictures. The 60% of flair as well as T1CE images and their ground truth images are utilized for training CNN model. While the remaining 40% of the images and 100% of T1 and T2 are utilized for the testing purposes. For the dataset BRATS, the most accurate model was found to be FNN with accuracy of 97.36%, whereas SVM was 95.29%. Similarly, for BRATS dataset, FNN was best suited with accuracy rate of 94.96% and BRATS dataset, FNN was best suited with accuracy of 90.42%.

In this article [12], the objective was to detect brain tumor using computer-assisted-diagnosis with high precision. In this article, the authors have presented segmentation through U-net architecture with ResNet50 as a backbone on the Fig share data set and attained a level of 95.04% of the IoU or intersection over union. The dataset was taken from Fig Share source including 3,064 brain MRI slices obtained from 233 patients. For multi-classification purposes the researchers have applied pre-trained models such as ResNet50, DenseNet201, MobileNet V2, and InceptionV3. Thus, the outcomes of models MobileNet V2 was 91.8%, for Inception V3 it was 92.8%, for ResNet50 it was 92.9%, for DenseNet201 it was 93.1%, and for NASNet the accuracy was 99.6%. Among them, NASNet showed the highest accuracy.

The objective of the paper [13] is to raise the level and efficacy of MRI machines to classify brain tumors and identify their types. Thus, to do so, the authors have various CNN, and deep learning models like Xception, ResNet50, InceptionV3, VGG16, and MobileNet. The researchers have taken dataset from Kaggle website which contains 4480 images and used 50% of data for training and 50% for validation purposes. For training purposes 800 unseen images were used. The F1-scores for unseen images of Xception was 98.75%, whereas for ResNet50 it was 98.50%, for InceptionV3 it was 98.00%, VGG16 it was 97.50%, and for MobileNet it was 97.25% respectively.

In this article [14], the aim was to propose a hypothesis which suggests that the value of images which is boosted in pre-processing step will play a significant role in increasing the classification of execution of any statistical approach. Therefore, to support the concept, the authors used a better-quality image augmentation technique, consisting of three different sub-stages. These sub-stages consist of elimination of noise using median filter, secondly, contrast improvement using histogram equalization method and finally the image was converted from grayscale to RGB. Post image augmentation, the authors extract attributes from an enhanced MRI image of brain by means of a distinct wavelet transform. Further these features were reduced by color moments which consisted of mean, standard deviation, and skewness. The authors performed a cutting-edge deep neural network to classify the images as normal brain tumor images or pathological images. The method gained 95.8% which is greater than any other state-of-the-art procedures. The authors have taken dataset from Harvard medical school website containing 71 T2-weighted images of which 25 were abnormal while 46 were normal.

In this article [15], the aim was to identify brain tumors, one of the most lethal illnesses, with an extremely short life expectancy in their most severe form. Computer-aided tumor detection systems and convolutional neural networks presented success stories and made significant advances in machine learning. When collated with normal previous neural network layers, deep convolutional layers automatically extract critical and robust characteristics from the input space. In the proposed framework, the authors have conducted three experiments to identify brain cancers utilizing three architectures of convolutional neural networks. These architectures include Alex Net, Google Net, and VGGNet. Each research further investigates transfer learning approaches, like fine-tuning and freezing, with MRI slices of brain tumor. The researchers experimented on datasets available in Fig Share. The dataset contained 3064 MRI sliced aggregated from 233 patients. Data augmentation methods are applied to MRI images to simplify results, increase dataset samples, and lessen the likelihood of over-fitting. In suggested investigations, the fine-tuned VGG16 architecture attained classification and detection accuracy of up to 98.69%.

The paper [16] proposes a neoteric approach based on long short-term memory (LSTM) model using MRI. Firstly, the quality of multi-sequence MRI is boosted using N4ITK and Gaussian filters with size 5 × 5. The 4-layer deep LSTM model serves the purpose of classification. Ideal hidden units are nominated from each layer, like 200 HU, 225 HU, 200 HU as well as 225 HU, respectively. The selection of these unseen or concealed units is governed by extensive experiments performed for acquiring better results. Datasets BRATS and SISS-ISLES are used for the validation of the results. The Patch-based CNN model is assessed over BRATS challenge for classification of brain tumor. Average processing time on CNN model is 5.502 s, whereas for LSTM it is 0.1889s and achieved accuracy being 95% on BRATS Challenge dataset. The proposed model yielded 97% accuracy on BRATS 2015. This shows that the proposed LSTM model provides better and faster results and thus is used in place of the CNN model.

The paper [17] proposes a revamped deep learning mechanism called Dolphin-SCA based Deep CNN. It provides a mechanism to ameliorate accuracy and make efficient decisions in classification. The process involves pre-processing of the input MRI images, followed by subjecting them to the segmentation procedure. A fuzzy deformable synthesis model with Dolphin Echolocation based Sine Cosine Algorithm named Dolphin-SCA is used for the segmentation process. This is followed by a features extraction process which focusses on power LBP and other statistical features such as mean, variance and skewness. These features are utilized in DCNN for brain cancer detection using Dolphin–SCA algorithm. The results are shown by means of BRATS and SimBRATS databases. The sensitivity, specificity and accuracy are utilized for evaluation of the performances. The mentioned technique achieves a maximum accuracy of 95.3% and sensitivity and specificity of 97.7% and 95.3% respectively.

The authors [18] aim at diagnosing brain cancer through MRI images by using CNN models. They have used Resnet50 architecture is used as the base of the model with the slight modification that the last five layers have been replaced with ten new layers. The dataset used for the study was taken from Brain MRI Images for Brain Tumor Detection. It contains two folders with 98 images without brain tumors and the other folder has 155 images with tumors. The main layers involved in the proposed model are input layer, convolutional layer, dropout, fully connected, pooling layer, SoftMax, and classification layer. The developed hybrid model attained an accuracy of 97.01%. These pictures are also classified by using Alex Net, ResNet50, InceptionV3, Google Net, and Densenet201 models. They concluded that hybrid model is effective and operates very well, as is seen numerically.

The authors [19] have used Edge-based Contourlet Transformation to register various input images and their pre-processing and analyzing the region-of-interest of the region containing tumor. This segmentation algorithm provided precise boundaries and combined Center-Symmetric Local Binary Patterns (CSLBP) and Gray Level Run Length Matrix (GLRLM) to efficiently detect brain tumors. The classification of tumors is done through Adopting Neural Network (ANN) technique. The proposed system consists of two phases – the training and the testing phase. In the first phase, the images are trained to ANN classifier, following which areas containing tumor are stored. The model has the following procedures – registration carried out by an Edge-based Contourlet Transformation, followed by pre-processing using average filtering and a RGB to Gray conversion, segmenting the tumor regions, feature extraction using GLRLM and CSLBP and ending with a supervised ANN classifier. The dataset contained three MRI sequences, namely, T1-weighted images, T2-weighted images. and PD-weighted images and had over 200 input images. The proposed model classified the images into malignant, benign, and normal and had an accuracy of 94%.

The authors [20] proposed a model consisting of five layers, namely, linear contrast stretching using discrete cosine transform (DCT) and edge-based histogram equalization, followed by deep learning feature extraction using VGG16 and VGG19 CNN models. The third step included correntropy-based joint learning coupled with extreme learning machine (ELM). This was then followed by fusing partial least square-based robust covariant features into a singular matrix which was then used as input to the extreme learning machine for classification of brain tumors. The dataset used for the proposed model was BRATS. The system had an accuracy of 92.50% for the BRATS 2018 dataset.

In this article [21], the authors have used the most prevalent imaging approach for discerning atypical brain tumors, i.e., magnetic resonance imaging (MRI). MRI scans have traditionally been evaluated manually by radiologists to discover abnormal irregularities in the brain. Manually interpreting many photos takes time and is tough. As a result, computer-based detection aids in precise and rapid diagnosis. The researchers suggested a strategy in this article that leverages deep transfer learning to automatically categorize normal and pathological brain MR data. To train the model, the authors employed recent deep learning algorithms such as data augmentation, optimal learning rate finding, and fine-tuning. Six hundred thirteen MRI images were used to train and test the model. The model attained a 5-fold classification accuracy of 100%. The authors created a solution which is ready for testing on large databases and can aid radiologists with their daily MR image screening.

In this article [22], the objective was to examine MRI scans of the brain in traditional way for detecting brain cancers. This method is laborious and susceptible to human errors while dealing with big data and varied types of brain tumors. The authors sought to train a CNN model to detect the three most frequent forms of brain malignancies, namely gliomas, meningiomas, and pituitary tumors, in this article. In this study, they developed the simplest conceivable CNN architecture: one convolution, one max-pooling, and one flattening layer, following a complete connection by one hidden layer. A brain tumor dataset was used in training CNN. The dataset contained 3064 T-1 weighted CE-MRI images publicly available on Fig share. The authors were able to obtain a training accuracy of 98.51% and a validation accuracy of 84.19% using our basic architecture and no prior region-based segmentation.

The paper [23] deals with a 3-class classification problem to segregate the three most prominent types of tumors: glioma, meningioma, and pituitary. The projected system uses the idea of deep transfer along with already trained Google Net for extracting attributes from brain MRI images. It uses a patient-level five-fold cross-validation process from Fig Share on MRI dataset. The mean classification accuracy of the system is 98%. The dataset from fig share was a pool of 3064 brain MRI images of 233 patients. The MRI images were T1-CE MRI modality, comprising coronal, sagittal and axial views. The dataset was bifurcated into 3 sub-categories of data consisting of 1426 images of glioma, 708 images of ningioma, and the rest 930 images for pituitary- related cancer. All images are.mat files with size 512 × 512. Google Net is designed for color RGB images, with input layer of size 224 × 224 × 3. The models used in the process were transfer learned deep CNN, SVM, and KNN, each providing accuracy of 92.3%, 97.8%, and 98% respectively.

The paper [24] focuses on the utilization of already trained CNN architecture and block-wise fine-tuning strategy contingent on transfer learning to achieve accurate as well as precise brain tumor MRI image classification. The projected method is assessed on a T1-weighted contrast-enhanced magnetic resonance images (CE-MRI) benchmark dataset. The technique implemented in the paper is more generic, as it omits the usage of handcrafted attributes, needs least pre-processing and yields an accuracy of 94.82% in 5-fold cross-validation. The outcomes are compared with old-fashioned machine learning as well as CNN methods. Investigational results state that the proposed system outclasses state-of-the-art classification on the CE-MRI dataset. A pre-trained CNN VGG19 model is used, which is edified on a large ImageNet dataset. The weights of the CNN are initialized with pre-trained VGG-19, and block-wise fine-tuning is implemented to observe the performance enhancement on CE-MRI dataset to achieve enhanced classification results. The images in the dataset are each of size 512–512 pixels, provided in matrix form with each pixel size as 49 mm (about 1.93 in) × 49 mm.

The paper [25] proposes a hybrid method involving the Neutrosophy and Convolution Neural Network (NS-CNN). Its purpose is to segregate brain MRI images and classify them as benign or malignant. The first step is MRI image segmentation by means of the neutrosophic set, i.e., expert extreme fuzzy-sure entropy (NS-EMFSE) method. In the classification stage, the attributes obtained from the segmented brain images are gathered with the help of CNN and classified with the help of SVM and KNN classifiers. Experimental calculation supported out based on 5-fold cross-validation on 80 benign tumors and 80 malign tumors. The results indicated that CNN attributes show a great classification performance, having diverse classifiers and have an improved classification performance than SVM, which has a success rate of 95.62%. The Cancer Genome Atlas Glioblastoma Multiforme (TCGA-GBM) dataset was used to test the NS-EMFSE-CNN approach. An average of 500 samples were taken in the database from several types of cancer types for TCGA. The accuracy achieved using the NS-EMFSE-CNN methods are 95.62% and 90.62%, using classifiers SVM and KNN, respectively.

In this article [26], the authors developed the deep learning classifiers which were able to classify 66 different MRI images of brain tumors and classify them into four distinct categories. The classifier was blended with the discrete wavelet transform (DWT) and principal components analysis (PCA). The authors carried out image segmentation by using fuzzy c-means. The data was acquired from the Harvard medical school website which consisted of 66 normal brain MRI images and 44 abnormal images. While classifying five different algorithms were performed by the authors which include, DNN, KNN for K=1, and for K=3, LDA, and SMO. The DNN AUC was around 98.4% while for LDA the AUC was 98.3%, for KNN=1, the AUC was 96.7, for K=3, the AUC was 95.4%, and SMO was 93.9%.

In this article [27], the authors have worked on detecting COVID-19 at an early age to stop its spread in human lungs. A model based on artificial neural network (ANN) with a combination of the CAD system has been designed for detection for accurate judgement and overcoming the limits of manual approaches. This study suggests a CAD system for COVID-19 that uses Artificial Bee Colony (ABC) optimized ANN (ABCNN) to identify and categorize anomalies in lung CT images. The lung CT images gathered from the public datasets are used to assess the suggested ABCNN technique. The suggested ABCNN methodology outperformed existing methods with a classification accuracy of 92.37% when tested on a collection of 4?0 lung CT images.

4.3 METHODOLOGY

In this chapter, the authors have applied deep learning models along with Convolutional Neural Networks (CNNs) for detecting brain tumor images. The application of transfer learning and state-of-the art algorithms helps in constructing accurate models.

Convolutional Neural Networks are algorithms used to distinguish between images based on importance assigned to features that we may find in them. The added benefit of CNN is that the pre-processing required is significantly less than other classification algorithms. They consist of interconnected weighted node layers with individual thresholds, including an input layer, hidden layer(s), and an output layer.

Transfer learning is a popular approach used to apply gained knowledge from one task as the initial point of another task. It works on tasks where model features are common. Pre-trained model approach is a very common approach used for deep learning. Now, a pre-trained model is selected, reused as the starting point for a second task and it is tuned based on the requirements of the task to optimize results. Many pre-trained models are available at hand with varying parameters like – ResNet-50, InceptionV3, VGG16, etc.

In this chapter, pre-trained models like MobileNetV2, Vision Transformer, ResNet-50, InceptionV3, and VGG16 have been used for the detection of brain tumor based on various first-order features and texture features. The results are then compared with themselves based on validation and test accuracy, recall, F1 score. The workflow of the chapter is described in Figure 4.1.

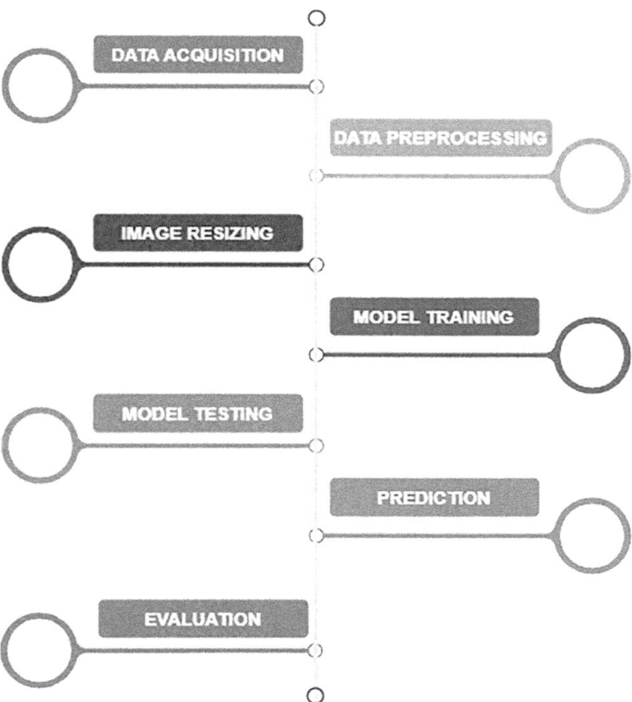

Figure 4.1 Workflow of the research.

The workflow of this chapter is described as follows:

1. **Data acquisition:** The dataset has been acquired from Kaggle, a subsidiary of Google LLC. The dataset contains five first-order features and eight texture features containing about 3764 images.
2. **Data pre-processing:** The data was cleaned and reduced including removing null values and then it was split in the ratio 70:30 for training and testing, respectively. Images were resized to 150 × 150 × 3.
3. **Model training:** The models used in this chapter are MobileNetV2, Vision Transformer, ResNet-50, InceptionV3, and VGG16.
4. **Model testing:** Based on model training, their categorical accuracy was predicted.
5. **Prediction:** The models predicted whether there was a tumor, represented by 1, or not, represented by 0.
6. **Evaluation:** All the pre-trained models' accuracy was compared.

4.3.1 Dataset

The dataset is extracted from Kaggle, a popular platform for data scientists and practitioners to publish, use, and build datasets and models. The dataset included 3764 images including both tumor and non-tumor images. The size of the data is 15 MB. and it was directly imported from the source, i.e., Kaggle to Kaggle notebook [28].

4.3.2 Applications used

Kaggle notebook is used for implementing, training, testing, and evaluation of the models. Accelerators such as GPU P100 and GPU T4x2 were used for the same provided by the Kaggle.

4.3.3 Models applied

In this chapter, the authors have used five different state-of-the-art algorithms to train, test, and evaluate the dataset. These models include VGG16, Vision Transformer, Inception V3, MobileNet V2, and ResNet50.

4.3.3.1 MobileNet V2

MobileNet V2 is a CNN architecture that is primarily made for efficiency on mobile devices. It has an initial convolutional layer comprised of 32 layers, which is succeeded by 19 layers in a bottleneck fashion. MobileNet V2 follows an inverted residual structure. The middle expansion layers use thin depth wise convolutions to filter attributes such as non-linearity. This is important to be done as it represents power in those layers [29]. The use of MobileNetV2 can be seen in Figure 4.2.

4.3.3.2 Vision transformer

The Vision Transformer, or ViT, employs the encoder part of Transformer architecture. It has been pre-trained on large datasets and can be applied on smaller datasets with high accuracy. It splits images into patches, flattens them, produces low-dimensional linear embedding from it and adds positional embedding which is then fed as input to the encoder

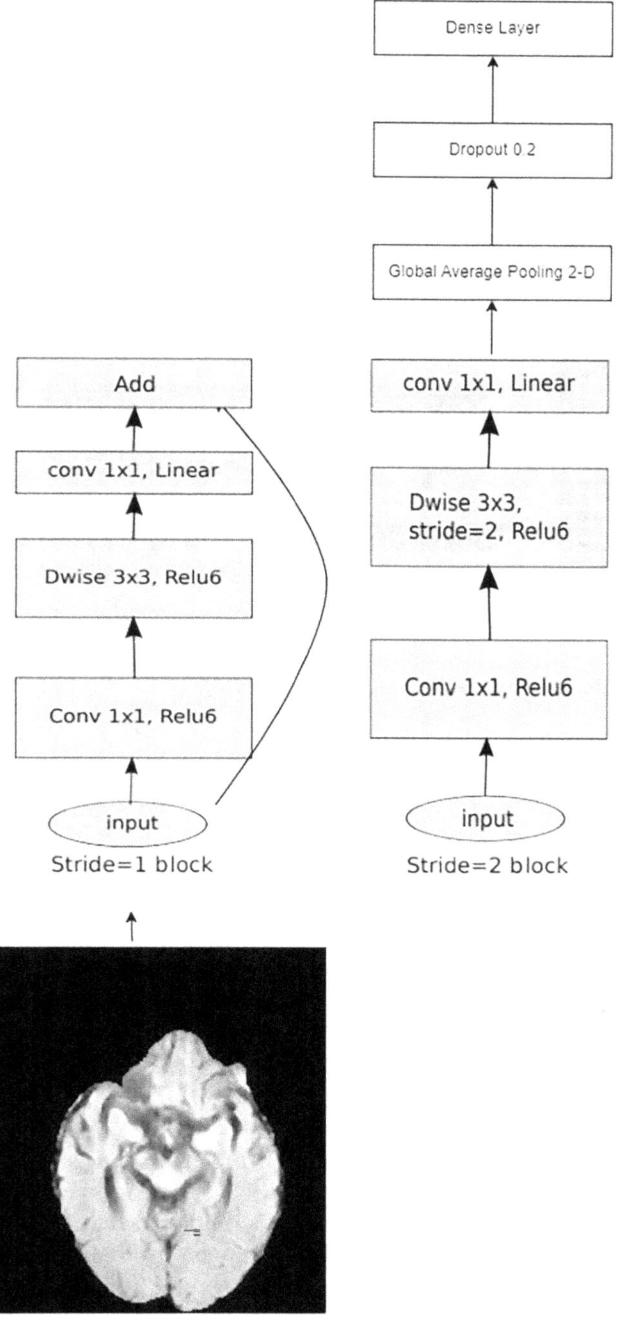

Figure 4.2 MobileNetV2 architecture applied in this chapter.

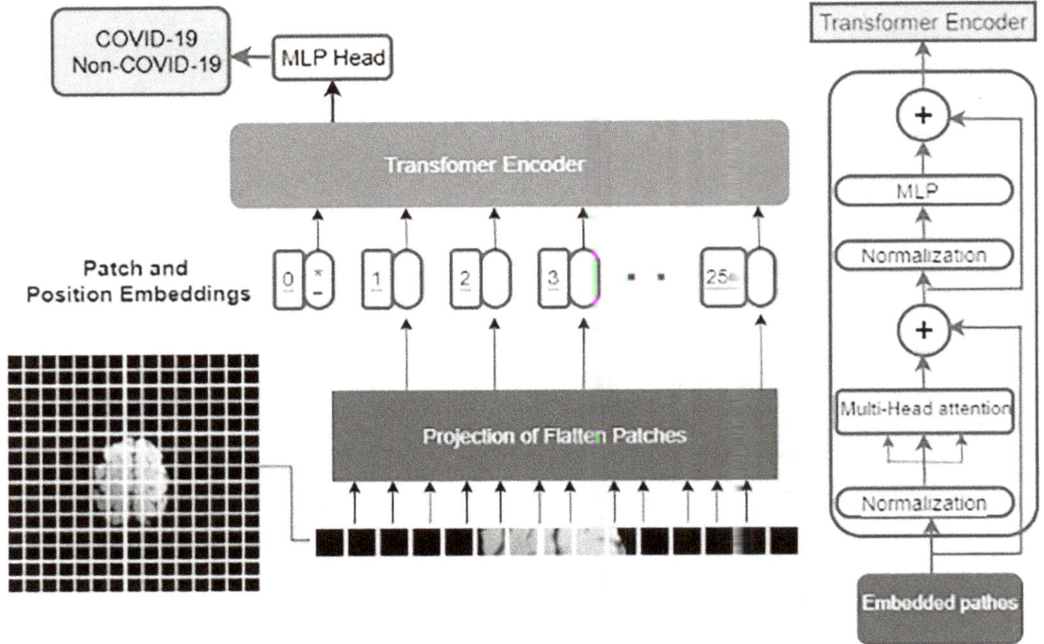

Figure 4.3 Vision transformer architecture used in this chapter.

after which it is pre-trained and fine-tuned. The use of Vision Transformer can be seen in Figure 4.3.

4.3.3.3 ResNet-50

ResNet-50 is a popular pre-trained model that is comprised of 50 layers, including convolutional layers, a MaxPool layer, and an average pool layer. It is a relatively heavier model of size 98 MB and 25.6 M parameters. It has a Top-5 accuracy of 92.1% and the highest accuracy of 74.9%. It has a bottleneck architecture which results in faster training in each layer [30]. The ResNet50 architecture can be seen in Figure 4.4.

4.3.3.4 InceptionV3

Inception V3 model is a commonly used model for image recognition and is comprised of several symmetrical as well as asymmetrical blocks. It is a moderately heavy model with a size of 92 MB and 23.9 M parameters. It has the highest accuracy of 77.9% and a Top-5 accuracy of 93.7% [31]. The Inception V3 can be seen in Figure 4.5.

4.3.3.5 VGG16

VGG 16 is an outstanding vision model architecture for detecting and classifying images. This Convolution Neural Net layer has 16 layers and is a heavy model. It has a size of 528 MB and a large network comprised of 138.4 M parameters. The topmost accuracy is 71.3% and has a Top-5 accuracy of 90.1%. The VGG16 can be seen in Figure 4.6.

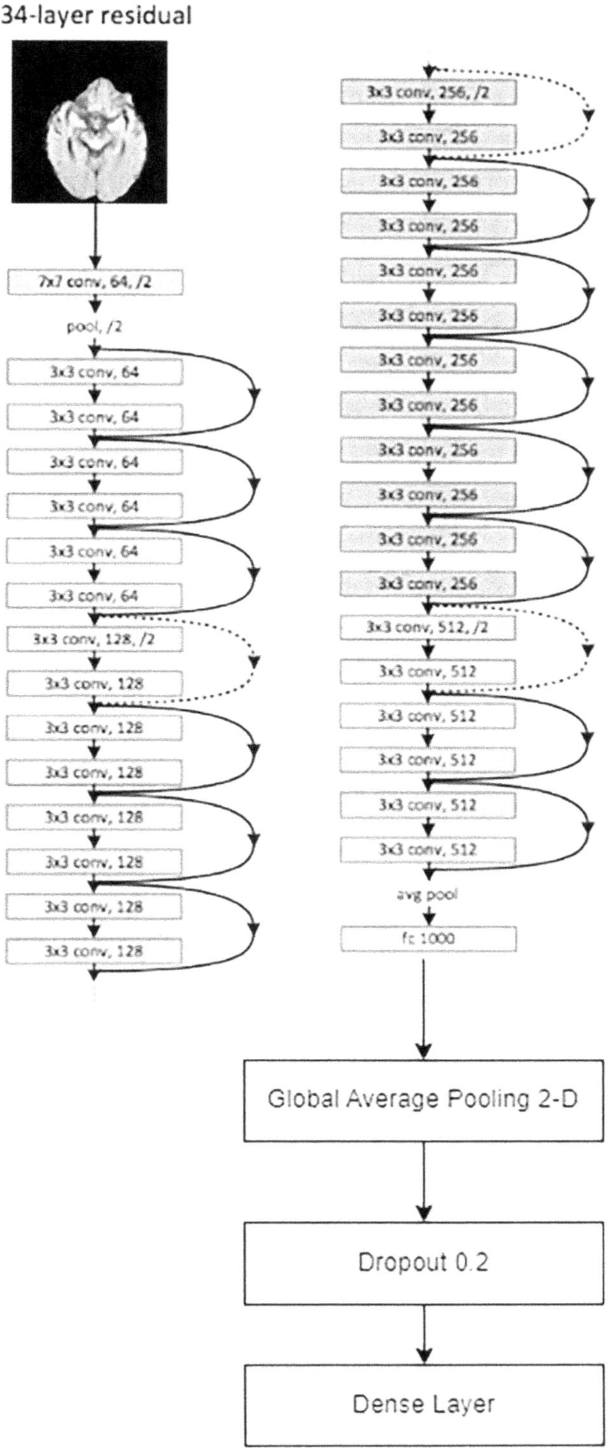

Figure 4.4 The ResNet50 architecture was used in this chapter.

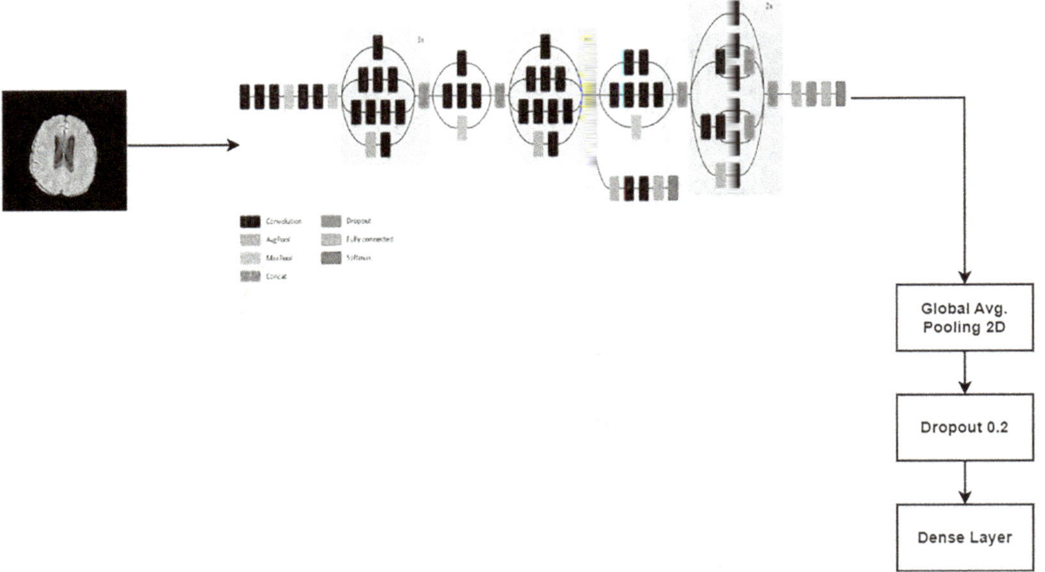

Figure 4.5. The InceptionV3 architecture is used in this chapter.

4.4 RESULTS AND DISCUSSION

In this chapter, the authors have used five models and compared the accuracy among them. In the vision transformer, the input size of the image used was 240 × 240 × 3. The train and test images were split in the ratio of 70:30 consisting about 2633 images for training and 339 images for testing. Further, the validation and test were split into a 70:30 ratio consisting of 790 images. The learning rate was 0.001 with weight decay of 0.0001. The batch size used while training this model was 32 with 100 epochs. Every image was divided into patches, with a patch size of 16 as shown in Figure 4.7. Thus, the total number of patches were according to the formula mentioned here.

Data augmentation was done by flipping the image horizontally, random rotation of 0.02, and random zoom with height and width factor of 0.02. Further, an Adam optimizer with loss function as binary cross-entropy is applied.

The confusion matrix of validation and test accuracy of vision transformer can be visualized in Figure 4.8. It shows the confusion matrix of validation accuracy, with only 12 images falsely predicted and 776 images correctly predicted.

Figure 4.9 shows the confusion matrix of test accuracy, where only seven images were misinterpreted while the rest were correctly predicted.

For the other four models, including MobileNetV2, Inception V3, ResNet50, and VGG16, the input size of the image was 224 × 224 × 3. Batch size of 32, optimizer Adam with epsilon 0.01, loss function as binary cross-entropy and metrics as Binary accuracy were applied.

From Figure 4.10, it was found that vision transformer was the best performing model among all the five models with an accuracy of 98.5%. As can be visualized, accuracies of ResNet50 and VGG16 lie between 85–90%, while that of Inception V3 and MobileNetV2 lied slightly above 90%, whereas Vision Transformer was above all represented in blue color.

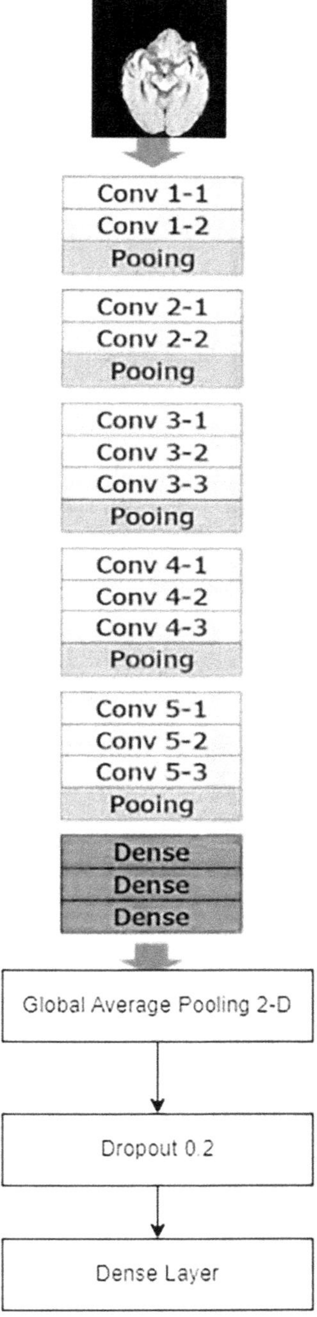

Figure 4.6 VGG16 architecture used in this chapter.

Similarly, the vision transformer had the least loss value of around 0.015 as compared to other models. VGG16 and ResNet50 lied between 0.3–0.4%, while that of MobileNetV2 and InceptionV3 lied between 0.2–0.3%, whereas the least loss was of the vision transformer as shown in Figure 4.11.

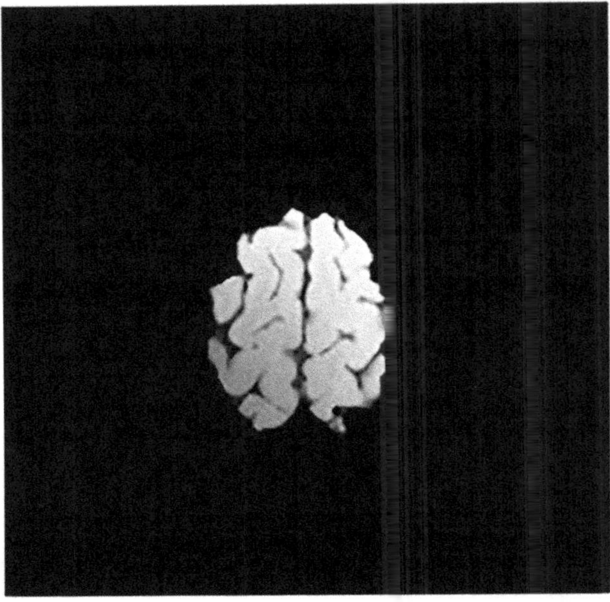

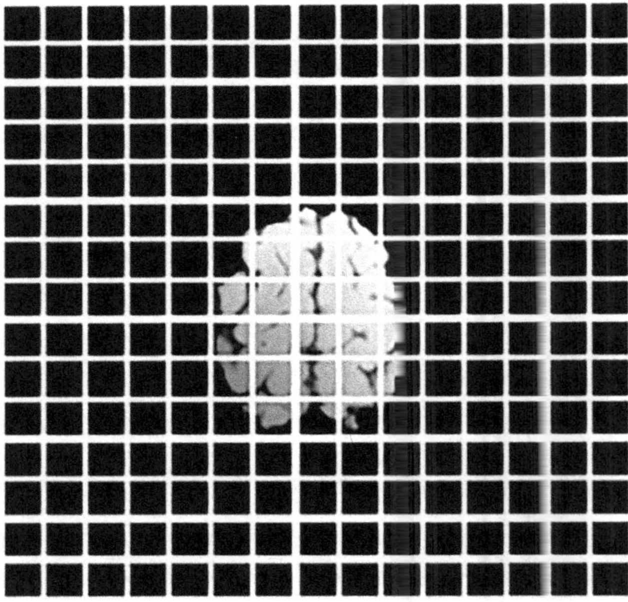

Figure 4.7 The patches in which every image was segregated into patch sizes of 16.

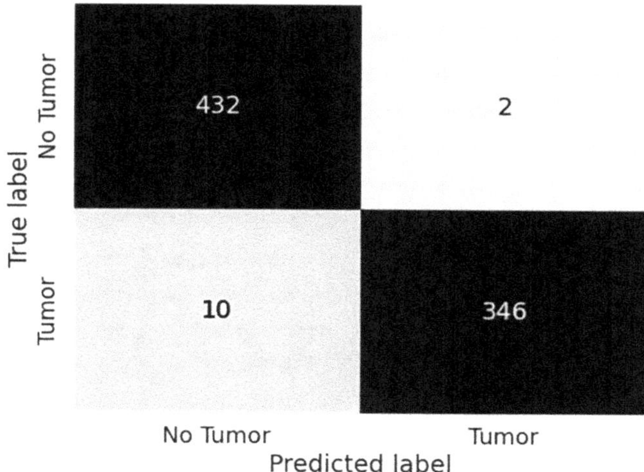

Figure 4.8 Confusion matrix of validation accuracy of vision transformer.

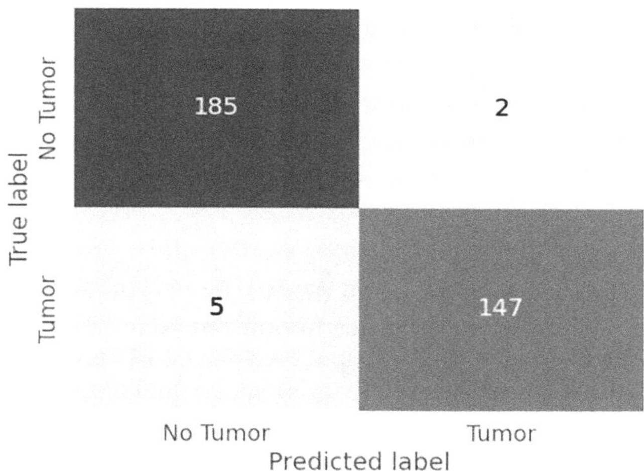

Figure 4.9 Confusion matrix of test accuracy of vision transformer.

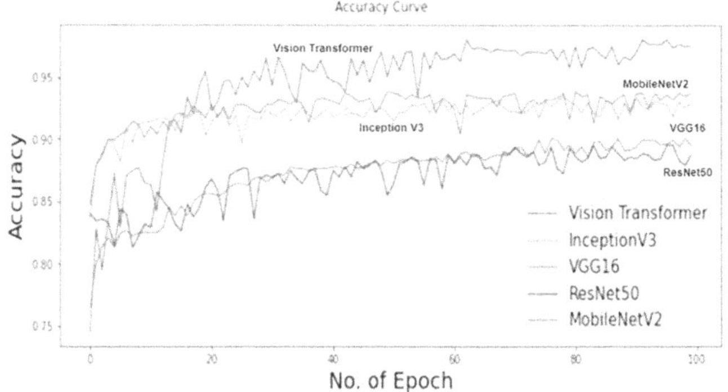

Figure 4.10 Accuracy curve of all 5 models against no. of epochs.

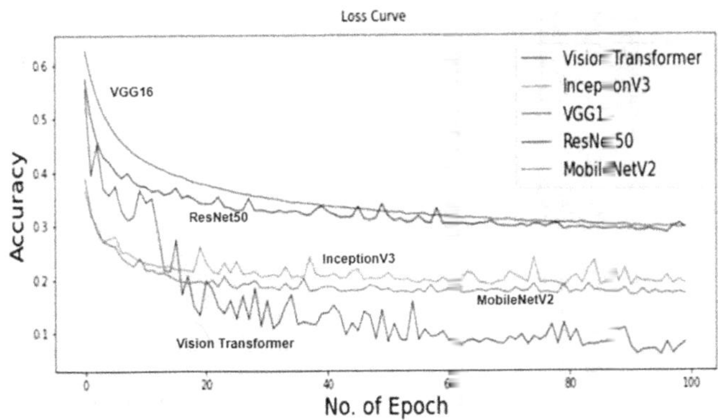

Figure 4.11 Loss curve of all five models against no. of epochs.

Table 4.1 Represents accuracies, precision recall, and F1-score of five models used in this chapter

Model name	*Validation accuracy*	*Test accuracy*	*Precision*	*Recall*	*F1-score*
MobileNetV2	0.942	0.944	0.942	0.942	0.942
Inception V3	0.936	0.936	0.936	0.936	0.936
VGG16	0.902	0.903	0.906	0.903	0.902
ResNet50	0.887	0.880	0.894	0.894	0.896
Vision Transformer	**0.985**	**0.985**	**0.988**	**0.982**	**0.985**

The validation and test accuracy, precision, recall, and F1-score can be seen in Table 4.1 . From the table it is clearly understandable that Vision Transformer has outperformed the other four models in all attributes. The validation and test accuracy of Vision Transformer is 98.5%, each with precision of 98.8%, recall of 98.2%, and F1-score of 98.5%. The second best performing model was MobilenetV2, with validation and test accuracies of 94.2% and 94.4% respectively, with precision, recall, and F1-score of 94.2% each. These outcomes can be combined with IoT devices in the future, which can later be used by medical professionals and doctors such as [32].

4.5 CONCLUSION

Brain tumors are one of the deadliest and most complex diseases in the history of humanity. While non-malignant tumors can be cured through surgeries, malignant tumors are the ones that need more attention and are not curable. MRI is one of the best techniques used by doctors, neurologists, and physicians to validate the occurrence of brain tumors. In this chapter, the objective was to detect the brain tumor using recent deep learning models such as a vision transformer and compare the end results with other models used in this chapter. In this chapter, the authors have collected datasets from Kaggle to conduct their research. The authors used five different models to compare the end results. Among all the five models applied, it was found that the vision transformer was the best performing model, with validation accuracy of 98.5%, precision of 98.8%, and F1 score of 98.5%.

The challenge while conducting the research was to find the correct accelerator or GPU so that the runtime of the code was not slow at all. Running the code online at times can take hours to compile and thus slow down the process. This was reduced by working on Kaggle and GPUs provided by them. The model proposed in the article consisting of vision transformer-based detection of brain tumors can be used in MRIs. This will give doctors a precise result and help them classify and make judgments about tumors more efficiently.

REFERENCES

1. 'Brain Anatomy and How the Brain Works | Johns Hopkins Medicine'. https://www.hopkinsmedicine.org/health/conditions-and-diseases/anatomy-of-the-brain (accessed Mar. 26, 2023).
2. 'Brain Tumor: Types, Risk Factors, Symptoms, and Treatment'. https://www.healthline.com/health/brain-tumor (accessed Dec. 22, 2022).
3. 'Brain Tumor: Symptoms, Signs & Causes'. https://my.clevelandclinic.org/health/diseases/6149-brain-cancer-brain-tumor (accessed Dec. 22, 2022).
4. 'Brain Tumor Facts'. https://braintumor.org/brain-tumors/about-brain-tumors/brain-tumor-facts/ (accessed Dec. 22, 2022).
5. 'World Brain Tumour Day 2022 "Together we are stronger", Health News, ET HealthWorld'. https://health.economictimes.indiatimes.com/news/industry/world-brain-tumour-day-2022-together-we-are-stronger/92078118 (accessed Dec. 22, 2022).
6. D. R. Nayak, N. Padhy, P. K. Mallick, M. Zymbler, and S. Kumar, 'Brain Tumor Classification Using Dense Efficient-Net', *Axioms*, vol. 11, no. 1, p. 34, Jan. 2022, doi: 10.3390/axioms11010034.
7. K. Sharma, K. Khanna, S. Gambhir, and M. Gambhir, 'Study on Brain Tumor Classification Through MRI Images Using a Deep Convolutional Neural Network', *Int J Inf Retr*, vol. 12, no. 1, pp. 1–19, Jan. 2022, doi: 10.4018/IJIRR.289610.
8. S. Rinesh *et al.*, 'Investigations on Brain Tumor Classification Using Hybrid Machine Learning Algorithms', *J Healthc Eng*, vol. 2022, pp. 1–9, Feb. 2022, doi: 10.1155/2022/2761847.
9. R. Nanmaran *et al.*, 'Investigating the Role of Image Fusion in Brain Tumor Classification Models Based on Machine Learning Algorithm for Personalized Medicine', *Comput Math Methods Med*, vol. 2022, pp. 1–13, Feb. 2022, doi: 10.1155/2022/7137524.
10. U. Zahid *et al.*, 'BrainNet: Optimal Deep Learning Feature Fusion for Brain Tumor Classification', *Comput Intell Neurosci*, vol. 2022, 2022, doi: 10.1155/2022/1465173.
11. A. Rehman, M. A. Khan, T. Saba, Z. Mehmood, U. Tariq, and N. Ayesha, 'Microscopic Brain Tumor Detection and Classification Using <scp>3D CNN</scp> and Feature Selection Architecture', *Microsc Res Tech*, vol. 84, no. 1, pp. 133–149, Jan. 2021, doi: 10.1002/jemt.23597.
12. T. Sadad *et al.*, 'Brain Tumor Detection and Multi-Classification Using Advanced Deep Learning Techniques', *Microsc Res Tech*, vol. 84, no. 6, pp. 1296–1308, Jun. 2021, doi: 10.1002/jemt.23688.
13. A. Saleh, R. Sukaik, and S. S. Abu-Naser, 'Brain Tumor Classification Using Deep Learning', in *2020 International Conference on Assistive and Rehabilitation Technologies (iCareTech)*, IEEE, Aug. 2020, pp. 131–136. doi: 10.1109/iCareTech49914.2020.00032.
14. Z. Ullah, M. U. Farooq, S. H. Lee, and D. An, 'A Hybrid Image Enhancement Based Brain MRI Images Classification Technique', *Med Hypotheses*, vol. 143, p. 109922, Oct. 2020, doi: 10.1016/J.MEHY.2020.109922.
15. A. Rehman, S. Naz, M. I. Razzak, F. Akram, and M. Imran, 'A Deep Learning-Based Framework for Automatic Brain Tumors Classification Using Transfer Learning', *Circuits Syst Signal Process*, vol. 39, no. 2, pp. 757–775, Feb. 2020, doi: 10.1007/s00034-019-01246-3.
16. J. Amin, M. Sharif, M. Raza, T. Saba, R. Sial, and S. A. Shad, 'Brain Tumor Detection: A Long Short-Term Memory (LSTM)-Based Learning Model', *Neural Comput Appl*, vol. 32, no. 20, pp. 15965–15973, Oct. 2020, doi: 10.1007/s00521-019-04650-7.

17. S. Kumar and D. P. Mankame, 'Optimization Driven Deep Convolution Neural Network for Brain Tumor Classification', *Biocybern Biomed Eng*, vol. 40, no. 3, pp. 1190–1204, Jul. 2020, doi: 10.1016/j.bbe.2020.05.009.
18. A. Çinar and M. Yildirim, 'Detection of Tumors on Brain MRI Images Using the Hybrid Convolutional Neural Network Architecture', *Med Hypotheses*, vol. 139, Jun. 2020, doi: 10.1016/j.mehy.2020.109684.
19. M. Mudda, R. Manjunath, and N. Krishnamurthy, 'Brain Tumor Classification Using Enhanced Statistical Texture Features', *IETE J Res*, 2020, doi: 10.1080/03772063.2020.1775501.
20. M. A. Khan *et al.*, 'Multimodal Brain Tumor Classification Using Deep Learning and Robust Feature Selection: A Machine Learning Application for Radiologists', *Diagnostics*, vol. 10, no. 8, Aug. 2020, doi: 10.3390/diagnostics10080565.
21. M. Talo, U. B. Baloglu, Ö. Yıldırım, and U. Rajendra Acharya, 'Application of Deep Transfer Learning for Automated Brain Abnormality Classification Using MR Images', *Cogn Syst Res*, vol. 54, pp. 176–188, May 2019, doi: 10.1016/j.cogsys.2018.12.007.
22. N. Abiwinanda, M. Hanif, S. T. Hesaputra, A. Handayani, and T. R. Mengko, 'Brain Tumor Classification Using Convolutional Neural Network', 2019, pp. 183–189. doi: 10.1007/978-981-10-9035-6_33.
23. S. Deepak and P. M. Ameer, 'Brain Tumor Classification Using Deep CNN Features via Transfer Learning', *Comput Biol Med*, vol. 111, p. 103345, Aug. 2019, doi: 10.1016/j.compbiomed.2019.103345.
24. Z. N. K. Swati *et al.*, 'Brain Tumor Classification for MR Images Using Transfer Learning and Fine-Tuning', *Computerized Medical Imaging and Graphics*, vol. 75, pp. 34–46, Jul. 2019, doi: 10.1016/j.compmedimag.2019.05.001.
25. F. Özyurt, E. Sert, E. Avci, and E. Dogantekin, 'Brain Tumor Detection Based on Convolutional Neural Network with Neutrosophic Expert Maximum Fuzzy Sure Entropy', *Measurement*, vol. 147, p. 106830, Dec. 2019, doi: 10.1016/j.measurement.2019.07.058.
26. H. Mohsen, E.-S. A. El-Dahshan, E.-S. M. El-Horbaty, and A.-B. M. Salem, 'Classification Using Deep Learning Neural Networks for Brain Tumors', *Future Comput Inform J*, vol. 3, no. 1, pp. 68–71, Jun. 2018, doi: 10.1016/j.fcij.2017.12.001.
27. S. Punitha, T. Stephan, R. Kannan, M. Mahmud, M. S. Kaiser, and S. B. Belhaouari, 'Detecting COVID-19 from Lung Computed Tomography Images: A Swarm Optimized Artificial Neural Network Approach', *IEEE Access*, vol. 11, pp. 12378–12393, 2023, doi: 10.1109/ACCESS.2023.3236812.
28. J. Bohaju, 'Brain Tumor', *Kaggle*. 2020. doi: 10.34740/KAGGLE/DSV/1370629.
29. M. Sandler, A. Howard, M. Zhu, A. Zhmoginov, and L.-C. Chen, 'MobileNetV2: Inverted Residuals and Linear Bottlenecks'. In *Proceedings of the IEEE conference on computer vision and pattern recognition* (pp. 4510–4520), Jan. 2018.
30. K. He, X. Zhang, S. Ren, and J. Sun, 'Deep Residual Learning for Image Recognition'. http://image-net.org/challenges/LSVRC/2015/ (accessed Mar. 26, 2023 [Online]).
31. C. Szegedy, V. Vanhoucke, S. Ioffe, and J. Shlens, 'Rethinking the Inception Architecture for Computer Vision'. In *Proceedings of the IEEE conference on computer vision and pattern recognition* (pp. 2818–2826), 2016.
32. D. P. Yedurkar, S. Metkar, F. Al-Turjman, N. Yardi, and T. Stephan, 'An IoT Based Novel Hybrid Seizure Detection Approach for Epileptic Monitoring', *IEEE Trans Industr Inform*, pp. 1–13, 2023, doi: 10.1109/TII.2023.3274913.

Chapter 5

Early detection of skin cancer through human-computer collaboration

Piyush Kumar[1], *Rishi Chauhan*[1], *Achyut Shankar*[2], *and Thompson Stephan*[3]

[1]Department of Computer Science and Engineering, Amity School of Engineering and Technology, Amity University, Noida, Uttar Pradesh, India

[2]WMG, University of Warwick, Coventry, United Kingdom

[3]Department of Computer Science and Engineering, Graphic Era Deemed to be University, Dehradun, Uttarakhand, India

5.1 INTRODUCTION

Skin cancer is a perilous disease due to which a lot of people suffer every year. The disease transpires on the skin of people and spreads all over the skin rapidly as shown in Figure 5.1. This occurs due to the peculiar growth of skin cells. Skin cancer is broadly classified into three distinct categories. These are basal cell cancer (BCC), squamous cell cancer (SCC), and melanoma. Melanoma is the most fatal of all the skin cancer types. It is difficult to detect melanoma from the naked eye.

Most people get affected by skin cancer due to being exposed to ultraviolet radiation. People who have lighter skin are more prone to suffer from this disease. Body parts like the torso, or upper extremities or lower extremities, etc. are severely affected by skin cancer. By the end of 2018, there were around 300,000 patients with skin cancer. Over 1 million people have been identified with BCC or SCC in 2018. If we talk about melanoma, the worldwide cases for melanoma alone were around 150,000 by the year 2020. People of Australia and New Zealand were found to be highly infectious as shown in figure 5.2 [1].

The melanoma rates of Australian and New Zealand males were significantly high compared to other countries as shown in Figure 5.3.

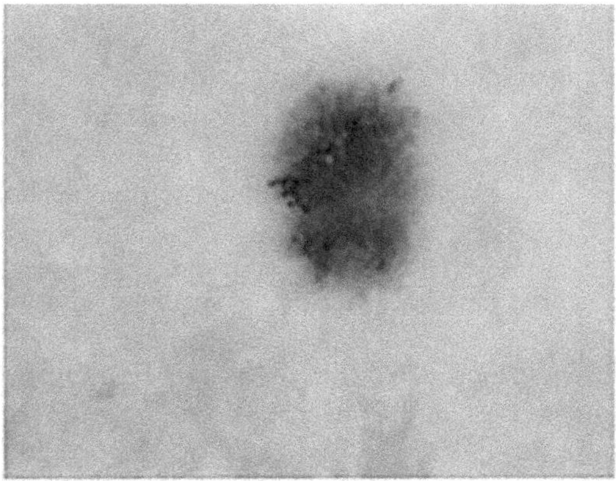

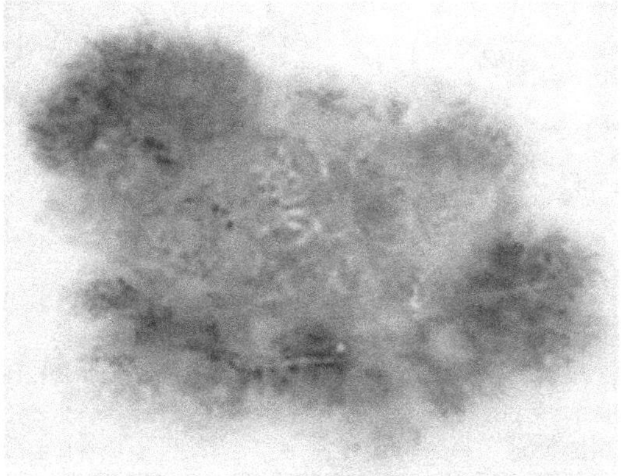

Figure 5.1 Skin cancer images; both images are Melanoma type.

DOI: 10.1201/9781003369059-7

Rank	Country	Number	ASR/100,000
	World	*324,635*	*3.4*
1	Australia	16,171	36.6
2	New Zealand	2,801	31.6
3	Denmark	2,886	29.7
4	The Netherlands	8,310	27.0
5	Norway	2,567	26.4
6	Sweden	4,265	23.3
7	Switzerland	3,357	21.6
8	Germany	31,468	20.5
9	Slovenia	735	19.7
10	Finland	2,090	19.5

Figure 5.2 Data showing total melanoma cases over the world and top 10 countries suffering from it [1].

Rank (men)	Country	Number	ASR/100,000
	World	*173,844*	*3.8*
1	Australia	9,463	42.9
2	New Zealand	1,541	34.8
3	The Netherlands	4,426	27.1
4	Denmark	1,382	26.2
5	Norway	1,298	25.8
6	Switzerland	1,822	22.8
7	Sweden	2,146	22.2
8	Germany	17,260	21.1
9	Slovenia	379	19.9
10	Finland	1,090	19.5

Figure 5.3 Data showing total melanoma cases for men over the world and top 10 countries suffering from it [1].

For females suffering from melanoma, Denmark ranked atop of Australia and New Zealand as shown in Figure 5.4.

Mortality of the entire world due to melanoma is around 57,000 in the year 2020. Of this, New Zealand people, i.e., around 472 people, have died due to melanoma skin cancer followed by Norway, i.e., 375 as shown in Figure 5.5.

Out of 472 New Zealand people, 321 were men while 151 were women. Thus, the ratio of male to female casualties in New Zealand is around 3:1. This can be seen in Figures 5.6 and 5.7.

Rank (women)	Country	Number	ASR/100,000
	World	*150.791*	*3.0*
1	Denmark	1.504	33.6
2	Australia	6.709	30.8
3	New Zealand	1.260	28.9
4	Norway	1.269	27.5
5	The Netherlands	3.890	27.4
6	Sweden	2.120	24.6
7	Belgium	1.951	22.6
8	Switzerland	1.535	20.8
9	Germany	14.208	20.4
10	Ireland	772	20.3

Figure 5.4 Data showing total melanoma cases for women over the world and top 10 countries suffering from it [1].

Rank	Country	Number	ASR/100,000
	World	*57.043*	*0.6*
1	New Zealand	472	4.7
2	Norway	375	3.2
3	Montenegro	32	3.0
4	Slovakia	317	2.8
5	Slovenia	127	2.6
6	Australia	1.408	2.4
7	Denmark	341	2.4
8	Croatia	236	2.4
9	The Netherlands	906	2.3
10	Serbia	393	2.3

Figure 5.5 Data showing total death cases due to melanoma over the world and top 10 countries suffering from it [1].

As said earlier, melanoma is the most dangerous type. It can appear anywhere on the body, whether the skin is healthy or where a tumorous mole is already present. However, the type of cancer, the patient's age, whether the cancer is chronic, and the stage of the disease all affect how the disease is treated. Various traditional methods of treating cancer are undergoing radiation therapy, topical chemotherapy, and cryotherapy.

In India it is found that the rate of skin cancer, specifically melanoma, is quite low when compared to countries in the Western Pacific and Europe. In India, mostly North Indians

Rank (men)	Country	Number	ASR/100,000
	World	*32,385*	*0.7*
1	New Zealand	321	6.7
2	Montenegro	20	4.0
3	Norway	207	3.8
4	Slovakia	177	3.8
5	Slovenia	76	3.4
6	Croatia	140	3.3
7	Australia	891	3.2
8	Serbia	242	3.1
9	North Macedonia	46	2.8
10	The Netherlands	543	2.7

Figure 5.6 Data showing total death cases due to melanoma for men all over the world and top 10 countries suffering from it [1].

Rank (women)	Country	Number	ASR/100,000
	World	*24,6[illegible]8*	*0.5*
1	New Zealand	1[illegible]1	2.8
2	Norway	1[illegible]8	2.6
3	Montenegro	[illegible]2	2.3
4	Slovakia	1[illegible]0	2.2
5	Denmark	1[illegible]4	2.1
6	The Netherlands	3[illegible]3	1.9
7	Slovenia	[illegible]1	1.9
8	Sweden	2[illegible]3	1.8
9	Australia	5[illegible]7	1.7
10	Serbia	1[illegible]1	1.7

Figure 5.7 Data showing total death cases due to melanoma for women all over the world and top 10 countries suffering from it [1].

have melanoma, where the male rate is 1.62 and the female rate is 1.21 [2]. With advancement in science and technology, new methods have been developed over the years for treatment of such complex diseases. With the assistance of artificial intelligence and machine learning, complex algorithms can be applied and used to make predictions. There is no such realm where AI and ML have not left their footprints. Algorithms like support vector machine (SVM), K-NN, random forest, decision tree, etc., are universally used nowadays in recent research works. Apart from this, the deep learning models, or pre-trained models for image processing like VGG19, VGG16, MobileNetV2, etc., are applied on the images to classify them based on their respective classes. Other applications like image segmentations or computer vision are also applied using these methods. These transfer learning models and state-of-the-art algorithms require high computational power, GPUs, VRAMs, and memory. Due to these GPUs, time required to implement these complex models is reduced. Today, there are several companies like NVIDIA, AMD, TESLA, etc. who have developed GPUs with high VRAMs, high computational power, and high memory allocation space [3].

In medical grounds, computer-aided diagnosis (CAD) has become immensely popular over the years. Tele-medicine is now becoming a trend. Patients can interact with their doctors and consult them from far distances [4]. Even, sometimes, with the assistance of tele-medicine, doctors perform certain complex surgeries. There are a lot of mobile applications that have been developed over the years where skin cancer patients can interact with their dermatologists. These interactions can be termed Human-Computer Interaction (HCI).

About 60% of the total world population uses mobile phones. There are over 332 million people who have become inexperienced users over the last year [5]. Thus, mobile phones are highly in demand and, apart from just browsing the internet, playing games, or watching Netflix, people use their device as a tool for diagnosis of their disease.

There are more than 229 skin cancer-related applications that are relevant to melanoma or non-melanoma skin cancer [6]. All apps include various functionalities like academic aid, references, self-observation, tele-dermatology, analytical tools, etc. [6]. All applications are free of cost, while there are some paid applications whose price ranges from $1 to $135 [6]. There are various IoMT applications that can be explored, while detection of skin cancer can be automated in the web application. In this article [7], the authors have programmed analysis for sustainable smart cities for the future. Although, due to COVID-19, even doctors and practitioners are emphasizing remote and automated detection of diseases so that the spread of viruses is minimum and patients get the best treatment [8].

This chapter's goal is to offer a web application that can detect the type of skin cancer and assist the cancer patients in knowing their cancer type at an early stage. During this pandemic, when the world is fighting against SARS-CoV-2, it is nearly impossible for cancer patients to visit their consultants for their regular treatment. Thus, during this pandemic, the web application will assist the doctors in detecting skin cancer at early stage.

5.2 LITERATURE REVIEW

The experts in this article [4] trained the Alex Net model using the HAM10000 dataset. The clinicians interacted via web application mode. Students at the Medical University of Vienna developed the platform that functioned as an interface for doctors to evaluate and measure the processed image. The model provides results that are 80.3% accurate, with a 95% Confidence Interval (CI).

In this article [9] the graph-cut algorithm was used by researchers for segmentation purposes. Naive Bayes classifier is used for classification of disease. ISIC 2017 dataset was used in this paper. Median filers were used to remove noise from the images. The authors have applied GLCM technique for feature extraction. Around 23906 images were used. After the model was implemented the accuracy for benign, melanoma and keratosis were 94.3%, 91.2%, and 92.9% respectively. Melanoma is poisonous skin cancer.

The research for this article [10] recommended a method based on Fourier Spectral analysis. In this process, filters such as the conventional, inverse, and k-law nonlinear filters are used. The Centenario Hospital in Hidalgo and the National Cancer Institute provided the data (INcan). The images are converted to grayscale before classification is performed. Seventy-two photos of benign lesions were included in the dataset of 332 dermatological images of skin cancer. The model resulted in the confidence level of 95.4%.

Further, in this article [11], the academics proposed methods based on deep neural networks. The images were cleaned and pre-processed using a deep Convolutional Neural Network. The dataset was extracted from the DermaQuest Database. The database had 126 images, of which 66 were of melanoma and the remaining 60 were not. The ratio of training to testing is 75% to 25%. Three different matrices, namely sensitivity, specificity, and accuracy, are employed for the numerical evaluation. The model's sensitivity, specificity, and accuracy were, respectively, 91.2%, 98.9%, and 93.5%.

In this paper [12], the SVM and ANN are used to detect melanoma skin cancer. The collection, which includes 320 photos overall, was extracted from Dermweb. 220 of the 320 images are melanoma skin lesions, while 100 of them are non-melanoma skin lesions. During the pre-processing phase, the median filter is employed. During the pre-processing stage, hairs are removed from the photos using the Dull Razor software.

In this article [13], melanoma skin cancer is detected using RCNN. This RCNN along with the use of fuzzy C-means clustering was made. In this study, the ISIC-2016 dataset was utilized. One thousand two hundred seventy-six photos totaled in the dataset; 900 were utilized for training, and 376 were used for testing. The model achieved 94.17% specificity, 97.81% sensitivity, and 94.8% accuracy.

In this paper [14], SVM is applied for classification purposes. Principal Component Analysis or PCA is done for trait extraction and TDS score metric was used. The Skin Cancer Picture-2016 provided on the Skin Vision website is just one example, the ISIC-2016 dataset was used in this study. Here, the median filter was used to clean the data. In this paper, picture segmentation is accomplished using Region of Interest (ROI) clustering. The accuracy achieved at the end was 92.1%.

In this paper [15], the watershed algorithm is used as segmentation process. K-NN, SVM, and Random Forest are used as classifiers. ABCD rule and GLCM method were combined for feature extraction. The ISIC dataset was used, where 1000 sample images were taken. As a result, it was discovered that Support Vector Machine performs better in terms of score than the Random Forest algorithm and K-Nearest Neighbor classifiers. Of the SVM's results, 89.43% were accurate while using the ABCD rule. The findings were 76.87% and 69.54% accuracy when compared to random forest and K-NN, respectively.

In this article [16], the researchers have designed a CNN model for detecting cancer. They used the HAM10000 dataset and MATLAB software tool for conducting their research. In their work, the researchers used deep learning models including MobileNetV2, Google Net, VGG16, DarkNet19, Shuffle Net, InceptionV3, Xception, SqueezNet, Resnet18, ResNet50, NasNet large, and NasNet Mobile. Among all these models, the Xception acquired the highest precision of 96.66% to classify cancer.

An original [17] idea has been applied in this paper to identify skin cancer. The authors of this paper have ensembled CNN with Multilayer perceptron for analyzing skin cancer images. The researchers have used HAM10000 dataset for detecting skin cancer and analyzing the images, which was then compared with results of other architecture. The suggested hybrid model in this article is unique in that it has a network structure that can manage both structured data. Overall top-1 and top-2 accuracy for the seven groups is 86%, 95%, and 96%, respectively, according to the findings.

In this article [18], the authors have created an automated framework which will extract key attributes from skin cancer images using CNN model for detection of melanoma.

During their research, the authors also investigated the consequences for boundary localization and normalization techniques for detecting cancer. They used 4 datasets namely, PH^2, ISIC 2016, and HAM10000, ISIC 2017. Results demonstrate that the DenseNet-121 with Multi-Layer Perceptron (MLP) performs better in terms of accuracy when compared to other CNN models and novel approaches, scoring 98.33%, 80.47%, 81.16%, and 81% on the PH, ISIC 2016, ISIC 2017, and HAM10000 datasets, respectively.

This study [19] offers a machine learning-based automatic image-based technique for identifying and classifying skin issues. The image will be analyzed, processed, and relegated using computational methods. To consider the many various features of processed photos, computational methods will be used to evaluate, process, and relegate image data. Skin photos are processed to improve the general clarity of the image after being first filtered to eliminate unwanted noise from the image. Advanced methods, such as Convolutional Neural Network (CNN), can be used to take features from an image, categories the image using the SoftMax classifier's algorithm, and produce a diagnostic report. This application will be a more effective and reliable system than the traditional method for diagnosing dermatological illnesses because it will give findings more quickly and accurately than the previous approach.

In this research [20], the sparrow search algorithm, a meta-heuristic optimizer, is suggested as a threshold-based automatic method for skin cancer detection, classification, and segmentation. The segmentation procedure is carried out using five U-Net versions in various combinations. In addition, the optimization of the hyperparameters is carried out by the meta-heuristic SpaSA algorithm using eight pre-trained CNN models. The dataset is compiled from five publicly available sources, where two distinct kinds of datasets are produced. The results reported for UNet++ with DenseNet201 with accuracy of 94.16% as accuracy, 91.39% as F1-accuracy.

In this article [21], to recover the damaged region from a skin cancer picture, a unique MFO-Fuzzy U net segmentation approach has been developed in this study. Raspberry Pi-connected IoT has been used for all picture processing. Bilateral filtering is used during the pre-processing of the photos to get rid of any unnecessary noise artefacts. Fuzzy U-net is used to overlap the skin region using the pre-processed photos as input. In order to segment the images, they are therefore sent into a fuzzy u-net, and May Fly Optimizer is employed to boost the accuracy range. To compare the efficacy of the current technique, accuracy, precision, specificity, recall, and F1 score were taken into consideration. Traditional networks like YOLO net, seg net, Mask RCNN, and U-net perform less accurately than the Fuzzy u-net. Using fuzzy u-net, the high accuracy ranges of 97.57% are maintained. For LinkNet-B7, U-net, and FCNs, the suggested MFO-Fuzzy U net model improves overall accuracy by 3.43%, 0.83%, and 9.21%, respectively.

In this article [22], the authors have found that in several fine-grained object classes, deep convolutional neural networks (CNN) have demonstrated excellent separability. To categorize dermoscopy pictures into benign or malignant lesions, this research proposes two brand-new hybrid CNN models with an SVM classifier at the output layer. Concatenated features from the first and second CNN models are sent to the SVM classifier, which classifies them. The labels acquired from a knowledgeable dermatologist are used as a benchmark to assess how well the suggested model performs. On the publicly accessible ISBI 2016 dataset, the suggested models outperformed the most recent CNN models. The proposed models' accuracy rates of 88.02% and 87.43% are still greater than those of the conventional CNN models.

5.3 METHODOLOGY

Advanced Convolutional Neural Networks (CNNs) and deep learning models are employed in this chapter to recognize and categorize various types of skin cancer pictures. Deep neural networks are quite different from supervised machine learning algorithms. It involves the utilization of RAM, GPUs, and hundreds of GBs of VRAM in GPUs. Hence, transfer learning is applied to build accurate models in a timely manner.

Transfer learning is an ability done to transmit knowledge. Every day, people learn something new that can be applied elsewhere to solve similar kinds of work. It can be said that transfer learning is the concept of overcoming remote learning models and applying data obtained for one work to solve the associated ones. In transfer learning models vital information such as weights of layers, features, etc., is extracted from the already trained models for training new models [23]. Now transfer learning is expressed in terms of the pre-trained model. These models are trained on large benchmark dataset to solve problems of a similar kind [24]. There are different pre-trained models that have distinct size, accuracy, depth, and parameters. For e.g., ResNet50, VGG16, VGG19, InceptionV3, etc.

5.3.1 Dataset

HAM10000 dataset is a popular dataset used in much research works in the field of classification of skin images. Hence, this dataset was used for classification and training the model. The dataset contains 10015 dermatoscopic images. All the images were of the domain of pigmented abrasions. The dataset consisted of seven distinct categories of skin cancers. The dataset also includes metadata that states that more than 50% of lesions are validated by histopathology, and the remaining occurrences are either confirmed by supplement examination, expert approval, or in-vivo confocal microscopy validation (confocal)The median age of patients is 40–50 years of age. Additionally, around 54% of them are males while 46% person are women. Further around 22% of patients have tumors on their backs while 21% have tumors on lower extremities [25,26].

5.3.2 Device/application used

The device used for the purpose of project was ASUS - ROG Zephyrus 15.6″ QHD Gaming Laptop with AMD Ryzen 9 of 16GB Memory with NVIDIA GeForce RTX 3070 and 1TB SSD. Jupyter notebook and Google Collaboratory was used for the purpose of training the model and projecting the kind of skin cancer. Visual Studio Code was utilized for innovation and the design of the web application.

5.3.3 ResNet – 50 architecture

The pre-trained deep learning model ResNet50, also known as the Deep Residual Network architecture, comprises around 25,636,712 parameters. The model is only 98 MB in size and has a top-5 accuracy of 92.1%. This accuracy refers to the model's performance on the ImageNet validation dataset. The ResNet50 architecture is divided into four stages. The input layer takes images having their height, width, and channels. The most common size during experiments is (224 × 224 × 3). Three here refers to the RGB color channels. There are initially two layers: a convolution layer with a 7 × 7 kernel size and a max-pooling layer with a 3 × 3 core size. Phase 1 contains three residual blocks, each including three layers with a convolutional size of 64, 64, and 128. Phase 2 involves doubling the channel size and cutting the input in half. The ResNet50 architecture resembles a bottleneck. Three layers are stacked one on top of the other for each residual function. The three layers are a 1*1 convolution, 3*3, and 1. The 1*1 convolution layer achieves the size reduction and subsequent repair of the dimensions. The 3*3 layer remains a bottleneck even with decreased input or output proportions. The system boasts 1000 neurons in a completely connected layer after an average pooling layer [27-30].

5.3.4 Proposed architecture

In the proposed model, ResNet50 architecture is used to classify types of skin cancer images.

In the proposed model, Figure 5.8, a skin cancer image is taken and trained on the pre-trained ResNet50 architecture. Four extra layers were added to the architecture. Two of them were dropout layers, each of rate 0.5. The other two-layers were dense layers, of which one layer had 128 units with activation function as RELU and the other dense layer had units equal to the number of pigmented abrasions. In our case, it was 7. The activation function around the next dense layer is SOFTMAX. Both the dense layers contain L2-regularizer at the rate of 0.02. For the model, layers were not trained at first, moreover, their weights were used. Later, the layers were trained.

5.3.5 Flask framework/web application

The web application is designed on Visual Studio Code. The flask framework is a python-based web framework. The code of flask framework can be easily connected with the localhost 5000 in a browser when app.py is executed. The application is designed mostly using HTML 5 and CSS and consists of six to seven pages.

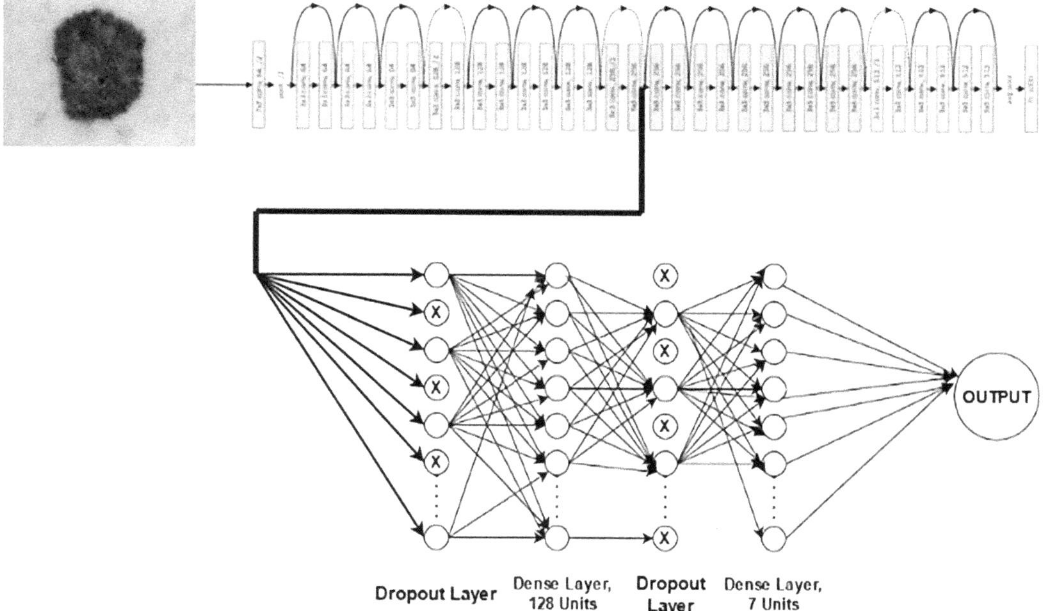

Figure 5.8 Proposed model architecture using pre-trained ResNet50 architecture along with 4 extra layers: 2 each of dense layer and dropout layer.

5.4 RESULTS AND DISCUSSION

The result section includes model implementation, where the model implementation is done to get necessary outcomes. In the initial phase, all the required libraries were installed in the jupyter notebook. The model was designed using Keras libraries. For the model training purposes, metadata was used. The image size taken for the experiment was 75 × 100. During the data cleaning process, it was found that the dataset is heavily biased. Thus, to balance the wights of each class, weights were applied. Feature and target variables were defined, and the images were converted from matrix to list. Following that, the list was then standardized by taking mean and standard deviation. The dataset was divided into a ratio of 80:20 with a random state of 3. Further, one-hot encoding was performed on the labels of both the training and testing dataset. One-hot encoding is necessary as integer encodes are removed and binary variables are added for every unique integer value. Now after the pre-processing is done, the model has been built.

The proposed architecture was designed. The pre-trained ResNet-50 architecture was loaded where the top was not included, and average pooling and weights were from IMAGENET taken. The input shape of the image was taken to be (75, 100, 3). The model was then constructed by adding several dropout and fully connected layers with ReLU as their activation function. The model was then compiled. Adam optimizer was used at a rate of 0.001 along with categorical cross-entropy as the loss function and the measure "Accuracy." Adaptive Rate Annealer was made up to track the validation accuracy with three levels of patience, a 0.5 factor, and a 0.00001 minimum learning rate. Data augmentation was carried out too. Numerous augmentation techniques were used including rotation range, zoom range, width shift range, and height shift. Now, after the data augmentation, the model was fit. The batch size used in this chapter was 10. After training the model for 30 epochs, the model achieved an accuracy of 90.61% and validation accuracy was obtained as 93.47%.

The curve of model accuracy and model loss is shown in Figure 5.9. It reflects accuracy per epoch of both training and validation data. It can be clearly visualized that, with the increase in number of epochs, the model accuracy is increasing, and loss is constantly decreasing. Accuracy touched the 90% mark by the 30th epoch while the loss decreased below 0.4 by the last epoch. For the test data, similar kinds of pre-processing techniques of standardization were done using mean and standard deviation.

Now, Figure 5.10, represents the confusion matrix of the model. Nine hundred ten images of *df*" is predicted as dermatofibroma, while 841 images of melanoma were truly predicted. Further, 792, 795, 787, 828, and 916 were truly classified images of classes "*akiec*", "*bcc*", "*bkl*", "*nv*", "*vasc*" respectively.

Figure 5.11 shows a table that illustrates the model's categorization report. In this chapter, the metrics used were precision, recall, f1-score, and support.

Precision is the metric to find the total number of positive predictions made. On the other hand, Recall signifies the number of correct cases the classifier correctly forecasted; F1 score is applied to find the value by combining both precision and recall. Last, support is how many samples of correct predictions are present in a particular clas [31–32].

With a support count of 2003, the model's estimated accuracy is 83%. Further, each class has a precision of above 90%, and classes like "*akiec*", "*df*", and "*vasc*" achieved a precision score of 100%. The f1 score of every class is 80% and above except the "*bkl*" category.

The whole prediction was integrated with the web application. The "*.h5*" file was taken from the jupyter notebook and saved in the directory of visual studio code where the web application was designed.

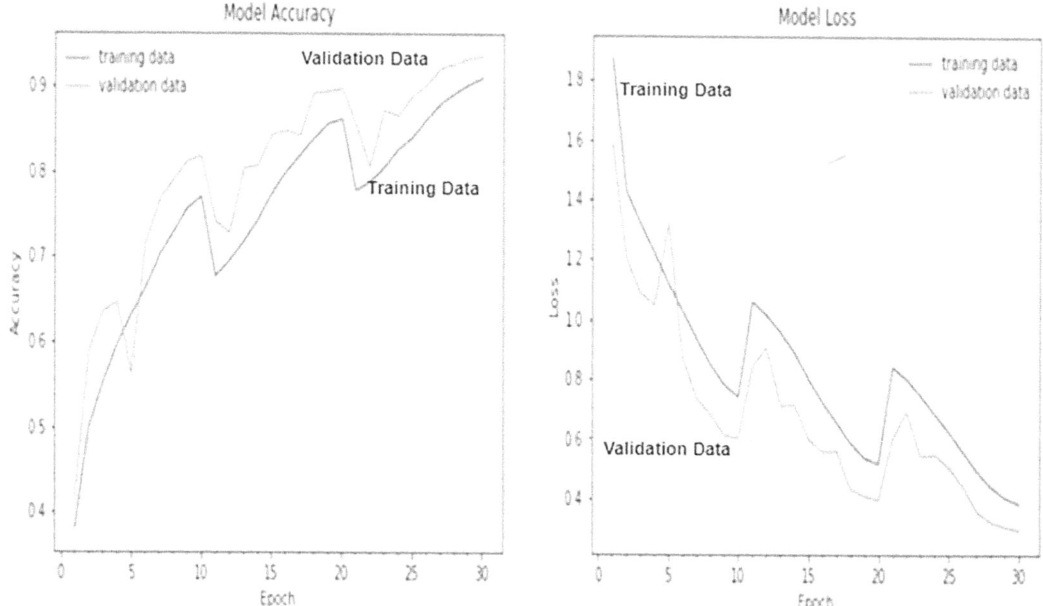

Figure 5.9 Graph represents the model accuracy and model loss.

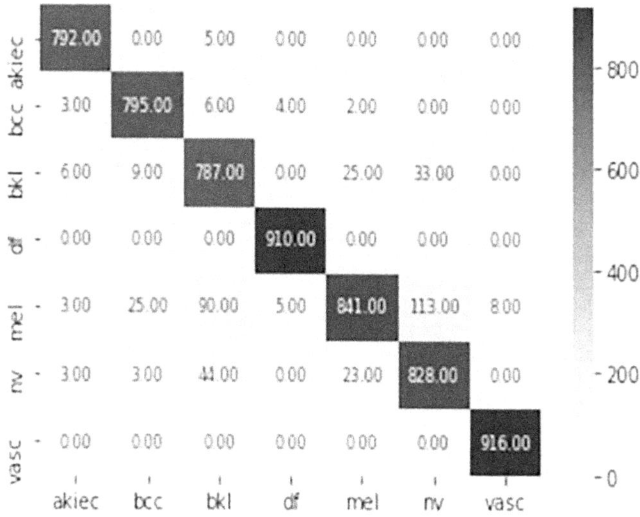

Figure 5.10 Depicts the model's confusion matrix.

Figure 5.12 shows the home page of the web application designed using HTML5 and CSS with the assistance of flask framework.

In Figure 5.13, the image represents the predicted class as *"akiec"* in the web application. Thus, the prediction was successfully integrated with the web application.

Similarly, in Figure 5.14, the image represents the predicted class as *"df"* in the web application.

```
Classification Report
              precision    recall  f1-score   support

       akiec       1.00      0.94      0.97        70
         bcc       0.97      0.[illegible]9      0.81       149
         bkl       0.96      0.[illegible]0      0.66       381
          df       1.00      0.[illegible]7      0.80        33
         mel       0.77      0.[illegible]9      0.87      1051
          nv       0.91      0.[illegible]5      0.82       279
        vasc       1.00      0.[illegible]2      0.90        40

    accuracy                           0.83      2003
   macro avg       0.95      0.[illegible]      0.83      2003
weighted avg       0.86      0.[illegible]      0.82      2003
```

Figure 5.11 Represents the model's classification report.

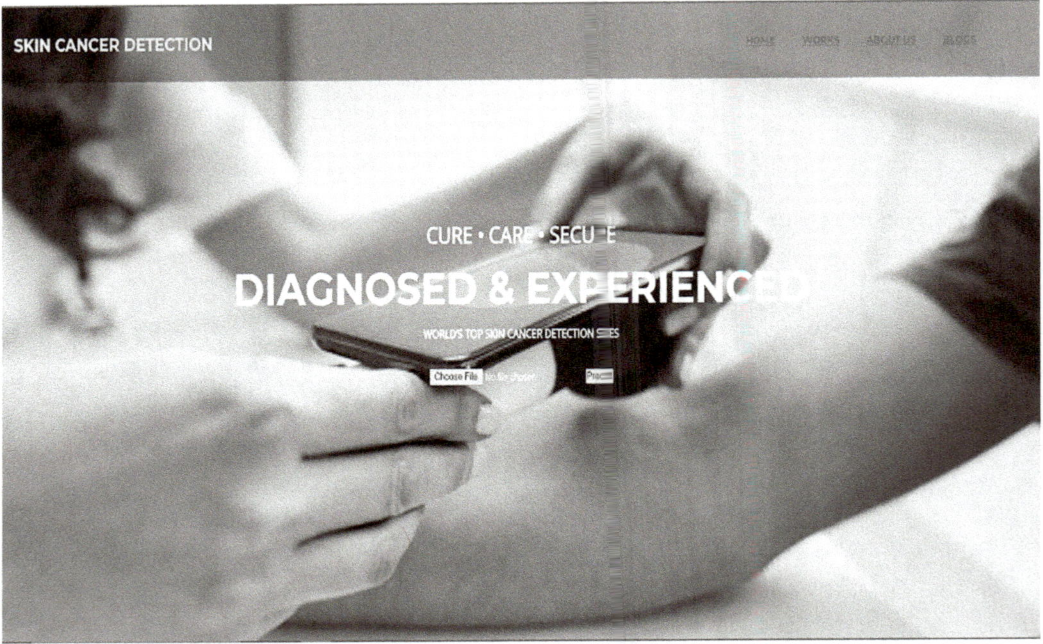

Figure 5.12 Represents a web application's home page.

The result of this paper was then compared with the already completed research work. These are as follows:

As it can be observed from Table 5.1 that, ResNet50 architecture applied in this chapter outperforms already completed research work. However, there were certain challenges while handling the data. The researchers faced over-fitting issues while calculating predictions. Different models, optimizers, and learning rate were tested, and finally in the last layer, the L2 regularizers (0.02) were applied. Other challenges were data storing and GPU runtime. On various occasions, the model was first stored in google drive and was tested on Google colab using in-built GPUs, but they weren't sufficient. Thus, it was then run in tthe ASUS ROG Zephyrus laptop containing AMD Ryzen 9 and NVIDIA GeForce RTX 3070, which gave outcomes in hours as compared to Google colab which used to get show errors such "run-time error" and "100% GPU used."

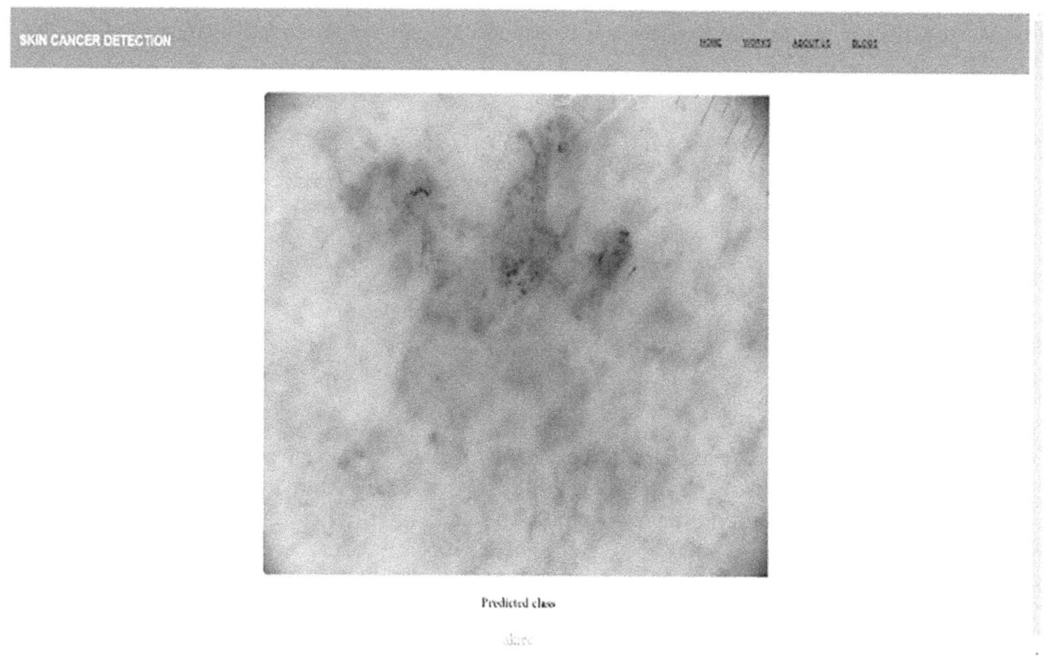

Figure 5.13 Represents the predicted image in the web application with prediction class as "*akiec*".

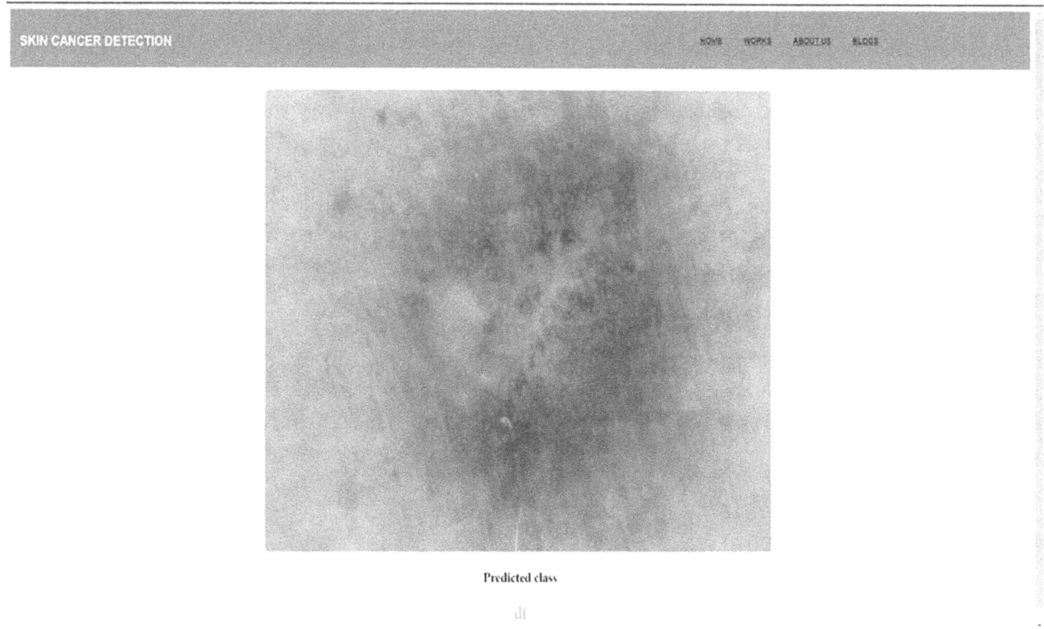

Figure 5.14 Represents the predicted image in the web application with prediction class as "*df*".

Table 5.1 Represents comparison between this research work and previous completed research

Paper title	*Dataset*	*Model/Algorithm used*	*Accuracy achieved*
This research work	**HAM10000**	ResNet50 architecture	93.47%
[4]	HAM10000	FlexNet architecture	80.3%
[32]	Real time data was recorded using sensors	CNN architecture	82.4%
[33]	4361 Dermoscopic images acquired by SMP	Inception V2, K-means algorithm and sonification	81%

5.5 CONCLUSION

In this chapter, the aim was to design a web application that will be beneficial for skin cancer patients to click pictures and share with doctors for early-stage treatment. Thus, in this chapter, the authors designed a deep learning and state-of-the-art algorithm with the help of ResNet50 architecture. This proposed architecture has an accuracy of 93.47% and classifies distinct types of skin cancer. The precision of the three classes, i.e., *"akeic,"* "df," and *"vasc,"* is 100%, while for others it is above 90%. Similarly, metric recall is above 80% for all classes except the *"bkl"* class. The flask framework was used to host the web application on the local server. The architecture was then integrated with the web application designed using HTML5 and CSS. The web application predicts accurately every class of image. Hence, it was observed that the proposed model using ResNet50 architecture outperforms the previously studied model.

The web application holds a lot of potential in it, which can be improvised in future. The application can be interlinked with patients living in remote and urban areas. If in case of emergency, doctors and ambulances for patients will be available at the nearest hospital. The major challenge that the researchers faced during this work was that the data was biased. Thus, not all categories had the same number of images, and there were overfitting issues that were removed by using regularizers. In conclusion, this paper will serve the skin cancer patients of urban cities but will also help the people living in rural areas by connecting patients to doctors. Although melanoma is difficult to detect with the unaided eye, these intricate techniques are used to accurately predict illness in its preliminary stages, allowing for timely treatment and the possibility of saving lives. However, it can be difficult for patients to travel to the clinic for treatment and routine checkups during an ongoing COVID-19 pandemic. Thus, in the future, skin cancer can be detected using these applications on smartphones or tablets. In order to incorporate this, researchers across the globe must explore more deep learning models, and even try to apply them on different diseases and make these applications real-time by providing a platform for doctors and patients to interact with each other.

REFERENCES

1. 'Skin cancer statistics | World Cancer Research Fund International'. Accessed: Mar. 27, 2023. [Online]. Available: https://www.wcrf.org/cancer-trends/skin-cancer-statistics/
2. 'Why Some Parts of India Have Higher Rates of Skin Cancer: Study | The Swaddle'. Accessed: Mar. 27, 2023. [Online]. Available: https://theswaddle.com/study-shows-higher-rates-of-skin-cancer-in-some-parts-of-india-heres-why/

3. R. Kaymak, C. Kaymak, and A. Ucar, 'Skin lesion segmentation using fully convolutional networks: A comparative experimental study', *Expert Syst Appl*, vol. 161, p. 113742, Dec. 2020, doi: 10.1016/J.ESWA.2020.113742.
4. P. Tschandl *et al.*, 'Human–computer collaboration for skin cancer recognition', *Nat Med*, vol. 26, no. 8, pp. 1229–1234, Jun. 2020, doi: 10.1038/s41591-020-0942-0.
5. 'Digital Around the World — DataReportal – Global Digital Insights'. Accessed: Mar. 26, 2023. [Online]. Available: https://datareportal.com/global-digital-overview
6. E. Chao, C. K. Meenan, and L. K. Ferris, 'Smartphone-based applications for skin monitoring and melanoma detection', *Dermatol Clin*, vol. 35, no. 4, pp. 551–557, Oct. 2017, doi: 10.1016/j.det.2017.06.014.
7. D. B. Shivanna, T. Stephan, F. Al-Turjman, M. Kolhar, and S. Alturjman, 'IoMT-based automated diagnosis of autoimmune diseases using multiStage classification scheme for sustainable smart cities', *Sustainability*, vol. 14, no. 21, p. 13891, Oct. 2022, doi: 10.3390/su142113891.
8. T. Stephan, F. Al-Turjman, M. Ravishankar, and P. Stephan, 'Machine learning analysis on the impacts of COVID-19 on India's renewable energy transitions and air quality', *Environ Sci Pollut Res*, vol. 29, no. 52, pp. 79443–79465, Nov. 2022, doi: 10.1007/s11356-022-20997-2.
9. V. R. Balaji, S. T. Suganthi, R. Rajadevi, V. Krishna Kumar, B. Saravana Balaji, and S. Pandiyan, 'Skin disease detection and segmentation using dynamic graph cut algorithm and classification through Naive Bayes classifier', *Measurement*, vol. 163, p. 107922, Oct. 2020, doi: 10.1016/J.MEASUREMENT.2020.107922.
10. E. Guerra-Rosas and J. Álvarez-Borrego, 'Methodology for diagnosing of skin cancer on images of dermatologic spots by spectral analysis', *Biomed Opt Express*, vol. 6, no. 10, pp. 3876–3891, Oct. 2015, doi: 10.1364/BOE.6.003876.
11. M. H. Jafari *et al.*, 'Skin lesion segmentation in clinical images using deep learning', *Proc Int Conf Pattern Recognit*, vol. 0, pp. 337–342, Jan. 2016, doi: 10.1109/ICPR.2016.7899656.
12. E. Jana, R. Subban, and S. Saraswathi, 'Research on skin cancer cell detection using image processing', *2017 IEEE International Conference on Computational Intelligence and Computing Research, ICCIC 2017*, Nov. 2018, doi: 10.1109/ICCIC.2017.8524554.
13. N. Nida, A. Irtaza, A. Javed, M. H. Yousaf, and M. T. Mahmood, 'Melanoma lesion detection and segmentation using deep region based convolutional neural network and fuzzy C-means clustering', *Int J Med Inform*, vol. 124, pp. 37–48, Apr. 2019, doi: 10.1016/J.IJMEDINF.2019.01.005.
14. H. Alquran *et al.*, 'The melanoma skin cancer detection and classification using support vector machine', *2017 IEEE Jordan Conference on Applied Electrical Engineering and Computing Technologies, AEECT 2017*, vol. 2018-January, pp. 1–5, Jul. 2017, doi: 10.1109/AEECT.2017.8257738.
15. A. Murugan, S. A. H. Nair, and K. P. S. Kumar, 'Detection of skin cancer using SVM, random forest and kNN classifiers', *J Med Syst*, vol. 43, no. 8, pp. 1–9, Aug. 2019, doi: 10.1007/S10916-019-1400-8/METRICS.
17. S. Tajjour, S. Garg, S. S. Chandel, and D. Sharma, 'A novel hybrid artificial neural network technique for the early skin cancer diagnosis using color space conversions of original images', *Int J Imaging Syst Technol*, vol. 33, no. 1, pp. 276–286, Jan. 2023, doi: 10.1002/IMA.22784.
16. S. Shaaban, H. Atya, H. Mohammed, A. Sameh, K. Raafat, and A. Magdy, 'Skin cancer detection based on deep learning methods', vol. 164, pp. 58–67, 2023, doi: 10.1007/978-3-031-27762-7_6.
18. H. K. Gajera, D. R. Nayak, and M. A. Zaveri, 'A comprehensive analysis of dermoscopy images for melanoma detection via deep CNN features', *Biomed Signal Process Control*, vol. 79, p. 104186, Jan. 2023, doi: 10.1016/J.BSPC.2022.104186.
19. S. Inthiyaz *et al.*, 'Skin disease detection using deep learning', *Adv Eng Softw*, vol. 175, p. 103361, Jan. 2023, doi: 10.1016/J.ADVENGSOFT.2022.103361.
20. H. M. Balaha and A. E. S. Hassan, 'Skin cancer diagnosis based on deep transfer learning and sparrow search algorithm', *Neural Comput Appl*, vol. 35, no. 1, pp. 815–853, Jan. 2023, doi: 10.1007/S00521-022-07762-9/TABLES/2.

21. A. Bindhu and K. K. Thanammal, 'Segmentation of skin cancer using Fuzzy U-network via deep learning', *Meas Sens*, vol. 26, p. 100677, Apr. 2023, doi: 10.1016/J.MEASEN.2023.100677.
22. D. Keerthana, V. Venugopal, M. K. Nath, and M. Mishra, 'Hybrid convolutional neural networks with SVM classifier for classification of skin cancer', *Biomed Eng Adv*, vol. 5, p. 100069, Jun. 2023, doi: 10.1016/J.BEA.2022.100069.
23. 'A Comprehensive Hands-on Guide to Transfer Learning with Real-World Applications in Deep Learning | by Dipanjan (DJ) Sarkar | Towards Data Science'. Accessed : Mar. 27, 2023. [Online]. Available: https://towardsdatascience.com/a-comprehensive-hands-on-guide-to-transfer-learning-with-real-world-applications-in-deep-learning-212bf3b2f27a
24. 'Transfer learning from pre-trained models | by Pedro Marcelino | Towards Data Science'. Accessed: Mar. 27, 2023. [Online]. Available: https://towardsdatascience.com/transfer-learning-from-pre-trained-models-f2393f124751
25. 'Skin Cancer MNIST: HAM10000 | Kaggle'. Accessed: Mar. 27, 2023. [Online]. Available: https://www.kaggle.com/datasets/kmader/skin-cancer-mnist-ham10000
26. P. Tschandl, C. Rosendahl, and H. Kittler, 'Data descriptor: The HAM10000 dataset, a large collection of multi-source dermatoscopic images of common pigmented skin lesions', *Sci Data*, vol. 5, pp. 2052–4463, Aug. 2018, doi: 10.1038/SDATA.2018.161.
27. 'Detailed Guide to Understand and Implement ResNets – CV-Tricks.com'. Accessed: Mar. 27, 2023. [Online]. Available: https://cv-tricks.com/keras/understand-implement-resnets/
28. 'ResNet and ResNetV2'. Accessed: Mar. 27, 2023. [Online]. Available: https://keras.io/api/applications/resnet/#resnet50-function
29. K. He, X. Zhang, S. Ren, and J. Sun, 'Deep Residual Learning for Image Recognition', Accessed: Mar. 26, 2023. [Online]. Available: http://image-net.org/challenges/LSVRC/2015/
30. Teemu Kanstrén, 'A Look at Precision, Recall, and F1-Score', Towards Data Science. [Online]. Available: https://towardsdatascience.com/a-look-at-precision-recall-and-f1-score-36b5fd0dd3ec#:~:text=F1%2Dscore%20when%20Precision%3D0.8%20and%20Recall%20%3D%200.01%20to%201.0&text=Here%20precision%20is%20fixed%20at,varies%20from%200.0%20to%201.0.
31. 'what does the numbers in the classification report of sklearn mean?', StackExchange. [Online]. Available: https://stats.stackexchange.com/questions/117654/what-does-the-numbers-in-the-classification-report-of-sklearn-mean#:~:text=The%20f1%2Dscore%20gives%20you,that%20lie%20in%20that%20class.
32. D. Połap, A. Winnicka, K. Serwata, K. Kęsik, and M. Woźniak, 'An Intelligent system for monitoring skin diseases', *Sensors*, vol. 18, no. 8, p. 2552, Aug. 2018, doi: 10.3390/S18082552.
33. A. Dascalu and E. O. David, 'Skin cancer detection by deep learning and sound analysis algorithms: A prospective clinical study of an elementary dermoscope', *EBioMedicine*, vol. 43, pp. 107–113, May 2019, doi: 10.1016/J.EBIOM.2019.04.055.

Chapter 6

Improved mass detection in mammogram images with Dual Tree Complex Wavelet Transform and Fourier Descriptors

M Kanchana[1], *R Naresh*[2], *C N S Vinoth Kumar*[2], *and P Pandiaraja*[3]

[1]Department of Computing Technologies, SRM Institute of Science and Technology, Kattankulathur, Chennai, Tamil Nadu, India

[2]Department of Networking and Communications, SRM Institute of Science and Technology, Kattankulathur, Chennai, Tamil Nadu, India

[3]Department of Computer Science and Engineering, M Kumarasamy College of Engineering, Thalavapalayam, Karur, Tamil Nadu, India

6.1 INTRODUCTION

The process of doing the examination using a mammogram is called mammography, which can be used for the detection and diagnosis of breast cancers in patients at an earlier stage. Mammography provides a better effective method of detecting breast cancer. The detection accuracy will be in the 80 to 90% range. Breast cancer has two separate indicators: masses and microcalcifications [1]. Right and left mammograms are the two distinct views of the mammograms, whereas Cranio Caudal (CC) and Medio Lateral Oblique (MLO) are the two different views of the mammograms. A limitation of DWT is that it has less directional selectivity and shift invariance, both of which DTCWT [2] has largely overcome. Here, a cutting-edge method of mass detection based on DTCWT that aids in overcoming the limitations of DWT is explored. Although it requires more work to implement, it produces results that are superior to those of the Discrete Wavelet Transform for mass cancer detection. This study demonstrates how DTCWT and ANN are used to detect mammography masses.

6.2 RELATED WORKS

CAD is proposed in [3] for mass detection in mammograms using wavelet transformed, region-based pixel-based segmentation, and the developed system is tested using 60 images. In this case, a feature extraction depending on regional growth is applied [4] to locate the mass lesion and create 83% as output with respect to ground truth. DTCWT is applied in [5] to detect microcalcification using MIAS database. DTCWT-based feature extraction is used in [6], and they used neural network to classify images using MIAS database. CAD for microcalcification detection is described in [7], which was built using a fuzzy neural network; the obtained classification accuracy is 83%. Mammographic mass detection is done using neural networks [8,9] and different feature types and also specified the significance of the various features. Various methods applied for mass detection and classification are described in [10] where they compared the methods. CAD for microcalcification detection illustrated in [11] is developed using DTCWT [12], PCA, and SVM, and the results were compared with the other standard wavelet transforms, and concluded that DTCWT provides competitive performance [13].

DOI: 10.1201/9781003369059-8

The work specified in [14] describes the review on various approaches used to detect mass in mammograms and also mentions the merits and demerits of the existing methods and compares existing methods for detection. Duel tree wavelet transform is presented in [15] for image resolution enhancement. In [2] the CAD system is proposed, in which DTCWT is utilized for feature extraction purposes, and SVM is utilized as a classifier to classify microcalcification, which produces an accuracy of 88.64%. DTCWT-based denoising method is proposed [16,17] for medical images. CAD model is proposed [18] for breast cancer classification using DTCWT and SVM. They achieved the accuracy of 87.94% and AUC value is 0.94. In [19] authors presented the technique to segment the medical images using DTCWT and CNN. They explained in [20] a technique to classify the sperm abnormality using DTCWT and SVM and they yield the accuracy of 82.33%, and proposed a method to obtain the denoised medical images using DTCWT [21]. They presented [22] an algorithm to detect the breast cancer using DWT and ANN and achieved an accuracy of 83.25%. Novel technique is described in [23] for breast cancer prediction using DTCWT and Random Forest Tree and achieved 0.74 as ROC.

Content-based image retrieval technique is implemented [24] for breast cancer classification using SVM classifier and tested mammogram images and results in classification accuracy of 76.91, 80.50, and 81.34 for SVM, Ada-SVM, and Cas-SVM, respectively. For detection of masses in mammograms, a novel hybrid method is discussed [25] using texture feature, decision tree, and multiresolution Markov random field models. A new method [26] is explored to detect the mass images using statistical measures and achieved a sensitivity of 80%. The authors tested their work using MIAS dataset. CAD for breast cancer identification is described using DTCWT and the obtained outputs are compared with SWT and Top-Hat transforms. The proposed work [27] analyzed fusion-based mammogram images by using the DTCWT method. They obtain the fused image by combining MRIs with X-ray mammogram images and concluded that the quality of image visualization is enhanced. Authors [28] explained the breast clinical diagnostic literature review employing machine learning techniques. The automatic breast cancer type classification approach [29] is explained using mammogram images. Breast cancer detection techniques were investigated [30] using fusion-based features, ELM, Convolutional Neural network, Deep learning, and SVM. In [31,32] subtraction of temporally sequential digital mammograms and machine learning-based CAD was proposed for the automatic segmentation and classification of masses in mammograms. They used different categories of features and various algorithms to classify the masses. They used [33] unified CNN to identify the mass in breast cancer using mammogram. They also used augmentation techniques and three different evaluation metrics in FFDM in order to predict masses and produced a detection accuracy of 85%. In [34] authors demonstrated Dual Fusion Mass Detector and Results-oriented Loss to classify the mass mammogram images with good detection accuracy.

6.3 PROPOSED METHODOLOGY

6.3.1 Dataset

There are 322 mammograms of the right and left breast in the MIAS database. Information is gathered from 161 patients, of whom 51 have images that have been determined to be malignant, 64 to be benign, and 207 to be normal. Microcalcifications (25 images), Circumscribed Masses (20 images), Architectural Distortion (20 images), Miscellaneous – as ill-defined masses (15 images), Asymmetry (17 images), and Speculated Masses are the different types of abnormalities (21 images).

Table 6.1 MIAS database information

Column no	*Description*
1st Column	MIAS Database Reference Number
2nd Column	Character of background Tissues F- Fatty G – Fatty-Glandular D – Dense - Glandular
3rd Column	Classes of Abnormality Present CALC-Calcification CIRC-Circumscribed Masses SPIC- Speculated Masses MISC-Other, ill defined Masses ARCH-Architectural Distortion ASYM-Asymmetry NORM-Normal
4th Column	Severity of Abnormality B-Benign M-Malignant
5th, 6th Column	X, Y image coordinates of centre of abnormality
7th Column	Approximate radius (in pixels) of a circle enclosing the abnormality

The image is 1024 × 1024 pixels in actual size. Background information, pectoral muscle, and various noises are typically present in MIAS database photos. 50% of the image has a lot of background noise. For a more accurate and thorough analysis and interpretation of breast pictures, all of those sounds must be eliminated.

The MIAS database is shown in Table 6.1, which includes data on the location of the anomaly (such as the centre of a circle enclosing the tumor), its radius, the position of the breasts (left or right), the types of breast tissues (fatty, fatty-glandular, and dense), and the type of tumor, if any, that is present (benign or malignant). Moreover, it has an information file with more details.

Table 6.2 provides the sample MIAS mammogram image with detailed description, which is chosen for the evaluation of the proposed computational framework. Figure 6.1 shows

Table 6.2 Sample MIAS mammogram image detailed description

Sl.No	*MIAS image information*
1	mdb001 G CIRC B 535 425 197
2	mdb003 D NORM
3	mdb005 F CIRC B 477 133 30
4	mdb013 G MISC B 667 365 31
5	mdb014 G NORM
6	mdb081 G ASYM B 492 473 131
7	mdb126 D ARCH B 191 549 23
8	mdb145 D SPIC B 669 543 49
9	mdb141 F CIRC M 470 759 29
10	mdb231 F CALC M 603 538 44

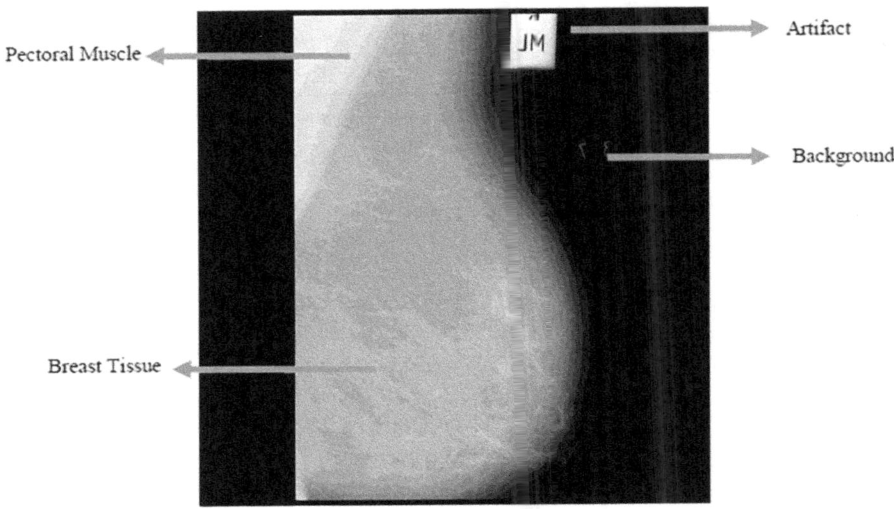

Figure 6.1 Sample mammogram image with artifacts (mdb 006).

sample original mammogram image (mdb 006) with artifacts background details like noises, labels, tape, and artifacts and the pectoral muscle.

6.3.2 Preprocessing

However, a mammogram is more reliable when it has contained a lot of noise in its background. In our proposed approach we are reducing the noise of the images through the application of average filters. The main function of this average filtering is that we can try substituting the mean amount of its spectators, including others, with the value of each pixel in the image. Median filtering seems to have the effect of preventing all number of pixels that are not representational of the circumstances. Figure 6.2 explains the overall architecture of the proposed study. Figure 6.3 (ROI Benign Image Mdb012) and Figure 6.4 (ROI Malignant Image Mdb028) show the ROI image (256 × 256) of Benign and Malignant images, respectively. Figure 6.5 (Filtered Benign Image Mdb01) and Figure 6.6 (Filtered Malignant Image Mdb028) shows the output images (256 × 256) after filtering process of benign and malignant, respectively.

6.3.3 Dual-tree complex discrete wavelet transform (DTCWT)

The basic as well as typical DWT includes drawbacks such as low unidirectional discrimination and lacking temporal information. In order to overcome these bottlenecks/restrictions, DTCWT is imported. In DTCWT [1,2,7,10], two real DWTs considered out of which one DWT produces a real part and the other gives an imaginary part of the transform. The DTCWT is a special category of DWT, made up of two parallel wavelet filter bank trees, which calculates complex coefficients to extract the real wavelet coefficients and imaginary wavelet coefficients separately.

In DTCWT, the upper DWT (Tree a) generates the real part wavelet coefficients and the lower DWT generates the imaginary part (Tree b) of the wavelet coefficients. Figure 6.7 depicts the block diagram of a 3-level DTCWT. DTCWT benefits are low computation time,

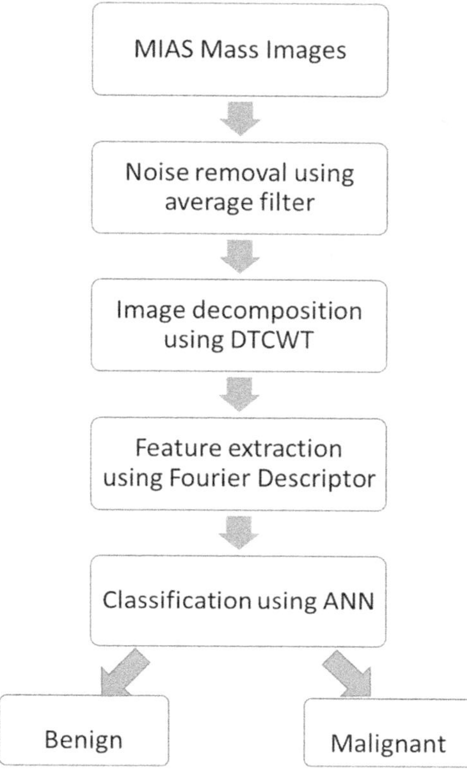

Figure 6.2 Architecture of the proposed study.

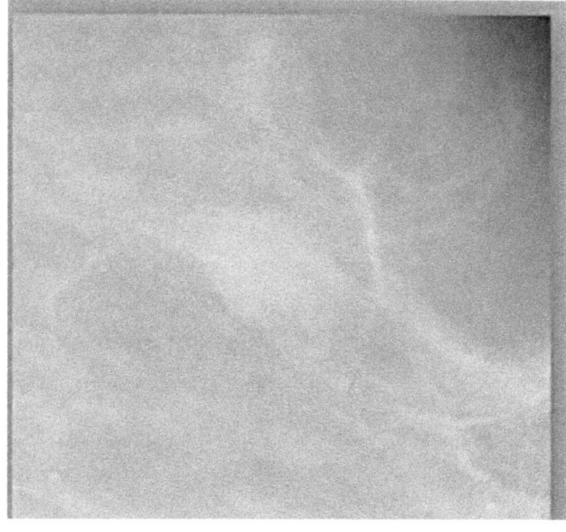

Figure 6.3 ROI Benign Image Mdb012.

limited redundancy, perfect reconstruction, good shift invariance, and directional selectivity. Figure 6.8 shows DTCWT decomposed resultant 12 subband of filtered Benign image Mdb012 (256 × 256), and Figure 6.9 shows the DTCWT decomposed resultant 12 subband of filtered Malignant image Mdb028 (256 × 256).

Figure 6.4 ROI Malignant Image Mdb028.

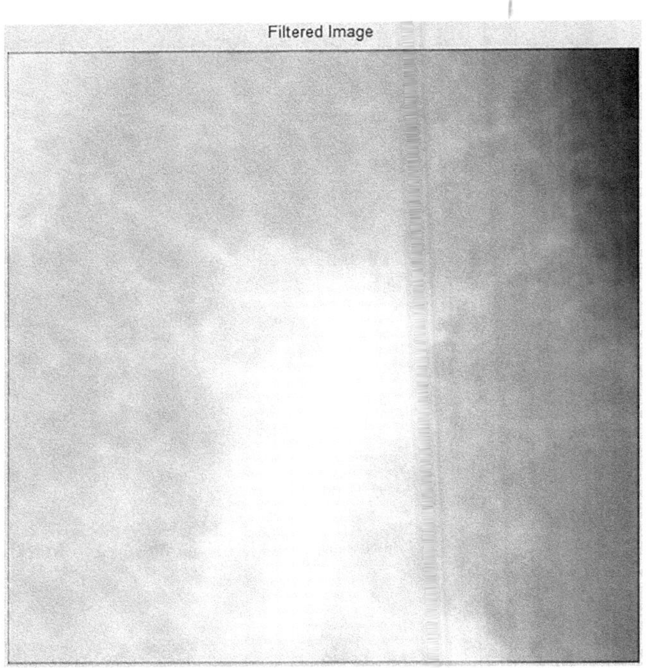

Figure 6.5 Filtered Benign Image Mdb012.

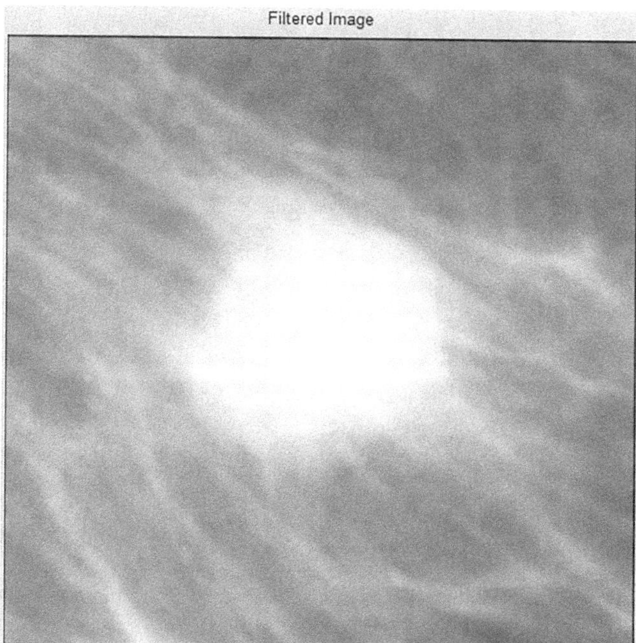

Figure 6.6 Filtered Malignant Image Mdb028.

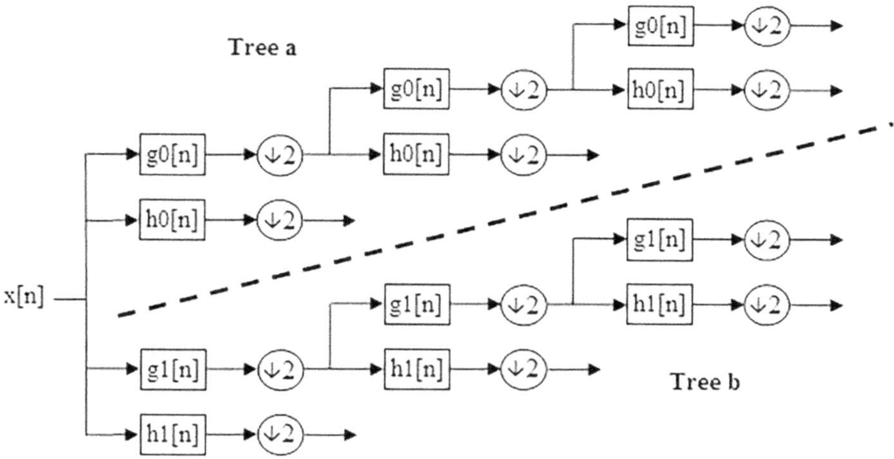

Figure 6.7 Block diagram for a 3-level DTCWT.

6.3.4 Feature extraction

For feature extraction purposes, the Fourier descriptor is used. The Fourier descriptor contains the Fourier decomposed coefficients [35]. In mammogram images the object edge is not easily visible, which may result in a significant change along the boundary due to noise or segmentation issues. Therefore, a suitable smoothing is needed to minimize these impacts. Fourier descriptors, a novel smoothing technique, are introduced in this chapter. It is easy to identify whether a tumor is

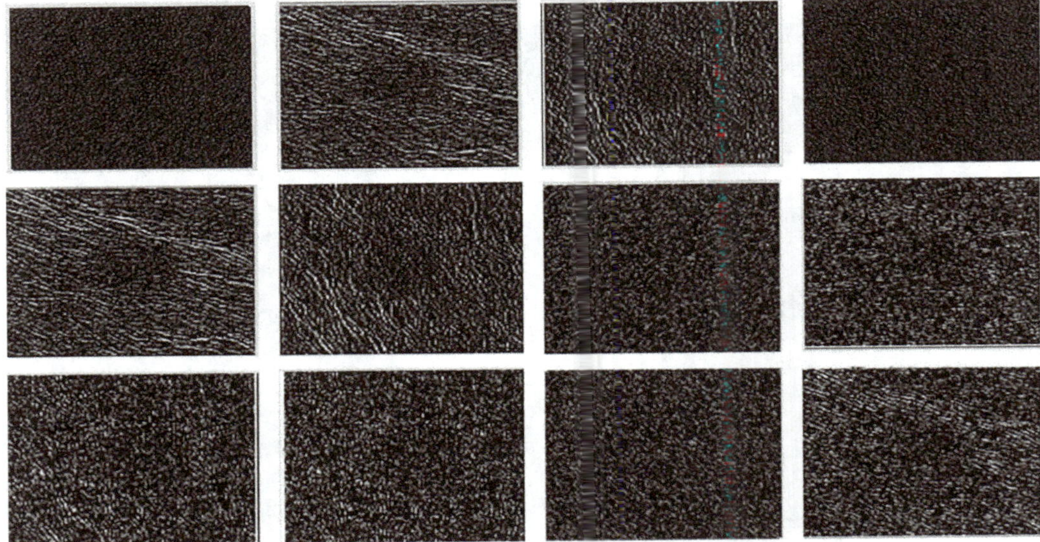

Figure 6.8 DTCWT decomposed resultant 12 sub band of Filtered Benign Image Mdb012 (256 × 256).

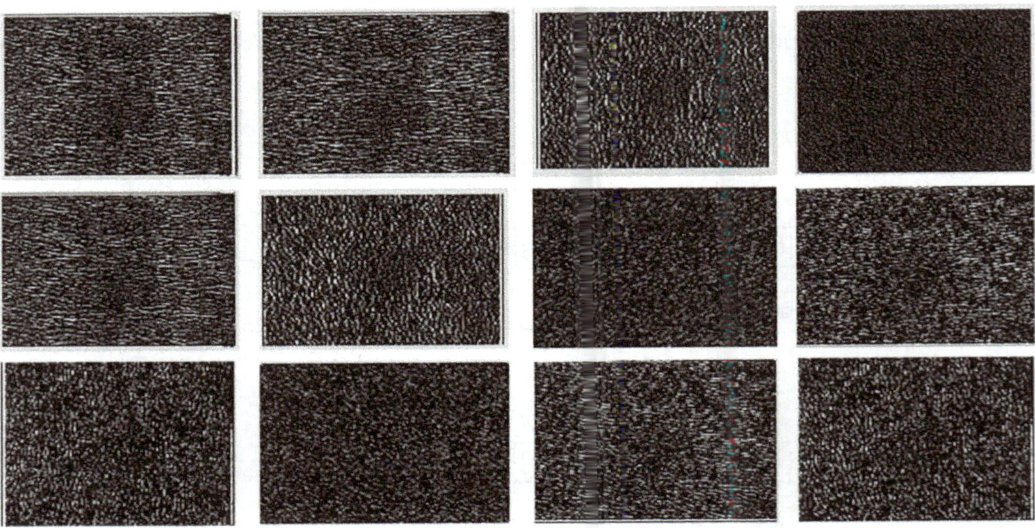

Figure 6.9 DTCWT decomposed resultant 12 sub band of Filtered Malignant Image Mdb028 (256 × 256).

normal or pathological based on its shape. Fourier descriptors are very helpful for pattern identification and are used to identify the shape of the tumor in mammograms. A Fourier-converted boundary serves as the foundation for Fourier descriptors. The shape is effectively represented by these characteristics, and it is not affected by rotation, translation, or scaling.

Fourier descriptor's are derived from Fourier transformations in which larger frequency values represent the fine details and smaller frequency values represent the global shape. Only a few Fourier descriptors are used to fully express a boundary. This contains shape-related data. Thus, these are employed to distinguish between various boundary shapes.

A complex number can be used to represent a digital boundary. Beginning at any location along the boundary marked by the coordinates (a0, b0), go clockwise. A complex number's x-axis represents the real number axis, and its y-axis represents the imaginary number axis. Due to the fact that it transforms a 2-dimensional issue into a 1-dimensional issue, this

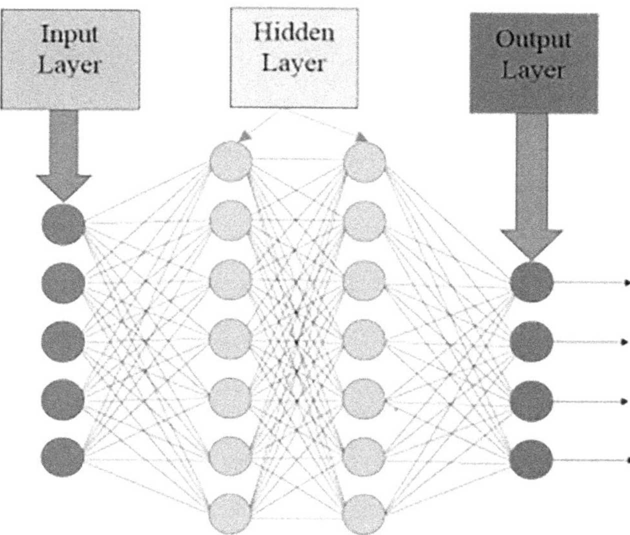

Figure 6.10 Artificial neural networks.

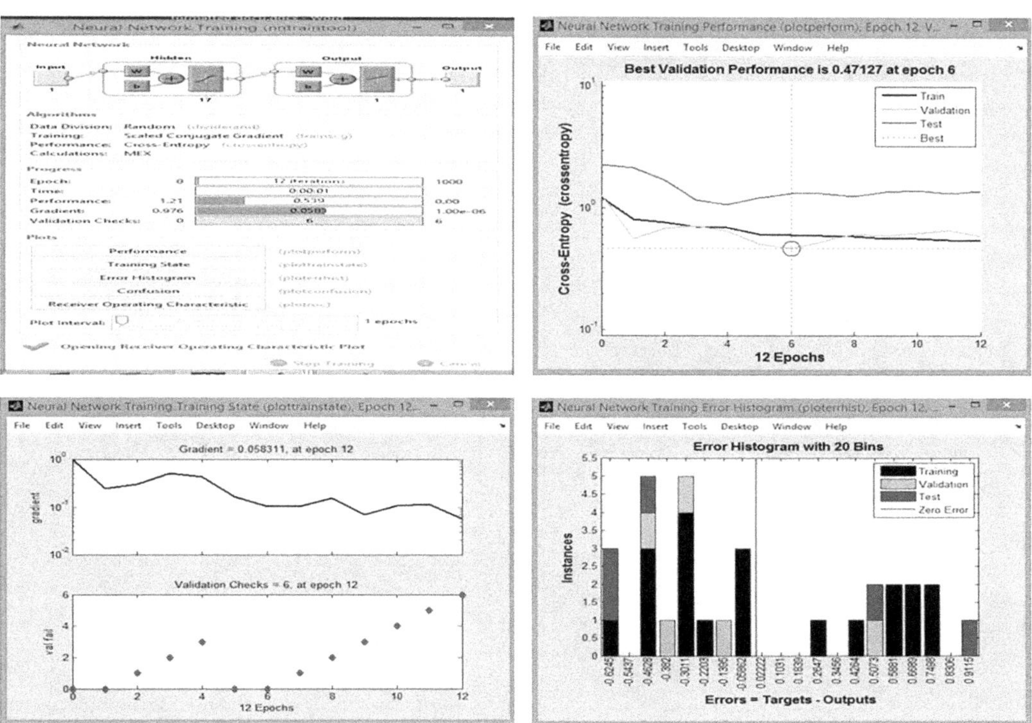

Figure 6.11 Various graphs of ANN classifier.

complex number offers a significant benefit. This complex co-efficient is nothing but a Fourier descriptor. A discrete Fourier is defined in equation 6.1.

$$F_n = \frac{1}{N} \sum_{i=0}^{N-1} s(i) \times e\frac{-j2\pi ni}{N} \tag{6.1}$$

where F_n is nth Fourier descriptor, S(i) is one-dimensional contour signal, N is total points of the contour, and i = 0,1,2,3 … ..N−1

FD's of size 'N' are calculated, which are invariant to translation. With the help of these Fourier descriptors, shape-based signatures are retrieved from either the deconstructed DTCWT imagery or a characteristic data is generated and it is the one input for the classification process.

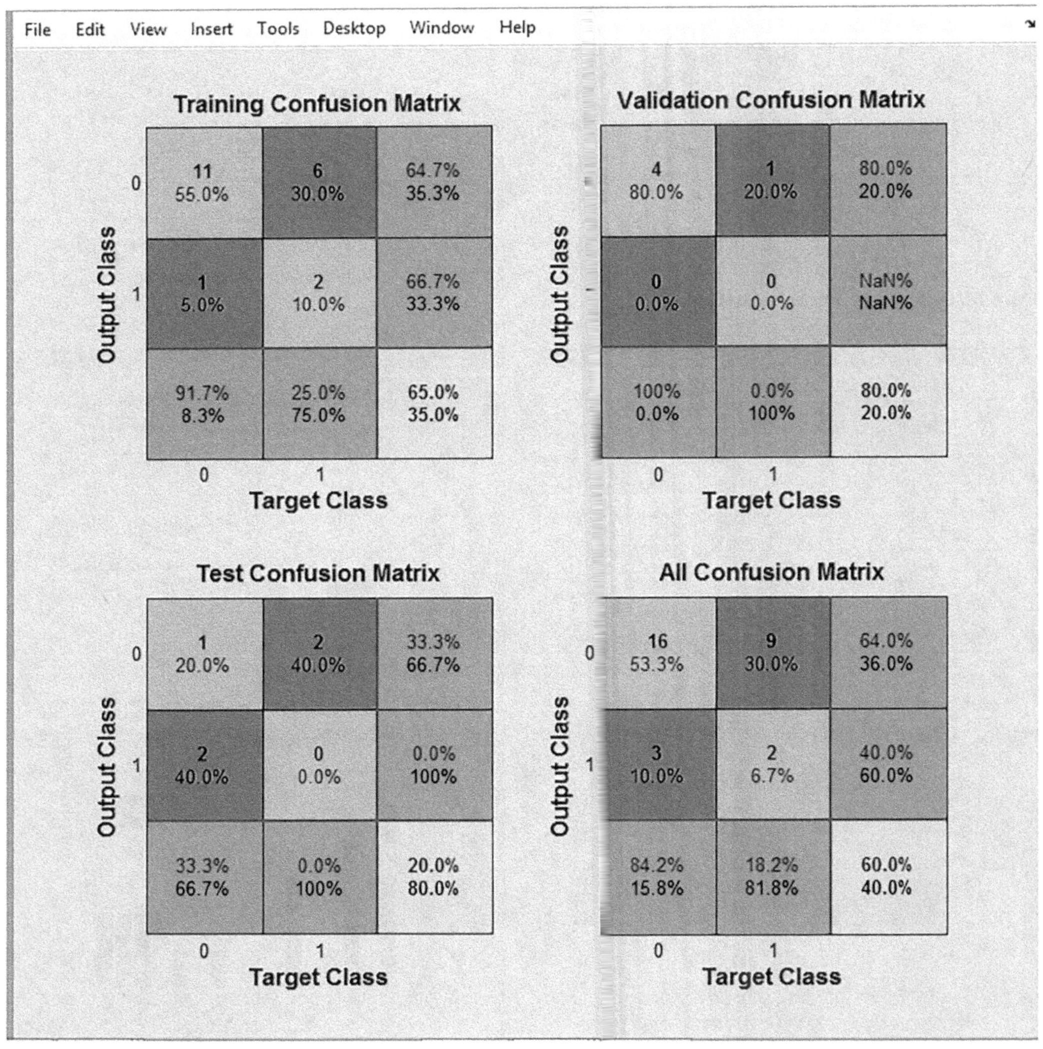

Figure 6.12 Confusion matrix.

6.3.5 Classification

The advantage of a neural network is that it can construct a system with the available set of data. An ANN with input, hidden, and output layers is shown in Figure 6.10. An ANN is suitable for a variety of tasks such as classification, prediction and visualization and it is also appropriate for multidisciplinary tasks. An ANN is taken into account for breast cancer medical images, which are a type of unstructured data. Learning procedures of the ANN will be based on the biological counterparts. ANN can be defined as a parallel distributed processor which has natural capability for storing the knowledge of experience. To calculate the likelihood of malignancy, we used a three-layer feed-forward neural network using Matlab and a back propagation learning technique. The layers contained an output layer with a single node generating the likelihood of malignancy for each finding, a hidden layer with 1000 hidden nodes, and an input layer with 32 mammographic descriptors. ANNs with

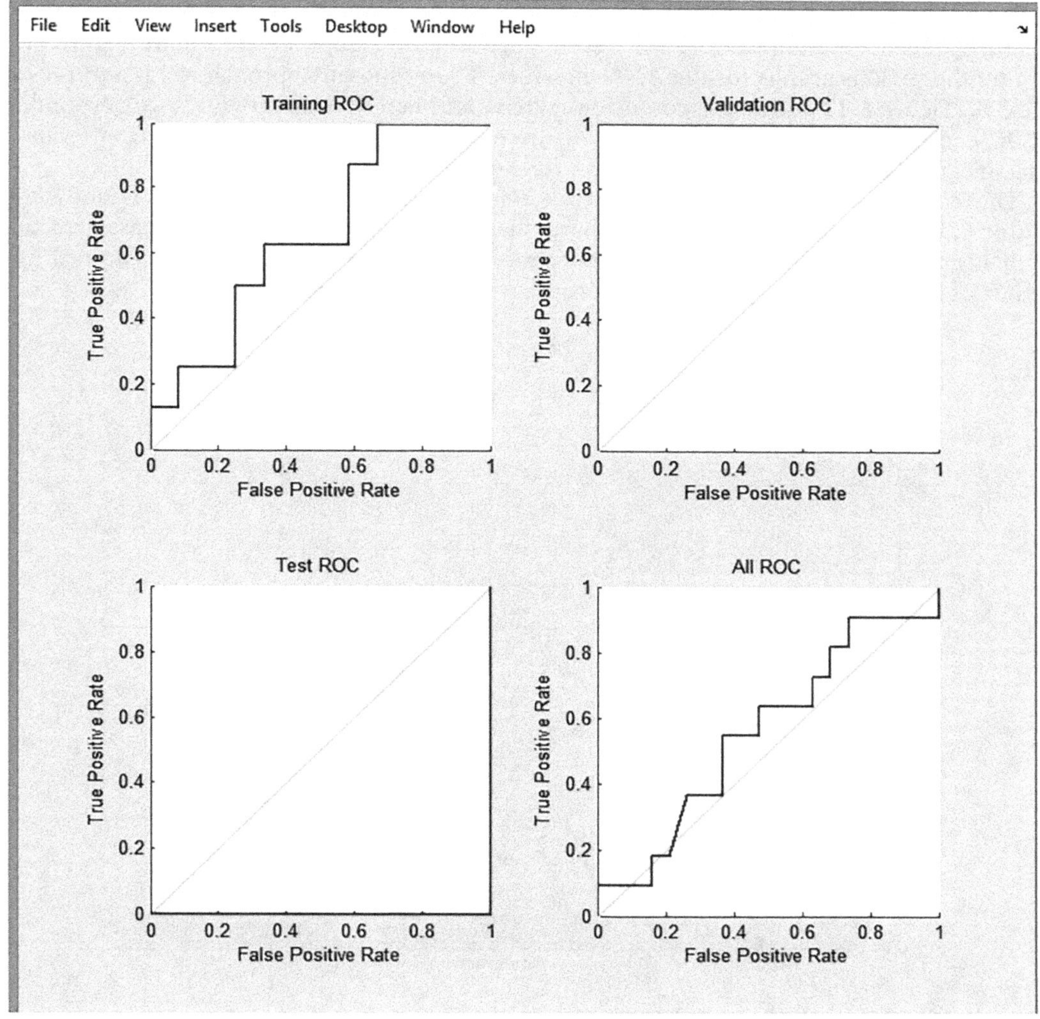

Figure 6.13 ROC curve.

a big number of hidden nodes generalize better than networks with a small number of hidden nodes when trained with back propagation.

We utilized ten-fold cross-validation, a common machine learning technique, to train and test our ANN. The data was split into ten subsets with about comparable sizes for ten-fold cross-validation. Nine of these subsets were pooled and used for training in the initial iteration. The final tenth set was utilized to evaluate how well our ANN performed in untested scenarios. Until all subsets had been tested once, we went through this process ten times.

6.3.6 Experimental setup and outputs

The proposed work is tested using the MIAS database. This MIAS database contains 322 images of 161 patients. Three hundred twenty-two images are divided into three categories, namely normal, microcalcification, and mass. In these databases are 207 normal images, 25 microcalcification images, and 90 mass images. In this approach, all the 90 mass images are taken for evaluation purpose. Among 90 images, for training and testing purposes, 60 photographs are examined, and for testing purposes, 30 samples were found. Figure 6.11 shows the various graphs for the ANN classifier. The proposed approach yields accuracy of 92.3%. Figure 6.12 shows the confusion matrix, and Figure 6.13 shows the corresponding ROC curves. Figure 6.14 depicts Performance evaluation of ANN effectiveness in terms of classification accuracy, sensitivities, and precision.

The comparison of the proposed work with the state-of-the-art works is shown in Table 6.3. Table 6.3 makes it evident that, when compared to other works, mass detection utilizing DTCWT produces greater classification accuracy. Better results are obtained as a result of DTCWT's strong directional property and shift invariance features.

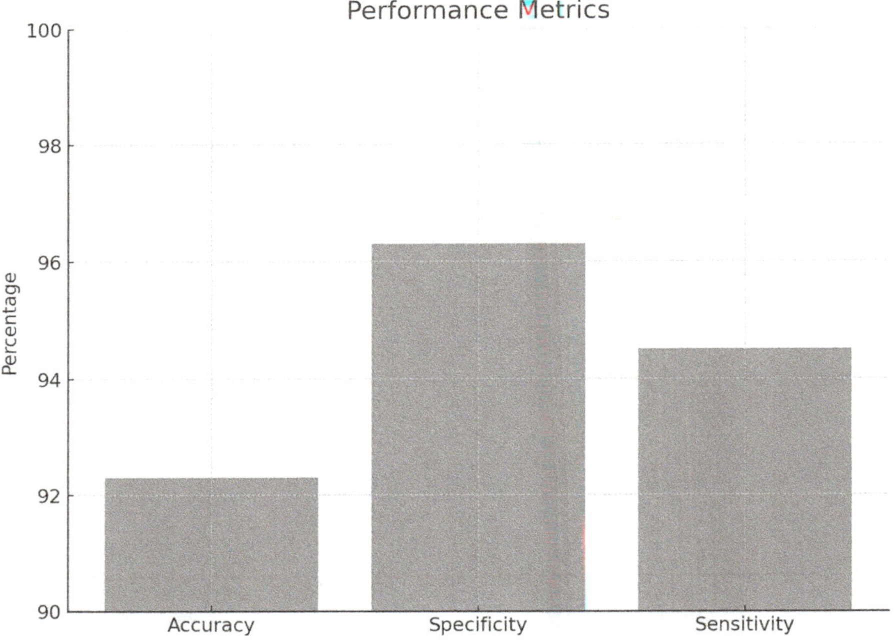

Figure 6.14 Performance evaluation of ANN.

Table 6.3 Comparison of proposed work with other existing methods

Sl. No	*Author details*	*Techniques used*	*Accuracy / AUR*
1	Verma B& Zakos J [7]	fuzzy neural network	83.3%
2	Wushuai Jian, Xueyan Sun, & Shuqian Luo [11]	DTCWT, PCA & SVM	83.5%
3	A. Tirtajaya and D.D.Santika [2]	DTCWT,SVM	88.64%
4	T.Wan, X.Liu, J.Chen & Z.Qin [18]	DTCWT, SVM	87.94%
5	Y.I.A.Rejani& S.T Selvi [22]	DWT,ANN	83.25%
6	Moschidis E,Chen X, Taylor C & Astley S.M [36]	DTCWT, Random Forest Tree	0.74 (Sensitivity)
7	Alfonso Rojas Domínguez & Asoke K Nandi [26]	statistical measures	80%
Proposed Work		DTCWT, Fourier Descriptor & ANN	92.3%

6.4 CONCLUSION

The purpose of this research is to compare DTCWT-based mass detection utilizing mammography with other methods already in use. Because of its low directional ability and shift variant property, the DWT approach for mass identification in mammograms only yielded limited results. This chapter concluded that our work results in 92.3% accuracy with the proposed method using DTCWT and ANN, due to the shift-invariance and better directional selectivity property of DTCWT. As compared to DWT-based methods, DT-CWT-based mass detection in mammograms yields good quality output. When data is highly dimensional, our suggested approach cannot produce satisfactory results. There are some areas where our future study may go that would be beneficial. In the future, the work is further extended by taking one or more other standard classifiers for the classification, and also the comparative analysis between the various classifiers will be done to find the best classifier with good classification accuracy. For improved prediction outcomes, the optimized features should be chosen from the extracted features. We intend to employ several deep learning models in the future for better outcomes.

REFERENCES

1. J. Hernández-Capistrán and J. F. Martínez-Carballido, "Thresholding methods review for microcalcifications segmentation on mammography images in obvious, subtle, and cluster categories," in *2016 13th International Conference on Electrical Engineering, Computing Science and Automatic Control (CCE)*, 2016, pp. 1–6.
2. A. Tirtajaya and D. D. Santika, "Classification of microcalcification using dual-tree complex wavelet transform and support vector machine," in *2010 Second International Conference on Advances in Computing, Control, and Telecommunication Technologies*, 2010, pp. 164–166.
3. J. Pragathi and H. T. Patil, "Multiresolution analysis for computer-aided mass detection in mammogram using pixel based segmentation method," in *2013 International Conference on Recent Trends in Information Technology (ICRTIT)*, 2013, pp. 214–220.

4. S. A. Hassan, M. S. Sayed, and F. Farag, "Segmentation of breast cancer lesion in digitized mammogram images," in *2014 Cairo International Biomedical Engineering Conference (CIBEC)*, 2014, pp. 103–106.
5. V. Alarcon-Aquino *et al.*, "Detection of microcalcifications in digital mammograms using the dual-tree complex wavelet transform (2009)," *Eng. Intell. Syst.*, vol. 17, p. 49, Mar. 2009.
6. L. Lowis, Hendra, and Lavinia, "The use of dual-tree complex wavelet transform (DTCWT) based feature for mammogram classification," *Int. J. Signal Process. Image Process. Pattern Recognit.*, vol. 8, pp. 87–96, Mar. 2015.
7. B. Verma and J. Zakos, "A computer-aided diagnosis system for digital mammograms based on fuzzy-neural and feature extraction techniques," *IEEE Trans. Inf. Technol. Biomed.*, vol. 5, no. 1, pp. 46–54, 2001.
8. R. Panchal and B. Verma, "Neural classification of mass abnormalities with different types of features in digital mammography," *Int. J. Comput. Intell. Appl.*, vol. 06, pp. 61–75, Nov. 2011.
9. W. Gu *et al.*, "High accuracy thyroid tumor image recognition based on hybrid multiple models optimization," *IEEE Access*, vol. 8, pp. 128426–128439, 2020.
10. H. D. Cheng, X. J. Shi, R. Min, L. M. Hu, X. P. Cai, and H. N. Du, "Approaches for automated detection and classification of masses in mammograms," *Pattern Recognit.*, vol. 39, no. 4, pp. 646–668, 2006.
11. W. Jian, X. Sun, and S. Luo, "Computer-aided diagnosis of breast microcalcifications based on dual-tree complex wavelet transform," *Biomed. Eng. Online*, vol. 11, p. 96, Dec. 2012.
12. N. Kingsbury, "Complex wavelets for shift invariant analysis and filtering of signals," *Appl. Comput. Harmon. Anal.*, vol. 10, no. 3, pp. 234–253, 2001.
13. I. W. Selesnick, R. G. Baraniuk, and N. C. Kingsbury, "The dual-tree complex wavelet transform," *IEEE Signal Process. Mag.*, vol. 22, no. 6, pp. 123–151, 2005.
14. A. Oliver *et al.*, "A review of automatic mass detection and segmentation in mammographic images," *Med. Image Anal.*, vol. 14, no. 2, pp. 87–110, 2010.
15. T. Celik and T. Tjahjadi, "Image resolution enhancement using dual-tree complex wavelet transform," *IEEE Geosci. Remote Sens. Lett.*, vol. 7, no. 3, pp. 554–557, 2010.
16. P. Luo, X. Qu, X. Qing, and J. Gu, "CT image denoising using double density dual tree complex wavelet with modified thresholding," in *2018 2nd International Conference on Data Science and Business Analytics (ICDSBA)*, 2018, pp. 287–290.
17. H. Naimi, A. B. H. Adamou-Mitiche, and L. Mitiche, "Medical image denoising using dual tree complex thresholding wavelet transform and Wiener filter," *J. King Saud Univ. – Comput. Inf. Sci.*, vol. 27, no. 1, pp. 40–45, 2015.
18. T. Wan, X. Liu, J. Chen, and Z. Qin, "Wavelet-based statistical features for distinguishing mitotic and non-mitotic cells in breast cancer histopathology," in *2014 IEEE International Conference on Image Processing (ICIP)*, 2014, pp. 2290–2294.
19. H. Lu, H. Wang, Q. Zhang, D. Won, and S. W. Yoon, "A dual-tree complex wavelet transform based convolutional neural network for human thyroid medical image segmentation," in *2018 IEEE International Conference on Healthcare Informatics (ICHI)*, 2018, pp. 191–198.
20. H. O. Ilhan, G. Serbes, and N. Aydin, "Dual tree complex wavelet transform based sperm abnormality classification," in *2018 41st International Conference on Telecommunications and Signal Processing (TSP)*, 2018, pp. 1–5.
21. C. Vimalraj, S. Esakkirajan, and P. Sreevidya, "DTCWT with fuzzy based thresholding for despeckling of ultrasound images," in *2017 International Conference on Intelligent Computing, Instrumentation and Control Technologies (ICICICT)*, 2017, pp. 515–519.
22. Y. Ireaneus Anna Rejani and S. Thamarai Selvi, "Digital mammogram segmentation and tumour detection using artificial neural networks," *Int. J. Soft Comp.*, pp. 112–119, 2008.
23. J. Bozek, M. Mustra, K. Delac, and M. Grgic, "A survey of image processing algorithms in digital mammography," in M. Grgic, K. Delac, and M. Ghanbari, Eds., *Recent advances in multimedia signal processing and communications*. Berlin, Heidelberg: Springer Berlin Heidelberg, 2009, pp. 631–657.

24. L. Wei, Y. Yang, and R. M. Nishikawa, "Microcalcification classification assisted by content-based image retrieval for breast cancer diagnosis," *Pattern Recognit.*, vol. 42, no. 6, pp. 1126–1132, 2009.
25. N. Szekely, N. Toth, and B. Pataki, "A hybrid system for detecting masses in mammographic images," in *Proceedings of the 21st IEEE Instrumentation and Measurement Technology Conference (IEEE Cat. No.04CH37510)*, 2004, vol. 3, pp. 2065–2070 Vol.3.
26. A. Rojas Domínguez and A. K. Nandi, "Detection of masses in mammograms via statistically based enhancement, multilevel-thresholding segmentation, and region selection," *Comput. Med. Imaging Graph.*, vol. 32, no. 4, pp. 304–315, 2008.
27. Vijayalakshmi G. *et al.*, "Image restoration on fusion of mammographs and mri breast images using dual tree complex wavelet transform," *Int. J. Adv. Sci. Technol.*, vol. 28, no. 17 SE-Articles, pp. 842–857, Dec. 2019.
28. D. Devakumari, Punithavathi V., "Study of breast cancer detection methods using image processing with data mining techniques,", *Int. J. Pure Appl. Math.*, vol. 118, no. 18, pp. 2867–2873, 2018.
29. F. Anwar, O. Attallah, N. Ghanem, and M. Ismail, "Automatic Breast Cancer Classification from Histopathological Images," *2019 International Conference on Advances in the Emerging Computing Technologies (AECT)*, Al Madinah Al Munawwarah, Saudi Arabia, pp. 1–6, 2020.
30. Z. Wang *et al.*, "Breast cancer detection using extreme learning machine based on feature fusion with CNN deep features," *IEEE Access*, vol. 7, pp. 105146–105158, 2019.
31. K. Loizidou, G. Skouroumouni, C. Nikolaou, and C. Pitris, "Automatic breast mass segmentation and classification using subtraction of temporally sequential digital mammograms", *Med. Imag. Diagn. Radiol.*, vol. 10, pp. 1801111–1801121, 2022.
32. K. Loizidou, G. Skouroumouni, G. Savvidou, A. Constantinidou, C. Nikolaou, and C. Pitris, "Benign and malignant breast mass detection and classification in digital mammography: The effect of subtracting temporally consecutive mammograms," *2022 IEEE-EMBS International Conference on Biomedical and Health Informatics (BHI)*, Ioannina, Greece, 2022, pp. 1–4, doi: 10.1109/BHI56158.2022.9926810.
33. P M Rajasree, A. Jatti, D. Santosh, U. Desai, and V. D. Krishnappa, " Breast masses detection and segmentation in full-field digital mammograms using unified convolution neural network," *Annu. Int. Conf. IEEE. Eng. Med. Biol. Soc.*, doi: 10.1109/EMBC48229.2022.9871866.
34. S. Liu, Z. Lai, H. Kong, and L. Shen, "Dual fusion mass detector for mammogram mass detection," *2022 IEEE 35th International Symposium on Computer-Based Medical Systems (CBMS)*, Shenzen, China, 2022, pp. 149–154, doi: 10.1109/CBMS55023.2022.00033.
35. K. Aznag, T. Datsi, A. El, and E. El Bachari, "Towards an improvement of Fourier Transform," *Int. J. Adv. Comput. Sci. Appl.*, vol. 11, no. 1, pp. 714–719, 2020.
36. E. Moschidis, X. Chen, C. Taylor, and S. M. Astley, "Texture-based breast cancer prediction in full-field digital mammograms using the dual-tree complex wavelet transform and random forest classification BT – breast imaging," International Workshop on Digital Mammography, Breast Imaging, IWDM 2014, Lecture Notes in Computer Science, vol. 8539, pp. 209–216, 2014.

Chapter 7

A deep learning-based model for early detection of COVID-19 using chest X-ray images

S Punitha, Vaishali R Kulkarni, and Thompson Stephan

Department of Computer Science and Engineering, Graphic Era Deemed to be University, Dehradun, Uttarakhand, India

7.1 INTRODUCTION

The COVID-19 virus has had a very serious impact on mankind. People suffering from COVID-19 have a vast range of symptoms from mild health problems such as cold, cough, and fever to respiration problems and sudden death. People have these symptoms after 2–14 days after getting exposed to the virus. The severity of the illness is varying from mild to serious health issues. Most people infected with the virus experience mild to moderate respiratory illness and recover without requiring special treatment. At the same time, many people became seriously ill and required medical attention. When old people were going through medical conditions such as cardiovascular disease, chronic respiratory disease, diabetes, etc, they may get sicker with COVID-19 [1].

When the COVID patient coughs, sneezes, speaks, or breathes heavily, and meets other people, the virus gets spread. The virus particles move in the form of large droplets to smaller aerosols. Droplets of the respiratory spreading. The prevention is done in the form of protection with the use of proper masks, use of sanitizer, frequent washing of hands, and the food items consumed. Following a social distance of at least one meter from others and getting vaccinated reduces the chances of infection. The main infection of COVID-19 is in the lungs. This infection can be treated using the proper X-ray scan results [2].

Deep learning (DL) is one of the methods in machine learning (ML) that is used in multiple applications to analyze images and perform classification based on some criteria. DL makes use of artificial neural networks (ANNs) layered architecture for filtering data and concluding some connections and relations of the data. The layers contact each other and learn to take decisions [3]. DL algorithms are used in deep neural networks (DNNs) based on the connections of human brain neurons. DNNs are like ANNs but work at a deeper level. The layers use formal methods for translating the raw data into meaningful output. There are additional layers that perform further refining of the output. There is tremendous potential for DL algorithms in the healthcare domain. Many healthcare diagnostics use convolutional neural networks (CNNs) which is yet another type of DNN for the classification of images obtained in various scans of patients [4]. The CNNs have been proved useful in improving the ability of the machines for recognizing and manipulating data. The healthcare, medical, and pharmacy fields have benefitted from CNN models as they can process large voluminous data. The data volume is increasing continuously due to different scan machines and the availability of digital data [5].

The DL methods have proven efficient in working on large data with specialized medical equipment. Some of the striking examples of DL methods in healthcare include determining

DOI: 10.1201/9781003369059-9

complicated case diagnoses in the fields of radiology, pathology, ophthalmology, and dermatology. With the use of the DL-based diagnosis, doctors are getting the benefit of a second opinion for the treatment. A similar DL model has been demonstrated in this study for the detection of COVID-19 fever using X-ray images [6]. The main contributions of this paper are:

1. Combination of DL and images from the COVID-19 Radiography Database from the Kaggle.
2. An end-to-end profound learning system that specifically predicts the COVID-19 malady from crude pictures without any requirement, including extraction.
3. A dataset of 10,192 normal images and 3,616 COVID images has been used in the ratio of 80:20 ratio for training and testing.
4. Data processing such as data augmentation, and application of the ImageNet has been used for training data.
5. Five models, namely VGG16, ResNet50, Dense-Net-121, DenseNet-201, and CNN, have been used for the classification of images and conclude the results of the diagnosis.

The rest of the chapter has been organized as follows: the related work of DL methods in healthcare is discussed in Section 7.2. The proposed methodology for COVID-19 detection is outlined in Section 7.3. The results of the experimentation are presented in Section 7.4, and finally, the conclusion and summary of this study are expressed in Section 7.5.

7.2 RELATED WORKS

In the past, there has been extensive research on intelligent medical image understanding. The diagnosis of the disease is not only by the experts but also with the assistance of different steps including classification, segmentation, detection, and localization in CNNs [7], an application of support vector machines.

An application of a CNN-based algorithm for image classification has been shown for various diseases such as pneumonia as given in [8]. In this study, the CNN models are compared with a linear support vector machine and the ORB method.

Healthcare applications and the advanced Internet of Things (IoT) are making quite revolutionary changes. With the effective use of IoT devices, CNN layered complexity can be large and the complexity analysis can consume more time. These drawbacks are overcome by using the discovery model of CNN for data classification. In this model, the first layer selects the important health-related factors, and later the positive and negative correlated factors are classified. This model is presenting the detection of the health problems such as blood pressure, diabetes, and overweight problems. The accuracy of the presented model is shown as a correlation of the three factors in the detection of the general health of people [9].

A review of different classification algorithms using DL concepts applied in the medical industry is presented in [10]. In this study, the accuracy, basic technologies, challenges, and available DL models are explored in detail.

A study that utilizes a memristive crossbar array (MCA) and a two-dimensional (2D) tunable Q-wavelet transform (TQWT) to decompose chest X-ray images from two datasets is introduced [11]. The method produced promising results with optimal peak signal-to-noise ratio and structural similarity index values at a quality factor of 4, oversampling rate of 3, and decomposition level of 2. The processed images were classified as COVID-19 or non-COVID-19 using ResNet50 and AlexNet convolutional neural network (CNN) models. The proposed approach achieved an average accuracy of 98.82% and 94.64% for the small and large datasets, respectively.

A novel learning framework for early diagnosis of COVID-19 patients using hybrid deep fusion learning models is proposed [12]. The proposed framework performs early patient classification based on collected samples of chest X-ray images and cough samples from potentially infected individuals. The captured cough samples are pre-processed using speech signal processing techniques, and deep convolutional neural networks extract Mel frequency cepstral coefficient features. Finally, the proposed system fuses extracted features using the weighted sum-rule fusion method to provide early diagnosis with an accuracy of 98.70% and 82.7% based on Chest X-ray images and cough (audio) samples, respectively.

A a method for automatic diagnosis of COVID-19, normal and pneumonia based on chest X-ray images is proposed [13]. The method involves training six classifiers using chest X-ray images and selecting the top five for both training and validation sets. The Bag of Features method is used to extract image features, and Majority Voting is used for image classification in both phases. The proposed model achieves an accuracy of 99.63%, with 99.86% accuracy in Phase 1 and 99.28% accuracy in Phase 2. The model also achieves high Specificity (%), Precision (%), Recall (%), F1 Score (%), AUC, and MCC values.

In [14], a classification model is presented for tri-stage COVID-19. The model is named as CXGNet that uses CNN, and two algorithms, namely grey-wolf optimizer and genetic algorithm, based on evolutionary computing. The different implementations of the model include 4-class, 3-class, and 2-class models.

An efficient method called deep feature fusion classification network is proposed to improve the accuracy of COVID-19 diagnosis [15]. The method comprises two modules: the deep feature fusion module and the multi-disease classification module. The network incorporates the spatial attention and channel attention modules to enhance the feature extraction capability of the model, and multiple-way data augmentation is applied to the chest X-ray images to increase the diversity of the samples. The Grad-CAM++ technique is used to make the features more intuitive and the deep learning model more interpretable. The proposed method achieves an accuracy of 99.89% in the triple classification of COVID-19, pneumonia, and healthy X-ray images on publicly available datasets, outperforming eight state-of-the-art classification techniques.

7.3 PROPOSED METHODOLOGY

A model with different phases used in this study is depicted in Figure 7.1. The steps such as data acquisition, data pre-processing, data augmentation, and model classification are mainly used in the detection of COVID and non-COVID patients.

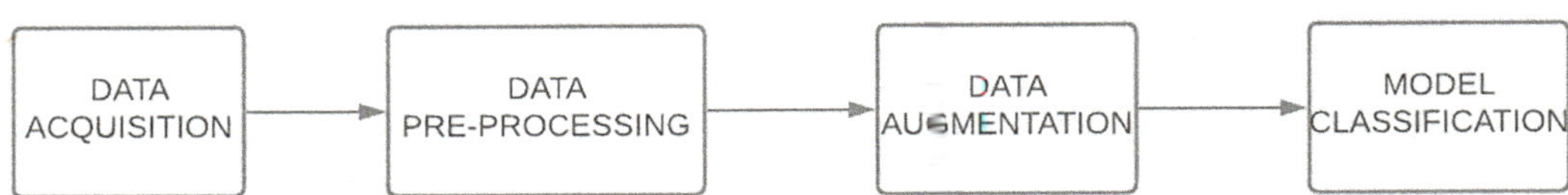

Figure 7.1 Model used for classification.

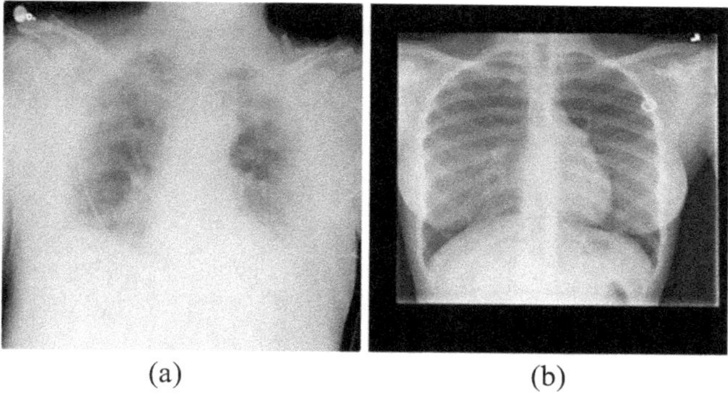

Figure 7.2 (a) COVID image, (b) Normal image.

7.3.1 Data acquisition

In the data acquisition step, the data has been collected from the COVID-19 radiography database from Kaggle. The images related to chest X-ray images are 13,808. The dataset has been divided into two classes namely covid and normal. In the database, there are 10,192 normal images and 3,616 covid images [13]. These chest X-ray images are stored in PNG format. Some of the normal and COVID-19-infected images are shown in Figures 7.2(a) and 7.2(b).

7.3.2 Data pre-processing

The data obtained from the Kaggle is in different sizes, and it is resized into one size in this step. All the images are formatted to fit into the size of 224*224 pixels.

7.3.3 Data augmentation

The imbalance of the data is overcome in this step by avoiding the overfitting model. The number of COVID-19-infected images is 3,616. A set of random images are subjected to flip, rotate, translate, and blur so that a greater number of images are generated for the COVID-19-infected images. Thus, at the end of this step, the number of normal and infected images is equal to 8,153. The resulting resultant images after augmentation are shown in Figure 7.3.

7.4 MODEL CLASSIFICATION

In model classification, a set of inputs is used in training to arrive at an essential conclusion. The classification model can be used to categorize or provide labels to the data. The data is utilized in a protected manner and is stored in different forms. Many predictions can be done by using the classification model. The different classification models such as CNN, recurrent neural networks (RNNs), Multilayer perceptron (MLPs), etc., are some of the examples of the DL models.

7.4.1 CNN

CNN has been an important network in the DL methods and has been applied in computer vision, natural language processing, etc., in the areas of both research and industry. CNNs are a subset of neural networks that utilize convolution rather than general matrix multiplication in at least one of their layers.

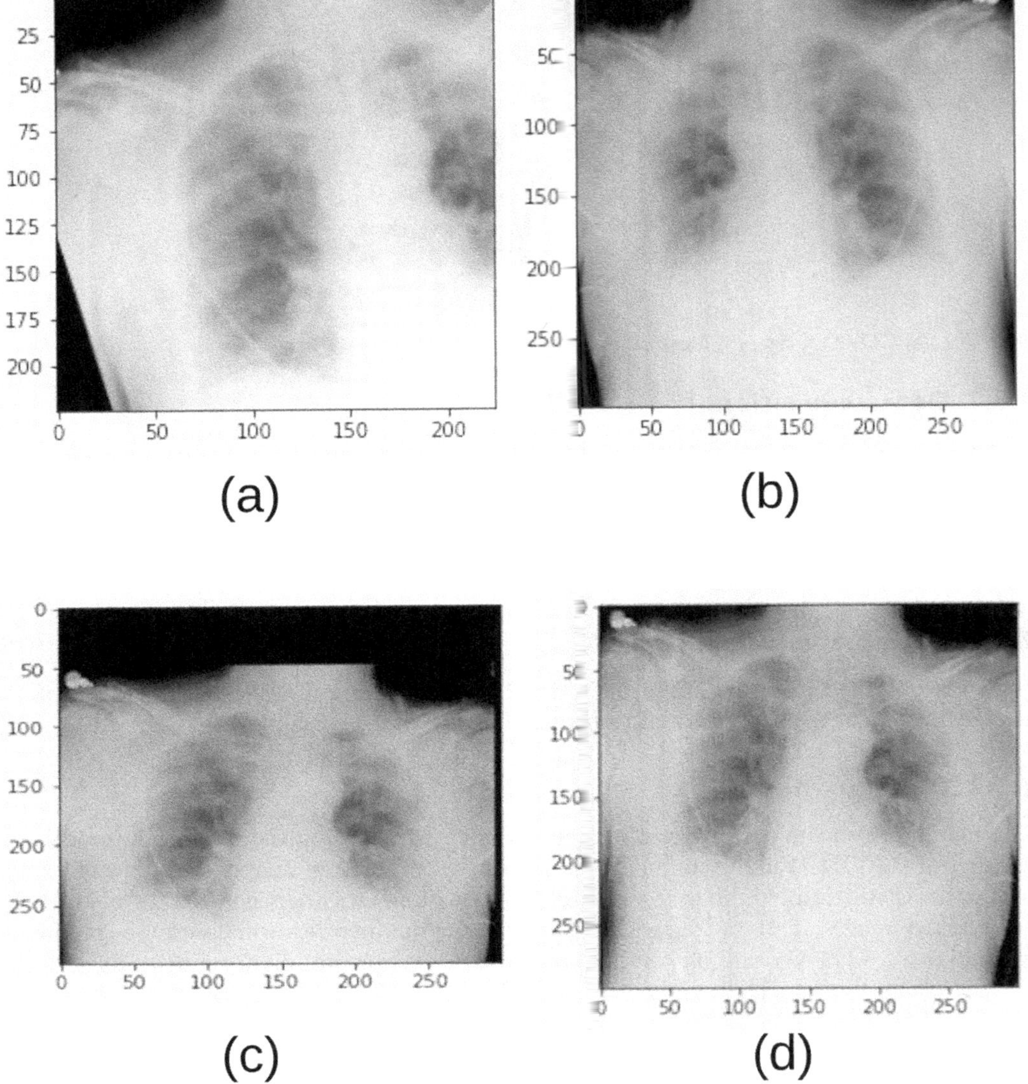

Figure 7.3 (a) Rotated image, (b) Flipped image, (c) Translated images, (d) Blurred image.

7.4.2 ResNet50

Residual Network (RN) is a CNN model with 50 layers. ResNet50 is a pretrained model that supports multiple CNN layers. It can be used for large datasets including images.

The ResNet50 uses filters for reducing the number of steps or to bypass the initial layers in the CNN. With the advantage of bypassing the layers the ResNet50 can work faster, and it is simpler compared to other CN models. The ResNet50 model architecture model is presented in Figure 7.4. The components of the ResNet50 are given as: 7 × 7 convolution kernel, max pooling, 9 layers, 12 layers, 18 layers, and 12 layers, and average pooling.

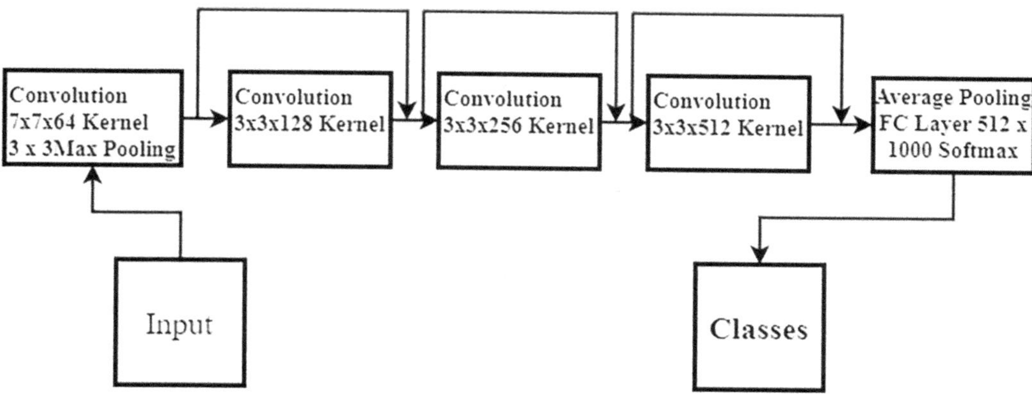

Figure 7.4 ResNet50 architecture.

7.4.3 DenseNet121 and DenseNet201

Another commonly used CNN is dense CNN (DenseNet). The path between the input and output is more, and it allows more members of network to access the path. DenseNet101 and DenseNet201 were similar, but DenseNet121 has 121 layers and DenseNet201 has 201 layers. The DenseNet architecture was shown in Figure 7.5.

It consists of many CNNs that are densely connected. The DenseNet model is used for more complex with large data and memory requirement.

7.4.4 VGG16

VGG16 stands for very deep convolutional networks for large-scale image recognition.

The important features of the VGG16 are as given:

1. Number of images in a dataset = 14 million
2. Number of groups = 1000
3. The accuracy = 92%
4. Multiple kernel-sized filters
5. It is better than Alex Net model.

The VGG16 architecture is shown in Figure 7.6.

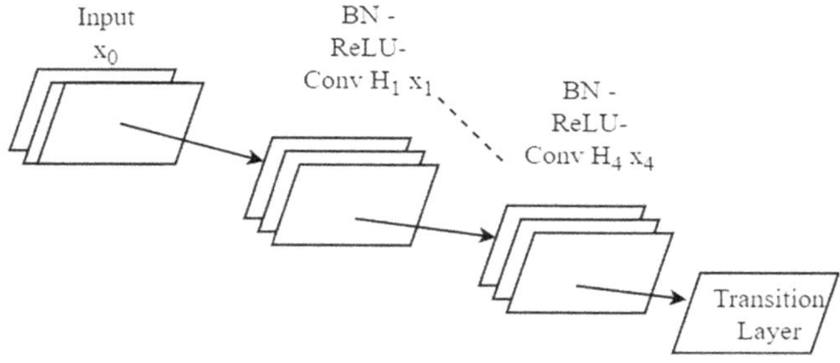

Figure 7.5 DenseNet architecture.

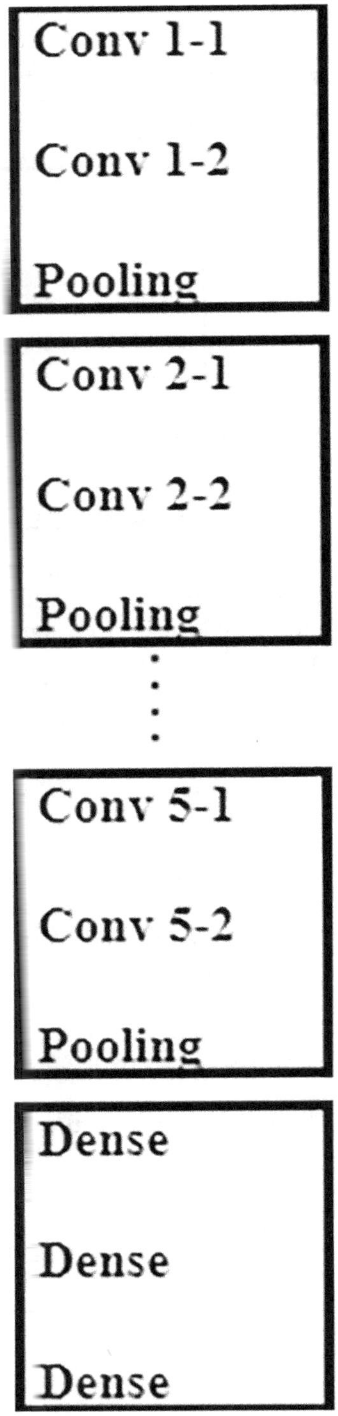

Conv 1-1
Conv 1-2
Pooling

Conv 2-1
Conv 2-2
Pooling

⋮

Conv 5-1
Conv 5-2
Pooling

Dense
Dense
Dense

Figure 7.6 VGG16 architecture.

7.5 EXPERIMENTAL RESULTS

The experimental results are given with the parameters such as the confusion matrix for all five models. The details of each result parameter are given as follows. The model has been evaluated.

7.5.1 Confusion matrix

A classification model output is presented using a confusion matrix table. It uses a collection of test data with known true values. A confusion matrix for each model used in this study is represented in Table 7.1. Figures 7.7–7.11 represent the confusion matrices of CNN, VGG-16, ResNet50, DenseNet121, and DenseNet201, respectively.

The terms used in confusion matrix are given as shown in Table 7.2.

Table 7.1 Confusion matrix

Cases	*Predicted 0*	*Predicted 1*
Actual 0	TN	FP
Actual 1	FN	TP

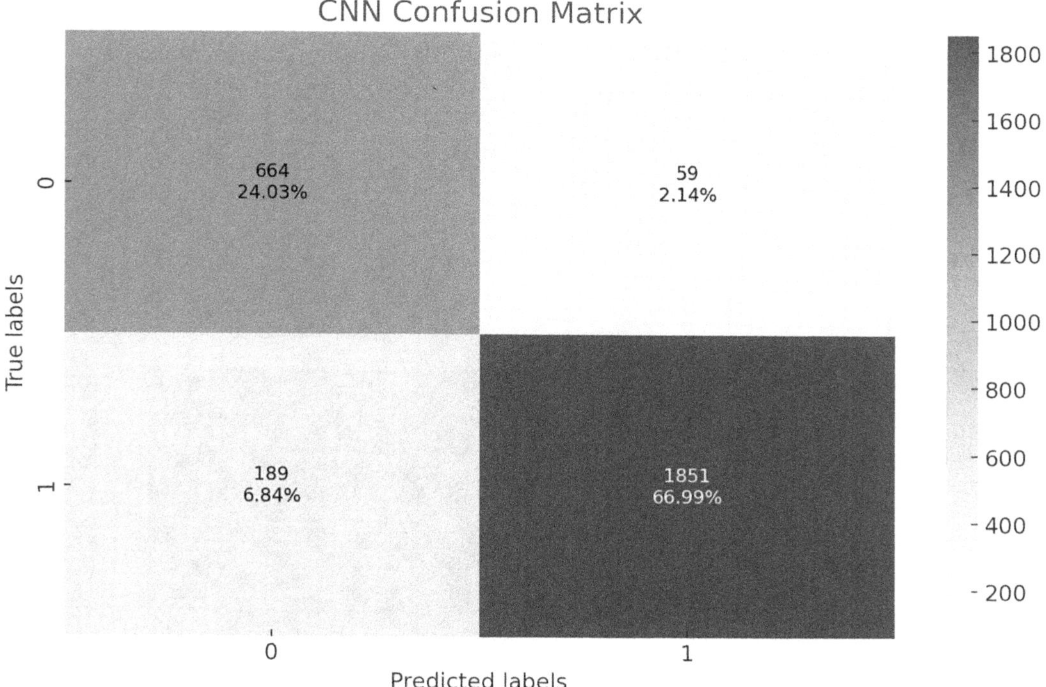

Figure 7.7 Confusion matrix of CNN.

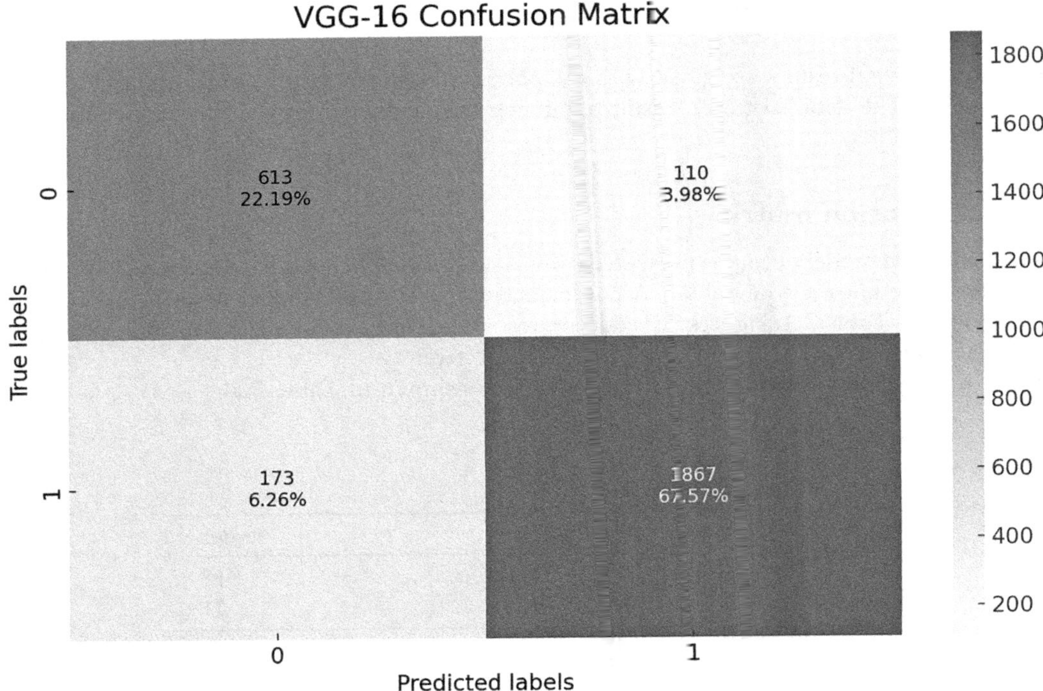

Figure 7.8 Confusion matrix of VGG-16.

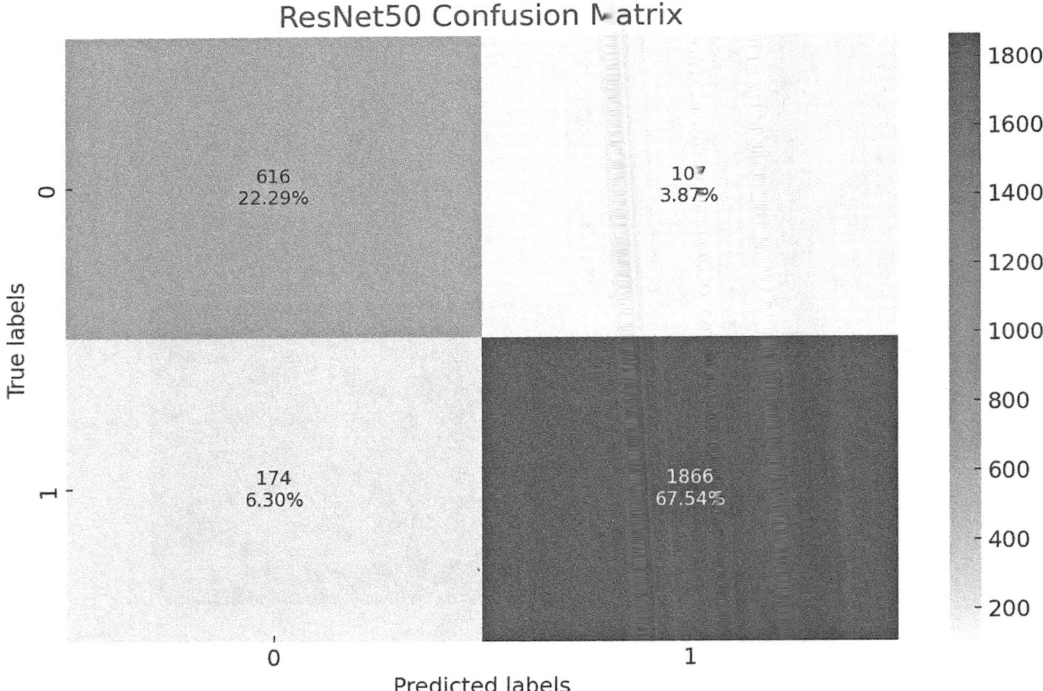

Figure 7.9 Confusion matrix of ResNet50.

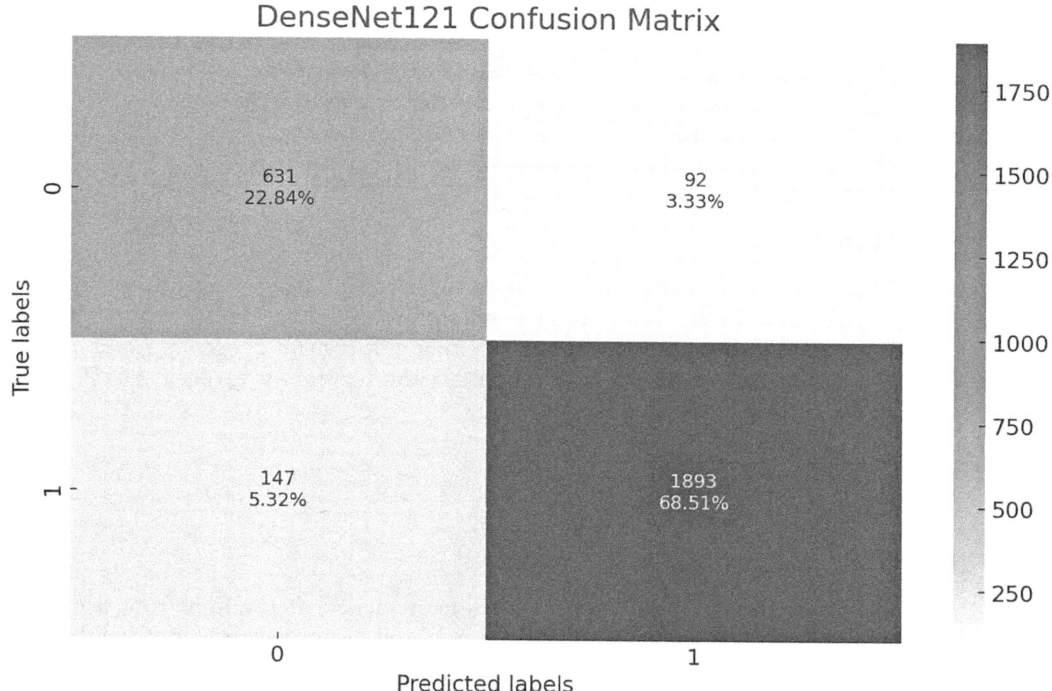

Figure 7.10 Confusion matrix of DenseNet121.

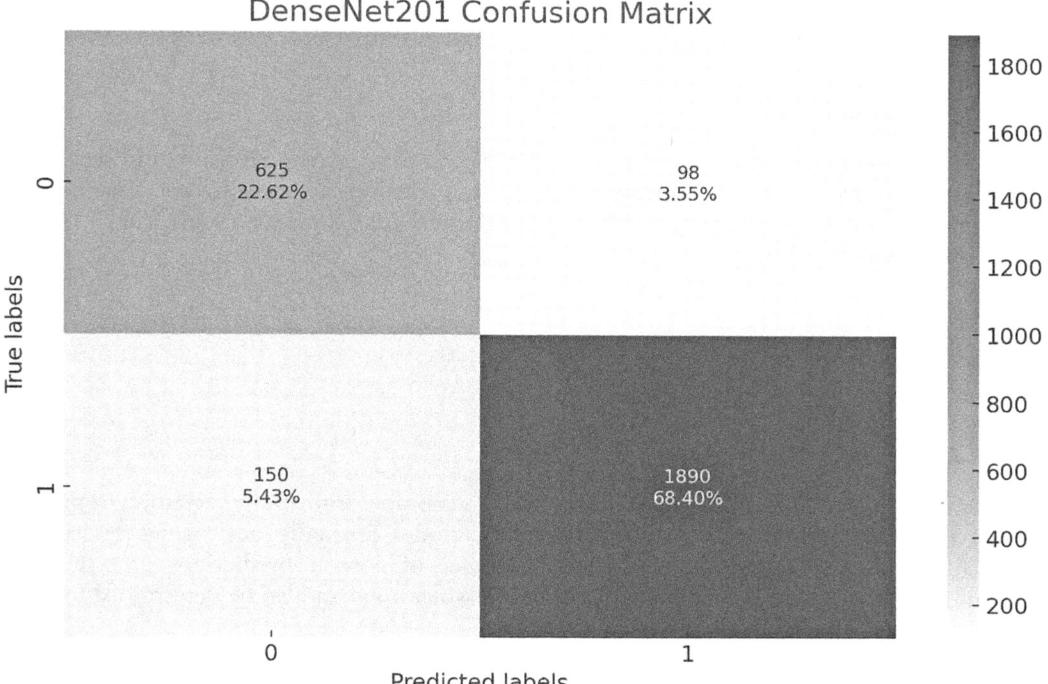

Figure 7.11 Confusion matrix of DenseNet201.

Table 7.2 Confusion matrix details

TRUE POSITIVE (TP) = these will predict 1, correctly classified as a positive class.
TRUE NEGATIVE (TN) = these will predict 0, correctly classified as a negative class.
FALSE POSITIVE (FP) = these will predict 1, incorrectly classified positive class.
FALSE NEGATIVE (FN) = these will predict 1, incorrectly classified negative class.

7.5.2 Precision

The quality of the predictions in the given records is expressed using precision. Precision is determined at a given threshold, taking into consideration only the topmost results returned by the method. Precision is the approximate chance that a document chosen at random from the pool of collected documents is relevant. The Precision formula is given in Eq. 7.1.

$$Precision = \frac{True\ Positive}{True\ Positive + False\ Positive} \tag{7.1}$$

7.5.3 Recall

The recall is the approximate chance that a document picked at random from a pool of application documents will be retrieved. Recall is computed using the number of valid results and the number of results that could have been returned. The recall is referred to as sensitivity in a binary grouping. The Recall formula is given in Eq. 7.2.

$$Recall = \frac{True\ Positive}{True\ Positive + False\ Negative} \tag{7.2}$$

7.5.4 F1 score

The highest possible value of an F1-score is 1.0, representing great precision and recall, and the lowest possible value is 0, indicating that either precision or recall is zero. The F1 score, also known as the Dice similarity coefficient, is another name for the F1 score (DSC). The F1 Score formula is Eq. 7.3.

$$F1 = 2\,\frac{Precision\ .\ recall}{Precision + recall} = \frac{TP}{TP + \frac{1}{2}(FP + FN)} \tag{7.3}$$

7.5.5 Accuracy

One metric for evaluating classification models is accuracy. Informally, accuracy represents the percentage of accurate predictions given by the model. Formally, accuracy is described as follows: accuracy is determined using the number of correct predictions and the total number of predictions. The accuracy of binary classification can also be determined in terms of positives and negatives, as seen in Eq. (7.4).

$$Accuracy = \frac{TP + TN}{TP + TN + FP + FN} \tag{7.4}$$

Table 7.3 Classification report

Model name	*Recall*	*F1 Score*	*Precision*
CNN	0.92	0.84	0.97
Vgg16	0.85	0.81	0.95
Resnet50	0.94	0.91	0.98
Densenet101	0.87	0.84	0.95
Densenet201	0.87	0.84	0.95

The details of precision, recall, F1 score, and accuracy details are given in Tables 7.3 and 7.4.

The performance metrics presented in Figure 7.12 indicate that all the models perform well, with the Resnet50 model slightly leading in terms of accuracy, and the CNN model closely matching its performance. The VGG16, while showing a modest decrease in performance compared to the CNN, still maintains a high level of precision.

Table 7.4 Classification report

Model name	*Recall*	*F1 Score*	*Accuracy*
CNN	0.91	0.94	0.91
Vgg16	0.91	0.93	0.90
Resnet50	0.96	0.97	0.95
Densenet101	0.93	0.94	0.91
Densenet201	0.93	0.94	0.91

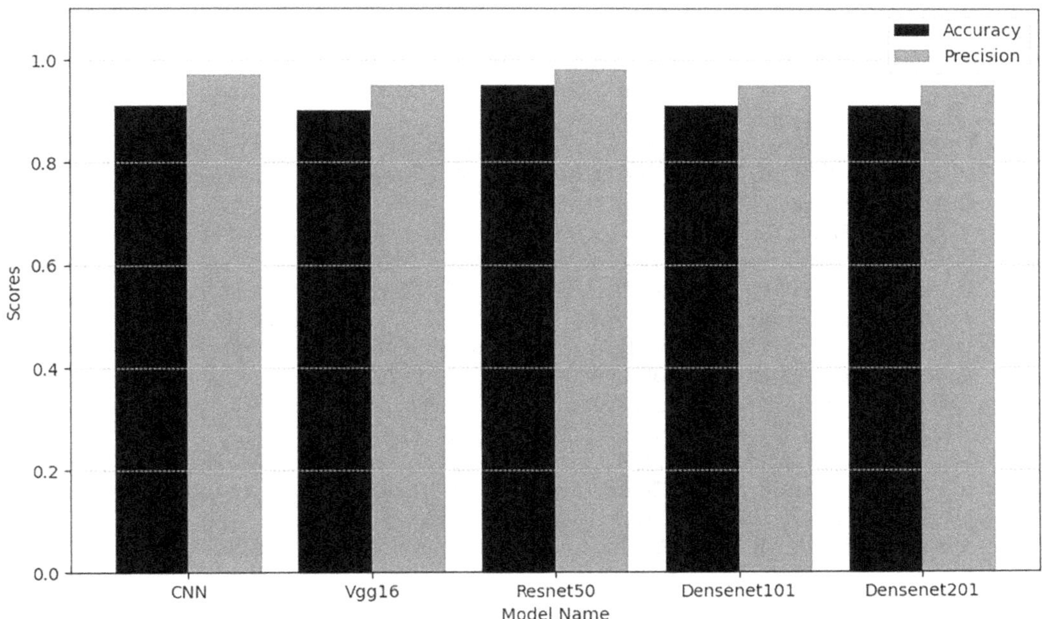

Figure 7.12 Comparative performance metrics of CNN models.

DenseNet101 and DenseNet201 display identical levels of accuracy and precision, which are solid, though not as high as those of the Resnet50 or CNN. This suggests that while there is a variance in the performance of the models, they all demonstrate a strong capability in correctly classifying positive instances as well as maintaining a high relevance in their positive predictions. Overall, the models exhibit a commendable balance between accuracy and precision, making them all suitable candidate for tasks requiring reliable classification performance.

7.6 CONCLUSION

Five pre-trained, fine-tuned models, including VGG16, ResNet50, CNN, DenseNet-121, and DenseNet-201 are used in this study for developing a DL system for early detection of COVID-19 from chest X-ray images. A dataset of 13,000 files has been created. Each model is assessed for its performance with parameters based on accuracy, precision, recall, and f1 score. The highest precision is for the model ResNet50, which is 98%. This is helpful in the accurate prediction and early detection of the COVID-19 disease. Improvement in the accuracy of classification and labeling data using various optimized deep learning models is the focus of future work.

REFERENCES

1. S. Minaee, R. Kafieh, M. Sonka, S. Yazdani, and G. Jamalipour Soufi, "Deep-COVID: Predicting COVID-19 from chest X-ray images using deep transfer learning," Med. Image Anal., vol. 65, no. 101794, p. 101794, 2020.
2. M. Z. Islam, M. M. Islam, and A. Asraf, "A combined deep CNN-LSTM network for the detection of novel coronavirus (COVID-19) using X-ray images," Inform. Med. Unlocked, vol. 20, no. 100412, p. 100412, 2020.
3. D. Apostolopoulos and T. A. Mpesiana, "Covid-19: automatic detection from X-ray images utilizing transfer learning with convolutional neural networks," Phys. Eng. Sci. Med., vol. 43, no. 2, pp. 635–640, 2020.
4. D. Haritha, N. Swaroop, and M. Mounika, "Prediction of COVID-19 cases using CNN with X-rays," in 2020 5th International Conference on Computing, Communication, and Security (ICCCS), 2020.
5. R. Jain, M. Gupta, S. Taneja, and D. J. Hemanth, "Deep learning-based detection and analysis of COVID-19 on chest X-ray images," Appl. Intell., 2020.
6. B. Sekeroglu and I. Ozsahin, "Detection of COVID-19 from chest X-ray images using convolutional neural networks," SLAS Technol., vol. 25, no. 6, pp. 553–565, 2020.
7. D. R. Sarvamangala and R. V. Kulkarni, "Convolutional neural networks in medical image understanding: A survey," Evol. Intell., vol. 15, no. 1, 2022.
8. S. S. Yadav and S. M. Jadhav, "Deep convolutional neural network based medical image classification for disease diagnosis," J Big Data, vol. 6, p. 113, 2019.
9. W. N. Ismail, M. M. Hassan, H. A. Alsalamah, and G. Fortino, "CNN-based health model for regular health factors analysis in internet-of-medical things environment," IEEE Access, vol. 8, pp. 52541–52549, 2020, doi: 10.1109/ACCESS.2020.2980938.
10. S. Shamshirband, M. Fathi, A. Dehzangi, A. T. Chronopoulos, and H. Alinejad-Rokny, "A review on deep learning approaches in healthcare systems: Taxonomies, challenges, and open issues," J. Biomed. Inform., vol. 113, p. 103627, 2021, ISSN 1532-0464, 10.1016/j.jbi.2020.103627.

11. K. Jyoti, S. Sushma, S. Yadav, P. Kumar, R. B. Pachori, and S. Mukherjee, "Automatic diagnosis of COVID-19 with MCA-inspired TQWT-based classification of chest X-ray images," Comput. Biol. Med., vol. 152, p. 106331, January 2023.
12. S. Kumar, R. Nagar, S. Bhatnagar, R. Vaddi, S. Kumar Gupta, M. Rashid, A. K. Bashir, and T. Alkhalifah, "Chest X ray and cough sample based deep learning framework for accurate diagnosis of COVID-19," Comput. Electr. Eng., vol. 103, p. 108391, October 2022.
13. K. M. Sunnetci and A. Alkan, "Biphasic majority voting-based comparative COVID-19 diagnosis using chest X-ray images," Expert Syst. Appl., vol. 216, p. 119430, 15 April 2023.
14. A. Gopatoti and P. Vijayalakshmi, "CXGNet: A tri-phase chest X-ray image classification for COVID-19 diagnosis using deep CNN with enhanced grey-wolf optimizer," Biomed. Signal Process. Control, vol. 77, p. 103860, August 2022.
15. J. Liu, W. Sun, X. Zhao, J. Zhao, and Z. Jiang, "Deep feature fusion classification network (DFFCNet): Towards accurate diagnosis of COVID-19 using chest X-rays images," Biomed. Signal Process. Control, vol. 76, p. 103677, July 2022.

Chapter 8

Detection of seizure activity in fMRI images using deep learning techniques

Abhishek Saigiridhari, Abhishek Mishra, Aditi Mahadware, Aarya Tupe, and Dhanalekshmi Yedurkar

Computer Science Department, MIT School of Engineering, MIT ADT University, Pune, India

8.1 INTRODUCTION

Since, there are over a million people in the world affected by seizures with underlying serious causes such as epilepsy, or PTSD, the numbers keep on increasing. With easy neuroimaging such as fMRI images, we can use deep learning techniques to detect the seizure pattern [1]. Seizures are a neurological disorder identified by abrupt electrical activity in the brain, which leads to a range of symptoms such as convulsions, spasms, unconsciousness,and sensory disturbances like sensations of tingling or seeing flashing lights. Epilepsy is the most common cause of seizures, affecting millions of people worldwide. While there are several methods available to diagnose seizures, such as EEG signals and heart rate monitoring, neuroimaging techniques such as fMRI images have emerged as promising tools for improving the accuracy of diagnosis and treatment. fMRI (functional magnetic resonance imaging) is a non-invasive neuroimaging method that scans activated neurons,brain activity and measures changes in blood flow without performing any surgery. By analyzing the patterns of neural activity in the brain, fMRI can provide valuable information about the location and type of seizure, which can help guide treatment decisions. However, interpreting fMRI images requires specialized knowledge and expertise, which can be a challenge for medical professionals. Therefore, developing automated tools and algorithms to analyze fMRI data could greatly boost seizure detection methods and diagnosis efficiency. In this project, we aim to develop deep learning models that can analyze fMRI images to detect seizures and classify them into different types. By training the models on large datasets of fMRI images, we hope to identify patterns and features that are specific to different types of seizures and can be used for accurate diagnosis and treatment. Our ultimate goal is to develop a user-friendly software application that can be used by medical professionals to quickly and accurately detect seizures and provide appropriate treatment. Such an application will definitely help bring about a change for millions of people globally having epilepsy and brain disorders by timely medical intervention, promoting better wellbeing and early detection [2].

8.2 FUNCTIONAL MAGNETIC RESONANCE IMAGING

8.2.1 fMRI images

fMRI (functional magnetic resonance imaging) is an approach to map out the brain activity based on alterations in blood circulation in response to various stimuli. This technique is based on the fact that when neurons become active, they require more oxygen and glucose, which is supplied to them by increased blood flow.

DOI: 10.1201/9781003369059-10

A magnetic field is used to align the body's hydrogen atoms during an fMRI scan, and radio waves are subsequently utilized to stimulate them, prompting them to emit signals that the scanner can pick up. By repeatedly measuring the signal over time, fMRI can generate a 3D image of the brain, showing which areas are active during a given task or in response to a stimulus [3,4].

fMRI images are significant in finding out neurological disorders, such as seizures, because they provide a detailed view of the brain's functional activity. Figure 8.1 shows the slices of the brain. By analyzing fMRI data, researchers can identify patterns of neural activity that are associated with specific tasks or conditions, which can help identify areas of the brain that may be affected by a disorder [5]. For example, in the case of epilepsy, fMRI by identifying brain regions that are causing seizure activity, allows for more precise treatment alternatives. fMRI can also be used to monitor the progression of the disorder and the effectiveness of treatment over time.

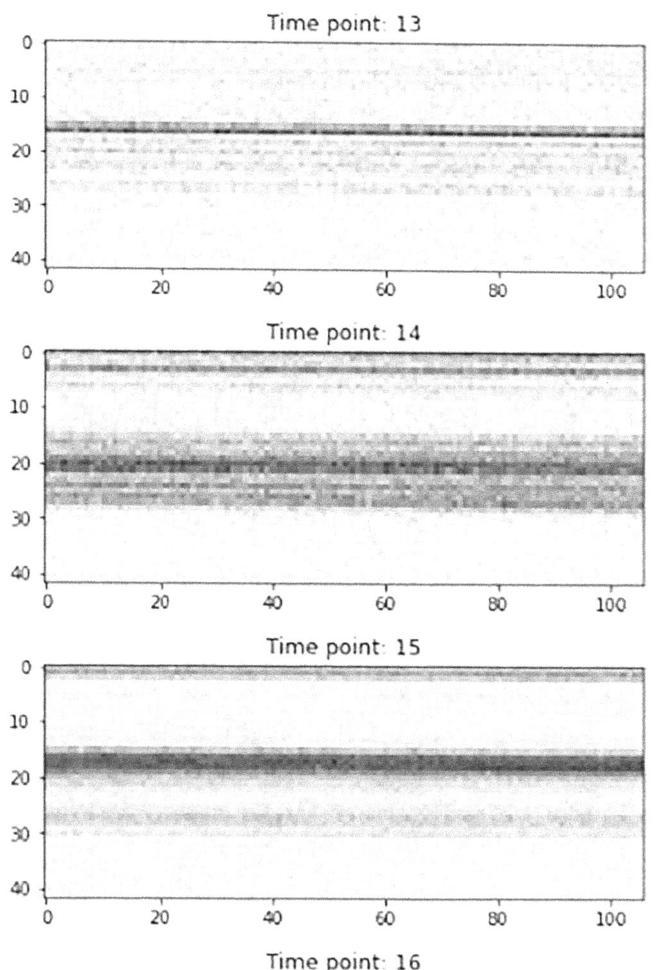

Figure 8.1 Slices of brain.

8.2.2 Seizures and epilepsy

An uncontrolled, sudden electrical disturbance in the brain known as a seizure can alter one's movement, level of consciousness, and behavior.

Seizures are symptoms of a neurological disorder, such as Epilepsy, but they can also be caused by other conditions such as brain tumors, head injuries, and infections.

During seizures, the brain's regular functions are interfered with, resulting in aberrant activity and symptoms such as loss of consciousness, convulsions, or sensory problems [6]. Figure [Figure 8.2] Highlights the raw fMRI images.

Surgical intervention or medication management are options for treating epileptic episodes, or seizures, depending on the underlying cause and severity of the disorder.

8.2.3 How seizures can be detected

Seizures can be detected through various methods, including:

- Electroencephalogram (EEG): A test known as an EEG can be used to evaluate the electrical activity of the brain in a non-invasive manner. During a seizure, there is a characteristic pattern of abnormal electrical activity that can be detected by an EEG.
- Video monitoring: Video monitoring is a technique that involves recording a patient's behavior during a seizure. This can help medical practitioners to detect and understand the type of seizure and the area of the brain that is affected.
- Magnetic resonance imaging (MRI): MRI is a medical diagnostic imaging technique that uses magnetic fields and radio waves to generate crisp pictures of the brain. MRI can help to identify structural abnormalities in the brain that may be causing seizures.
- Computed tomography (CT) scan: Computed tomography scan is a technique that creates comprehensive images of the brain and body. CT scan can help to identify structural abnormalities in the brain that may be causing seizures.
- Positron emission tomography (PET) scan: PET scan is a medical imaging that uses a radioisotope to create 3-D images of the brain. PET scan can help to identify areas of the brain that are affected by seizures, helps in the diagnosis and management of various neurological conditions.

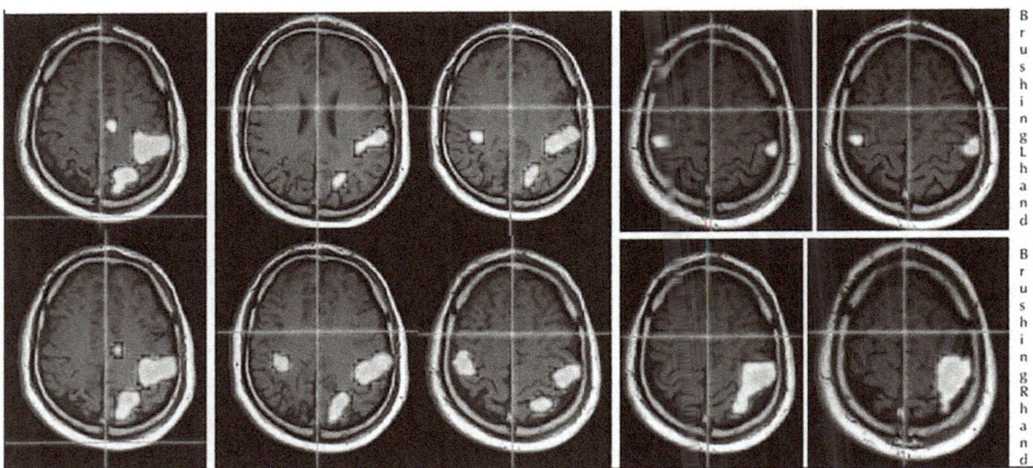

Figure 8.2 Raw fMRI noisy images [7].

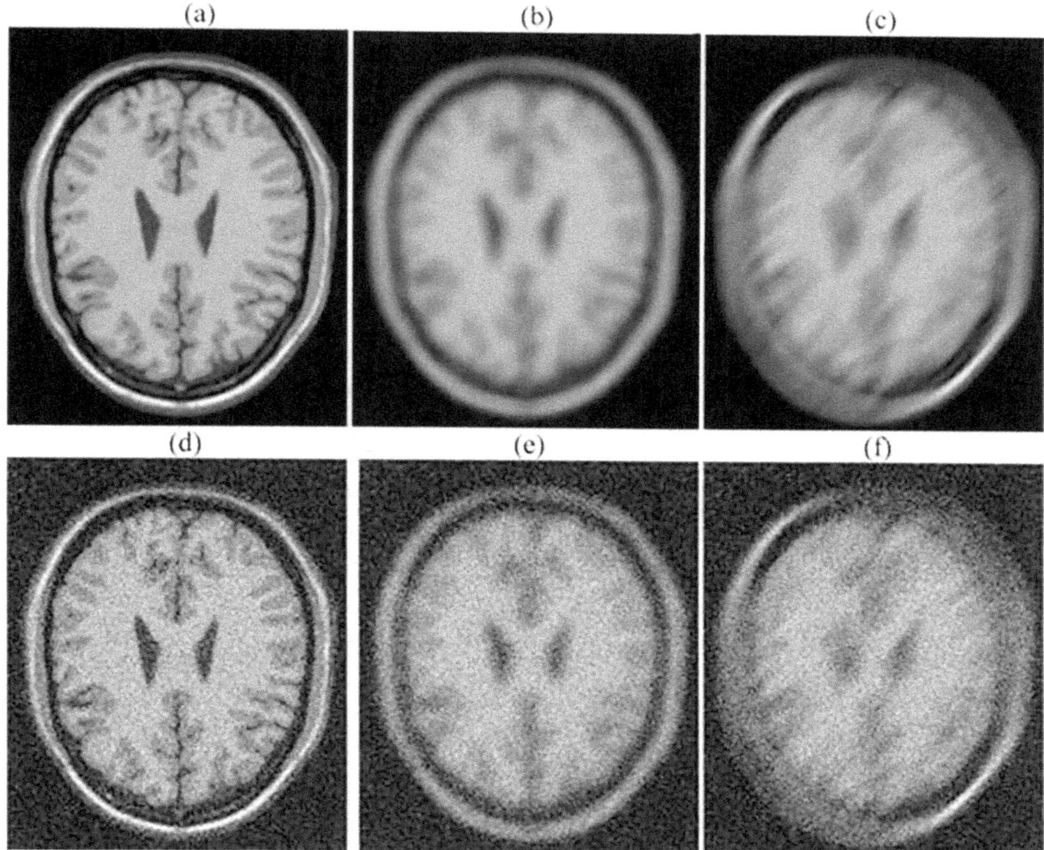

Figure 8.3 MRI brain image with blur and noise. (a) original image; (b) Gaussian blur; (c) Motion blur; (d) Rician noise only; (e) Guassian blur plus Rician noise; (f) Motion blur plus Rician noise [9].

Besides these methods, some modern techniques such as functional magnetic resonance imaging (fMRI) and magnetoencephalography (MEG) are being used to detect seizures and to determine the brain regions implicated in seizures. Figure 8.3 shows the seizure activity highlighted fMRI image [8].

It is important to work with a healthcare professional to understand the most accurate technique of detecting seizures based on the individual's specific symptoms and medical history.

8.2.4 Investigating the role of frontal and temporal lobes in epileptic seizures

Seizures can occur in different lobes of the brain, and functional magnetic resonance imaging (fMRI) can be used to determine the brain regions that are activated during a seizure. Here is a brief overview of how seizures can occur in different brain lobes:

- Frontal lobe seizures: Seizures that originate in the frontal lobe can cause symptoms such as abnormal movements, changes in behavior or mood, and difficulty speaking. During an fMRI scan, increased activity can be seen in the frontal lobe during a seizure.

- Temporal lobe seizures: Temporal lobe seizures are a type of seizure that starts in the temporal lobe of the brain and can cause symptoms such as acoustic delusions, sense of familiarity and recognition experiences as well as memory problems. During an fMRI scan, increased activity can be seen in the temporal lobe during a seizure.
- Parietal lobe seizures: Parietal lobe seizures can result in tingling feelings, numbness, and problems with spatial awareness, among other symptoms. The parietal lobe exhibits greater activity during a seizure on an fMRI scan.
- Occipital lobe seizures: Seizures that originate in the occipital lobe can cause symptoms such as visual disturbances, such as flashes of light or hallucinations. During an fMRI scan, increased activity can be seen in the occipital lobe during a seizure.

It is important to note that seizures can also involve multiple lobes of the brain, and the exact location of the seizure can vary from person to person.By identifying the precise regions of the brain impacted by a seizure, an fMRI scan can assist in directing the treatment and control of the condition.

8.2.5 Methodology of detecting seizures

Figure 8.4 explains the overall implementation steps for the seizure detection in fMRI images

Preprocessing is important in fMRI analysis as it remove noise from the data, standardizes the format for comparison across studies, and improves the signal-to-noise ratio. It corrects various types of artifacts and biases that can arise due to physiological processes, motion, and scanner artifacts. Overall, preprocessing is a crucial step that ensures the quality and reliability of fMRI data analysis.

PROJECT FLOW

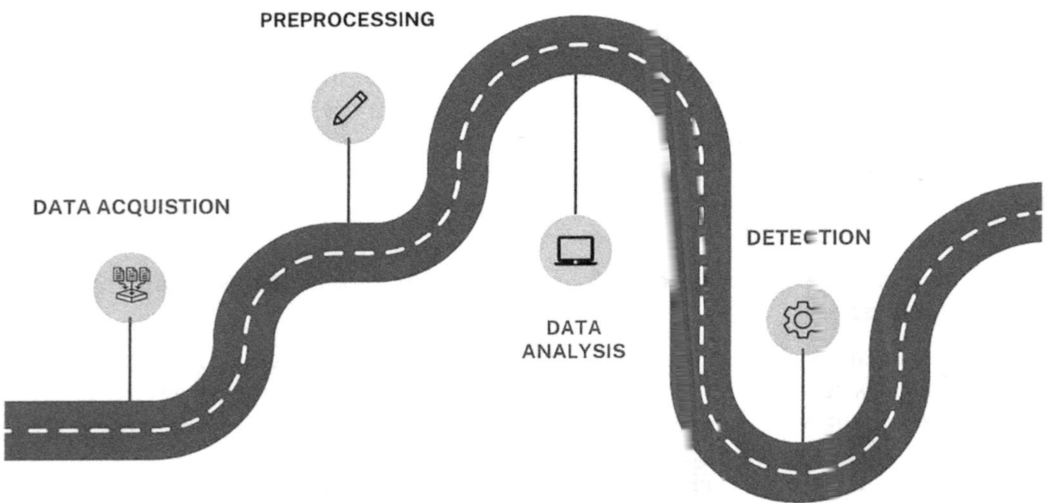

Figure 8.4 Flow of implementation steps.

8.2.5.1 Types of preprocessing techniques

Figure 8.5 showcases various steps used for the preprocessing of fMRI images.

- Slice Timing Correction:

During the fMRI scan, the MRI machine acquires images of the brain slice-by-slice. However, the slices are not acquired simultaneously, but rather sequentially over time. This can introduce a temporal offset between the slices, which needs to be corrected.

Slice time correction is comparable to album organization for photos. A moment in time is captured when we take a picture. Similar to this, multiple time slices are captured during a brain scan. However, there's a chance that these slices weren't photographed consecutively, much like photos in an album. We are able to arrange these slices in the right sequence with the aid of slice time correction, much like we would arrange the photos in our album. This makes it easier for us to understand what's going on in the brain at different times (Figure 8.6).

- Motion Correction:
  Participants may move during the fMRI scan, which can introduce unwanted variation in the data. To correct this, the images are aligned to a reference image (usually the first image in the sequence) to correct for head motion.

  Maintaining camera stability during photography is analogous to motion correction. You know how you have to keep the camera motionless while taking a picture in order

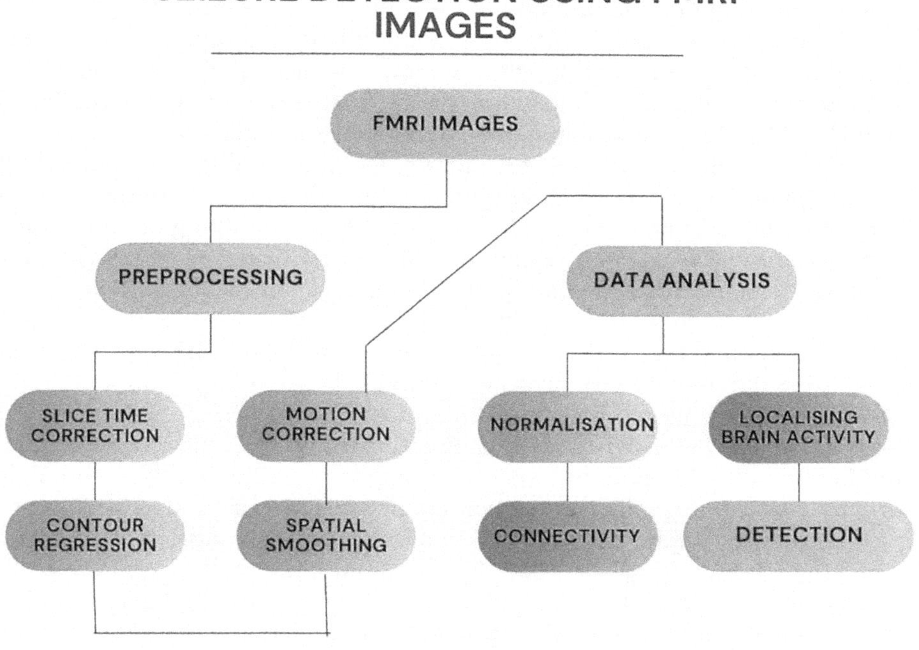

Figure 8.5 Flow of feature engineering.

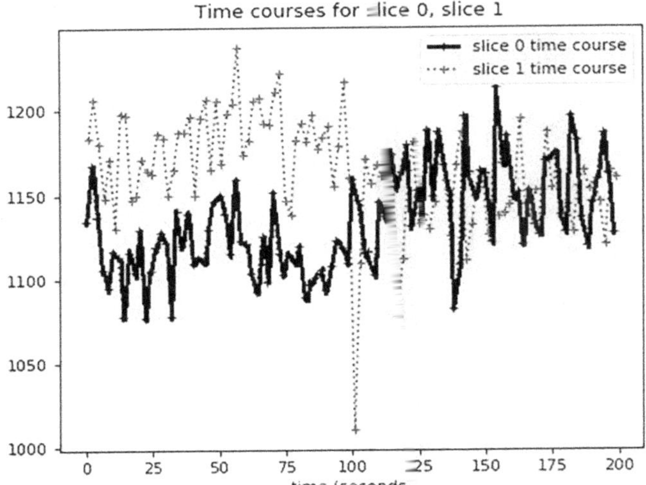

Figure 8.6 Time courses for Slice 0, Slice 1 – through preprocessing of FMRI images [5].

to prevent blurry images? This also holds true for employing fMRI technology to take images of your brain. People occasionally move slightly while within the machine, which might cause the images to appear fuzzy. Essentially, motion correction involves employing a specialized tool to ensure that the subject of the photograph remains motionless and very still during the whole process of taking it.

- *Skull Stripping:* The MRI image includes not only the brain, but also the skull and other tissues. To isolate the brain, a process called "skull stripping" is performed to remove the non-brain tissue.

  In fMRI, it means removing the skull from the brain image to make it clearer.
- *Spatial Smoothing:* The fMRI signal is noisy and spatially heterogeneous, so spatial smoothing is often applied to minimize the occurrence of noise and strengthen the SNR (Signal to Noise) Ratio, we aim to maximize the signal and reduce the noise as much as possible. This helps ensure that brain activity is depicted clearly in fMRI images.

  Spatial smoothing is like using a soft sponge to gently smooth out a rough surface. In fMRI, it means making the image less noisy by using a filter to average the signal across nearby pixels.
- *Normalization:* To compare fMRI data across participants or studies, it is often necessary to standardize the data to a customary space.

In fMRI, it means making sure that all the images are in the same format and can be compared across different people, scans, and studies.

- *High-pass Filtering:* fMRI data typically includes low-frequency noise (e.g., breathing and heart rate), which can be removed by applying a high-pass filter to the data.
- *Artifact Detection:* Finally, various sources of artifacts can be identified and removed, such as spikes in the data caused by head movement, scanner noise, or physiological noise.

Finding a hidden gem in a virtual world is how fMRI artifact detection works. When it comes to functional magnetic resonance imaging, it entails locating any abnormal features in the picture that may have happened accidentally, such a a person's head accidentally moving while being scanned. Figure 8.7 shows the noised and denoised image of the brain.

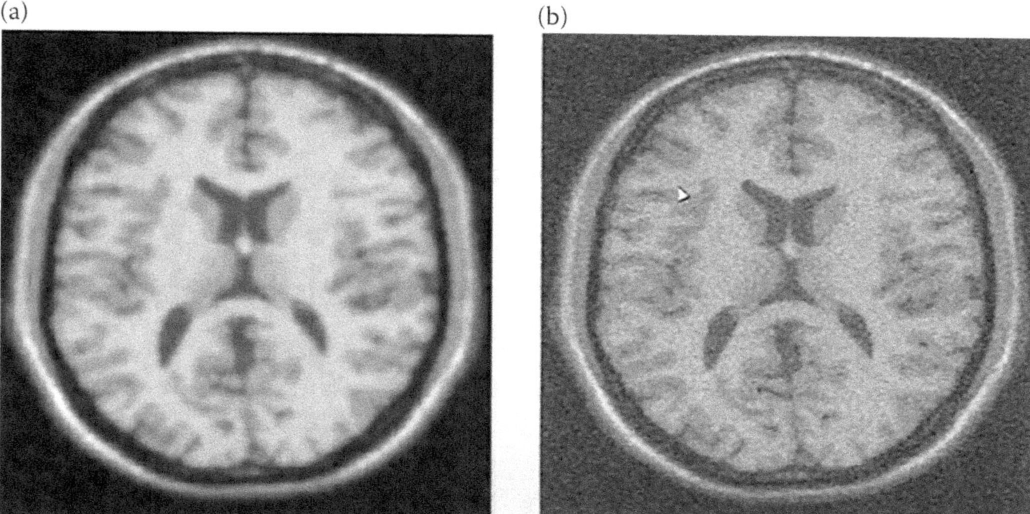

Figure 8.7 (a) De-noised, (b) Noisy image of brain.

8.3 DEEP LEARNING ALGORITHMS

8.3.1 Convolutional neural networks

Using fMRI images, CNNs (Convolutional Neural Networks) have proven to be quite successful at detecting seizures. In general, CNNs are hierarchical learning models that are used to solve problems pertaining to first identifying and subsequently categorization of the images based on their visual characteristics. They are made up of several convolutional layers that may categorize the input image into one of the available output classes by learning a hierarchy of features from raw image data, followed by fully connected layers.

In order to apply CNNs for fMRI seizure detection, the fMRI images can be preprocessed to extract relevant features.For fMRI data, common preprocessing methods include adjusting the motion artifacts that have been obtained. We also try to enhance the quality of the images by blurring them and also minimizing the unwanted signals that are present in the data. The fMRI data can be transformed into a 3D image stack after preprocessing, where each slice corresponds to a particular moment during the fMRI scan.

A series of fMRI pictures that have been classified as seizure or non-seizure images can subsequently be used to train the CNN model. The CNN gains the ability to identify pertinent elements from the input fMRI pictures that are most helpful for detecting seizures during training. Following that, new, unseen fMRI pictures are classified as seizure- or non-seizure-related using the learned features.

The ability of CNNs to understand intricate, nonlinear correlations between input characteristics and output classes is one of their advantages. Due to the fact that the patterns of cerebral processing linked to epilepsy can be extremely nonlinear and challenging to detect using conventional statistical methods, this is particularly helpful for detecting seizures using fMRI pictures.

Another benefit of CNNs is their capacity to extract spatially localized features from the input images, which can be used to pinpoint the locations in the brain that are responsible for such abnormal neurological activity. This may help determine the particular type of seizure or in directing surgical treatments for seizures.

Overall, CNNs have demonstrated considerable potential in detecting seizures using fMRI images, and they will surely refine our understanding of the diagnosis and management of epilepsy in the future.

8.4 PAPER SURVEY OF APPLICATIONS IN BRAIN DISORDER DETECTIONS USING FMRI IMAGES

8.4.1 Machine learning model to predict seizure susceptibility from resting-state fMRI connectivity [10]

In their study, [10] the objective was to create a machine learning model which was capable of forecasting the likelihood of seizures using Dynamic functional interactive data obtained from intrinsic task free fMRI) scans.

8.4.1.1 Methodology

The authors collected rs-fMRI data from 57 individuals with epilepsy and 38 healthy participants They used graph theory-based connectivity measures to construct functional connectivity networks for each participant. They then used a machine learning approach, specifically a support vector machine (SVM) classifier, to predict seizure susceptibility in the epilepsy group based on their rs-fMRI connectivity data.

The authors found that their SVM classifier achieved a high accuracy of 86% in predicting seizure susceptibility in the epilepsy group. They also found that the connectivity measures in the brain cortex were the most important features in predicting seizure susceptibility.

The authors used a support vector machine (SVM) classifier to predict seizure susceptibility in the epilepsy group based on their rs-fMRI connectivity data. They also used graph theory-based connectivity measures to construct functional connectivity networks for each participant [10].

Due to the inadequacy of data items in the dataset, the limitation of relevancy and generalizability was faced. The effects of medication on the rs-fMRI data, which may impact the accuracy of the classification, was not taken into consideration. Finally, the study did not validate their SVM classifier on an independent dataset, and future studies could explore the generalizability of their approach. Table 8.1 shows the comparison.

Table 8.1 Comparison of various algorithms for the seizure detection using fMRI

ML model	*Specificity*	*Accuracy*
SVM	0.723	67.5%
NEURAL NETWORK	0.715	69%
RANDOM FOREST	0.737	69%

8.4.2 An overview of deep learning techniques for epileptic seizures detection and prediction based on neuroimaging modalities: Methods, challenges, and future works

The paper outlines a comprehensive survey of deep learning methods that are utilized for the identification of abnormal spasms or attacks, using various neuroimaging techniques [11].

8.4.2.1 Review

The authors reviewed the literature to identify studies that employed advanced machine learning methods to identify and anticipate epileptic seizures through the use of Neuroimaging techniques. The studies were categorized according to the neuroimaging technique utilized, such as electroencephalography, which is based on recording the cerebral impulses by attaching electrodes to the scalp, magnetoencephalography which is developed for the detection of magnetic flux generated through the cerebral activity, and functional magnetic resonance imaging which quantifies the Oxygen carrying capacity of blood.

The authors found that deep learning techniques have demonstrated favorable outcomes in detecting and predicting epileptic seizures based on neuroimaging modalities. They also found that CNNs and RNNs are the most commonly used deep learning techniques for this purpose.

One limitation of this review is that other types of machine learning techniques and other modalities, such as EEG, were not included in this review. Additionally, the authors did not perform a meta-analysis or a systematic review, which could have provided a more rigorous evaluation of the studies. Finally, the authors did not discuss the limitations and challenges of the deep learning techniques reviewed, such as interpretability and generalizability.

8.4.3 Deep convolutional networks for automated detection of epileptogenic brain malformations

This review summarizes the current state-of-the-art in the use of deep convolutional networks for the automated detection of epileptogenic brain malformations [3]. We provide an overview of the methodology and algorithms used, the outcomes achieved, and the limitations of this approach.

Epileptogenic brain malformations are a common cause of epilepsy and can be difficult to detect using traditional methods. Automated detection using deep convolutional networks has the potential to maximize the speed and precision of the diagnosis. In this review[3], we aim to provide a comprehensive synopsis of the technological advancements in this area, including methodology, outcomes, and limitations.

The methodology used in each study was analyzed, including the types of networks used, the preprocessing steps, and the training and validation procedures [3].

The outcomes achieved by this project were evaluated which includes measures of accuracy, sensitivity, specificity, and other relevant metrics.

Various deep convolutional networks were used in the studies reviewed, including VGG, ResNet, and Inception. The networks were typically trained using large datasets of MRI scans with annotated labels indicating the presence or absence of epileptogenic brain malformations. Data augmentation was used in this project to increase the size of the training dataset which thereby helps in enhancing the working of the model when a new tuple/data is introduced to it.

Several limitations of the current approach were identified, including the lack of interpretability of the models, the need for large annotated datasets, and the potential for overfitting. Other limitations include the difficulty of detecting certain types of malformations, such as subtle cortical dysplasia, and the potential for misclassification due to imaging artifacts.

8.4.4 Deep-FMRI: End-to-end deep learning for functional connectivity and classification of ADHD using fMRI

The research paper [4] presents a deep learning method for analyzing the functional neural synchronization/connectivity and categorizing ADHD based on fMRI data.

The authors utilized a dataset consisting of 935 participants, including 315 ADHD and 620 typically developing controls, from the ADHD-200 competition. They applied preprocessing steps, including motion correction, spatial smoothing, and registration to the MNI space. They then used a deep learning approach that combines convolutional neural networks (CNNs) and feedforward neural networks (FNNs) to extract functional connectivity features from fMRI data and classify the participants as ADHD or controls.

The authors achieved exceptional outcomes in ADHD categorization using fMRI data, with an accuracy of 82.16%. They also found that the model captured brain regions and connections that are known to be associated with ADHD. They also utilized dropout regularization to prevent overfitting.

One limitation of this study is that it used a single dataset from the ADHD-200 competition, which could limit the relevancy aspect when compared with the rest of the population [4]. Additionally, the study did not compare the performance of the model with various machine learning or statistical models commonly used in fMRI analysis [4]. Finally, the study did not investigate the interpretability of the deep learning model, which is an important consideration in clinical settings [4].

8.4.5 The use of machine learning and deep learning algorithms in functional magnetic resonance imaging: A systematic review [6]

The authors [6] conducted an integrated and qualitative review published.in the past. They searched several databases and selected studies that used ML or DL algorithms to analyze fMRI data. Then based on the type of algorithm used, they categorized the observations, the type of fMRI data analyzed, and the clinical application of the study. They also assessed the quality of the studies using established criteria.

They found that the most commonly used algorithms were SVMs (support vector machines), neural networks, and decision trees. They also found that these algorithms have been used to analyze various types of fMRI data, including task-dependent fMRI, intrinsic based (without tasks) fMRI, and diffusion tensor imaging. Finally, they found that these algorithms have been applied in various clinical applications, including the identification and prediction of several neurological and psychosomatic/behavioral disorders.

The authors reviewed studies that used various algorithms, including support vector machines, neural networks, decision trees, random forests, and convolutional neural networks.

One limitation of this study is that it only reviewed studies published in the last decade, which may limit the scope of the review. Additionally, the authors only included studies that used machine learning or deep learning algorithms, and future studies could explore the use of other types of algorithms. Finally, the authors did not assess the quality of the fMRI data used in the reviewed studies, and the quality of the data may impact the accuracy of the results [6].

8.4.6 An empirical comparison of SPM preprocessing parameters to the analysis of fMRI data [5]

The authors [5], collected fMRI data from 10 healthy participants who underwent two identical motor tasks. They preprocessed the fMRI data using the Statistical Parametric Mapping (SPM) application and tested different combinations of preprocessing parameters, including realignment, normalization, smoothing, and high-pass filtering. To analyze the preprocessed data they used GLM (General Linear model) and compared the results using statistical tests.

Various pre-processing parameters were found to have a greater impact on the analysis of fMRI data. Specifically, they found that the combination of normalization and smoothing resulted in the highest statistical power for detecting task-related brain activity. They also found that high-pass filtering improved the detection of small activation clusters but could lead to false positives if the cutoff frequency was too low.

The authors used the SPM software to preprocess and analyze the fMRI data [5]. They used a GLM to model the relationship between the task-related stimuli and the brain activity and used statistical tests to assess the significance of the results.

One of the limitations of this study is the sample's small size that can limit the generalization of results. In addition, only a limited set of pre-processing parameters were tested, and future studies could explore the effects of other parameters, such as motion correction and outlier removal. Finally, the study only tested the effects of preprocessing parameters on a single type of motor task, and future studies could explore the generalizability of the results to other types of tasks and brain regions [5].

8.4.7 Classification of Alzheimer's disease using fMRI data and deep learning convolutional neural networks [8]

The authors [8] collected fMRI data from 160 participants, including 80 patients with AD and 80 healthy controls. A Convolutional Neural Network-based approach was used to derive characteristics from the fMRI dataset and classify participants as AD patients or healthy controls. They used various metrics, including accuracy, sensitivity, and specificity, to assess the model's functioning.

The authors found that the CNN-based approach achieved an accuracy of 95.6% in classifying AD patients and healthy controls. They also found that the medial temporal lobe, precuneus, and posterior cingulate cortex were the brain regions that were most important for the classification.

The authors used a CNN-based approach to extract features from the fMRI data and classify the participants as either AD patients or healthy controls [8]. The architecture of the CNN consisted of a duo of convolutional layers and a pair of fully connected layers.

They also used a technique called transfer learning, where the pre-tested and trained model was optimized to the specific task of AD classification.

One of the drawbacks of this study is that it only uses data from a single site, which may limit the generalizability of the research. Furthermore, the study only included a small number of participants, and future studies could explore the use of larger datasets. Finally, the study did not account for the effects of medication on the fMRI data, which may impact the accuracy of the classification [8].

8.4.8 Deep learning methods to process fMRI data and their application in the diagnosis of cognitive impairment: A brief overview and our opinion [12]

In order to diagnose cognitive impairment, functional magnetic resonance imaging (fMRI) data are processed using deep learning techniques. The authors [12], talk about the drawbacks of conventional techniques for analyzing fMRI data and how deep learning techniques can help to get around these drawbacks. Also, they offer a brief overview of prominent deep learning architectures (like CNNs and RNNs), and how these might be used in the processing of fMRI data.

The authors [12] then go into their own method for leveraging fMRI data and deep learning to identify cognitive impairment. They gathered fMRI data from Alzheimer's patients, people with mild cognitive impairment, and those who were healthy, and they utilized a CNN-based architecture to extract features from the data. They then divided the patients into three groups using a support vector machine (SVM).

The findings demonstrated that their system classified patients with cognitive impairment with high accuracy, highlighting the promise of deep learning techniques for data exploration on fMRI data in the diagnosis of Cognitive Impairment.

In summary, the research describes a potential strategy for the detection of cognitive impairment using fMRI data and gives a brief overview of analyzing fMRI data. The authors emphasize deep learning's potential in this area and propose that it might be applied to the creation of more precise and trustworthy diagnostic tools for cognitive impairment [12].

8.4.9 Overview of fMRI analysis

The Aim of fMRI (functional Magnetic Resonance Imaging) study [13] is to identify which parts of the brain are active (generating and sending electrical impulses for communication between the neurons) during a specific condition or while performing a specific task. The authors give a summary of the state of fMRI analysis at the moment and point out some issues that need to be resolved to increase the precision and dependability of fMRI results.

The fundamentals of fMRI analysis are covered in the paper [13], including how to evaluate changes taking place in neurological activities by measuring blood flow level by detecting changes in Intravascular Oxyhemoglobin concentration and how to identify brain regions that are noticeably active during a task using statistical approaches.

The authors of [13] discuss some of the difficulties that are now faced in fMRI analysis, including the necessity for reliable statistical techniques, precise spatial normalization of fMRI data, and the need to take into account physiological and motion distortions.

The paper also discusses some of the most recent developments in fMRI data analysis, including the use of multiple Machine Learning/ Deep Learning Algorithms to increase the precision and dependability of fMRI results and the use of multivariate analysis techniques to pinpoint brain activity patterns that are connected to particular cognitive processes.

The study ends by providing an overview of the current status of the fMRI analysis and a discussion of some of the issues that need to be resolved to increase the precision and dependability of fMRI results. According to the authors, more studies in this field may assist advance our comprehension of the brain and enhance our capacity to recognize and treat neurological and psychiatric problems.

8.4.10 Deep learning for brain disorder diagnosis based on fMRI images

A strategy based on deep learning is suggested by authors of [14], for the diagnosis of brain disorders using fMRI images. The study focuses on three important brain disorders that are challenging to diagnose with conventional imaging methods: Alzheimer's disease, schizophrenia, and depression.

The suggested method is using Convolutional Neural Networks (CNN), a deep learning model, to automatically extract characteristics from fMRI pictures and categorize them according to the type of brain illness. The study makes use of a collection of 388 fMRI pictures, comprising 100 images of healthy controls and 102 images of Alzheimer's disease, schizophrenia, and depression.

The findings show that the suggested method successfully diagnoses brain illnesses using fMRI images with good accuracy, sensitivity, specificity, and F1-score. The study (Wutao Yin et al., 2022) also shows how the proposed approach performs in comparison to other cutting-edge approaches, proving its superiority. According to Scientists,this method can be utilized as a powerful tool for the early diagnostics and treatment of brain disorders and illnesses, improving patient outcomes.

8.4.11 Post traumatic seizure classification with missing data using multimodal machine learning on dMRI, EEG, and fMRI

The study focused on three modalities of interest (fMRI, d-MRI, EEG) to classify late seizures into binary categories [15]. In terms of AUC, while the NB estimator performed better than the imputation-based individual modality-based learners, The experimental results showed that the IDSF algorithm outperformed the other methods in terms of performance. The multiple input modalities contained both shared and unique information, and the IDSF algorithm aimed to capture and utilize both types of information. fMRI alterations of the inferior temporal gyrus might be a perspective biomarker of LPTS, and finally, PTE.

There are certain drawbacks in this work and study. Since this study is still in progress, and the experiments are being carried out only on a limited number of subjects, for whom the necessary two-year follow-up data has been recorded.

EpiBioS4Rx has an expected enrolment of 300 subjects at completion. By increasing the sample size significantly, the proposed methods can be evaluated for their robustness, and it will also enable investigation of some of the contemporary techniques that can be applied [15].

8.4.12 Brain decoding using fMRI images for multiple subjects through deep learning

Neural mapping or decoding models like Convolutional Neural Networks and Variational Autoencoders are used for extracting vital attributes or features from brain images [16]. Other image classifiers fail in terms of performance while categorizing the image data being fed to the model. Detailed investigation allowed us to conclude that, once all the features and properties have been extracted, the model performs well in neural image classification. This indicates that comprehension of the various brain lobes and areas will be aided by the employed model.

The drawbacks we found are that, because CNN-based models are trained on GPUs, there is an additional requirement for more processing power and resources, which increases the cost and time involved. The decay of Gradient is also a matter of concern during optimization.

8.4.13 An IoT-based novel hybrid seizure detection approach for epileptic monitoring

The early detection of epileptic episodes using multichannel EEG data and IoT technology is a novel technique introduced in this paper [17]. The research goal is to create a seizure detection system that is precise.

The suggested system combines the convolutional neural network (CNN) method and Critical Spectral Verge (CSV) derived features from the Spike-Statistical (SS)-Flower Pollination Algorithm (FPA) for seizure detection. The study [17] achieves an average accuracy of 98.48% with the CNN classifier by using this method on the Temple University Hospital Electroencephalography Corpus (TUH EEG) dataset, which is a comprehensive open-source dataset for EEG signals.

The results show that the presented system performs better in terms of accuracy and specificity than other current strategies. When working with wearable medical technology, neuro experts find this strategy to be especially helpful.

Using multichannel EEG data and IoT technology, the research shows how well the SS-CSV-CNN method works for precisely detecting seizures. It offers valuable insights for the fields of neurology and wearable medical technology and offers a promising solution for the early detection of epileptic episodes.

8.4.14 Detecting COVID-19 from lung computed tomography images: A swarm optimized artificial neural network approach

In order to detect COVID-19 from lung CT images, a novel Swarm Optimized Artificial Neural Network (ABCNN-RP) is used for the first time in this study [18]. In comparison to current methods, the study's main goal is to achieve greater accuracy and less complexity.

This research study [18] uses the ABCNN-RP framework, which combines swarm intelligence and deep learning methods, to achieve this. The Internet of Medical Things (IoMT) is supported by cloud-based e-Healthcare application servers that are used to implement this framework. Large-scale COVID-19 dataset segmentation and classification are the main functions of the framework.

Findings show that the ABCNN-RP approach performs better in terms of accuracy than conventional Artificial Neural Networks (ANN) while maintaining a lower level of complexity. Additionally, the proposed framework exhibits promising results when compared to existing swarm intelligence approaches.

Overall, this study emphasizes the potential advantages of combining deep learning and swarm intelligence methods to identify COVID-19 in lung CT images. The study's findings show that the ABCNN-RP framework can produce precise and effective results, which makes it an important advancement in the field of medical imaging and the diagnosis of COVID-19.

8.5 DISCUSSION AND FURTHER DIRECTION

The aim of this research is to determine how well deep learning techniques can detect seizures on fMRI images. Millions of people suffer from seizures, a common neurological illness, and early detection can help spot underlying problems like epilepsy and possibly avert bodily injury. In order to understand how lesions contribute to the detection of seizures, the study will use tools to aid in the processing of fMRI data and retrieve information from the data.

The first step in the study involves preprocessing and manually analyzing the fMRI images to extract relevant features. This includes removing noise and artifacts(anomalies) from the images, segmenting the brain regions, and identifying abnormalities that could be related to seizures. This manual analysis will provide a baseline for comparison with the results obtained from deep learning techniques.

The next vital step involves application of various Deep learning algorithms, such as Convolutional Neural Networks (CNNs), Recurrent Neural Networks (RNNs), Autoencoders (AE), to the preprocessed fMRI images data.

Deep Learning models are built and the preprocessed data is fed to it to check and compare accuracies and efficiencies of different Models and not just accuracies but Loss and other factors are also considered. Then based on the results obtained, the Best Model is selected for Seizure Detection.

Complex patterns/trends in data and relationships among the attributes in the data can be learned by Deep Learning techniques and that is one of the advantages in using CNNs and RNNs which can be strenuous to identify manually. These techniques can also be trained on large datasets, allowing for better generalization and robustness in detecting seizures.

The study has several potential applications, including improving the accuracy and efficiency of seizure detection in clinical settings. This can help in identifying underlying issues such as epilepsy and potentially prevent harm to the body. Additionally, the study can aid in the evolution of new diagnosis tools and therapies or remedies for seizures and other neurological disorders.

However, there are also limitations to the study. One of the main challenges is obtaining a large, annotated dataset for training the deep learning models. Additionally, there may be variability in the fMRI images due to differences in imaging protocols and population of patients, which can affect the model's performance.

In conclusion, the study on seizure detection using fMRI images and deep learning techniques has the potential to improve the accuracy and efficiency of detecting the Seizures, aiding in the diagnosis and treatment of underlying neurological disorders. However, there are also challenges that must be overcome, including the need for large annotated datasets and addressing variability in imaging protocols and patient population.

8.6 LIMITATIONS OF FMRI

FMRI images aid in seizure detection by revealing abnormal brain activity and connectivity patterns, helping to identify and locate seizure foci. But the proposed research work has the following limitations:

- fMRI is a resource intensive technique that necessitates expertise and specialized equipment due to limited accessibility of its data. It becomes challenging to use it in medical facilities for monitoring seizure activity as a result.
- Deep Learning models depend a lot on annotated data for best performance.
- The analysis and interpretation of fMRI images for seizure detection frequently involve intensive computational resources and time requirements for performing inference due to the complex nature of fMRI data.
- Additionally, because fMRI measurements are indirect and depend on blood oxygenation levels, they might not be able to accurately detect the quick changes that take place during seizure activity. This could reduce the reliability of fMRI-based seizure detection.

8.7 CONCLUSION

fMRI is a promising technique for detecting seizures and studying their underlying mechanisms. The use of various fMRI approaches, such as BOLD signal changes, connectivity analysis, and graph theory, has enabled the identification of both focal and network-level changes associated with seizures. However, more research is required to establish the reliability and validity of fMRI as a clinical tool for detecting seizures. The development of standardized protocols and analysis methods, as well as larger and more diverse patient cohorts, will be crucial for advancing the field. fMRI analysis has the potential to enhance the modes of clinical practices. It could replace methods/procedures like intracranial EEG which are costly and also carry huge risks. It can also help in the development of personalized treatments by locating specific lobes in the brain where seizures are prevalent, thereby elevating the standards of patient care. We've applied CNN to retrieve features from the fMRI images dataset and have got the accuracy of 80%; we're still working on the model to increase its efficiency and also looking for various other models to get better results in the future.

REFERENCES

1. Garner, R., Ghariq, E., Vasavada, M. M., Singh, K. & Carney, P. R. (2021). Machine learning model to predict seizure susceptibility from resting-state fMRI connectivity. Frontiers in Neurology, 12, 715929.
2. Shoeibi, A., Khosravi, A., & Wang, X. (2021). An overview of deep learning techniques for epileptic seizures detection and prediction based on neuroimaging modalities: Methods, challenges, and future works. Frontiers in Neuroscience, 15, 650669. https://www.frontiersin.org/articles/10.3389/fnins.2021.650669/full
3. Gill, R. S., Hong, S. J., Fadaie, F., Caldairou, B., Bernhardt, B. C., Barba, C., ... & Bernasconi, A. (2021). Deep convolutional networks for automated detection of epileptogenic brain malformations: A review. Frontiers in Neurology, 12, 607136. https://www.frontiersin.org/articles/10.3389/fneur.2021.607186/full
4. Riaz, A., Asad, M., Alonso, E., & Slabaugh, G. (2021). DeepFMRI: End-to-end deep learning for functional connectivity and classification of ADHD using fMRI. Magnetic Resonance Imaging, 78, 56–66. https://www.sciencedirect.com/science/article/pii/S0730725X20304845
5. Della-Maggiore, V., Chau, W. K., Peres-Neto, P. R., & McIntosh, A. R. (2002). An empirical comparison of SPM preprocessing parameters to the analysis of fMRI data. Neuroimage, 17(1), 19–28. https://www.sciencedirect.com/science/article/pii/S1053811902912363
6. Rashid, M., Singh, H., & Goyal, V. (2021). The use of machine learning and deep learning algorithms in functional magnetic resonance imaging – A systematic review. Magnetic Resonance Imaging, 78, 101–116. https://www.sciencedirect.com/science/article/pii/S0730725X21001230
7. https://www.researchgate.net/figure/MRI-fMRI-and-SEEG-of-a-patient-with-epilepsy-originating-from-the-parietal-lobe-who-was_fig4_273782341
8. Sarraf, S., & Tofighi, G. (2016). Classification of Alzheimer's disease using fMRI data and deep learning convolutional neural networks. arXiv preprint arXiv:1603.08631. https://arxiv.org/abs/1603.08631
9. Chen, W., You, J., Pan, B., Liang, Z., & Chen, B. (2018). A sparse representation and dictionary learning based algorithm for image restoration in the presence of Rician noise. Neurocomputing, 286, 130–140. doi:10.1016/j.neucom.2018.01.066. https://www.researchgate.net/figure/MRI-brain-image-with-blur-and-noise-a-original-image-b-Gaussian-blur-c-Motion_fig2_322891462

10. Garner, R., La Rocca, M., Barisano, G., Toga, A. W., Duncan, D., & Vespa, P. (2019, April). A machine learning model to predict seizure susceptibility from resting-state fMRI connectivity. In 2019 Spring Simulation Conference (SpringSim) (pp. 1–11). IEEE.
11. Ibrahim, I., & Abdulazeez, A. (2021). The role of machine learning algorithms for diagnosing diseases. Journal of Applied Science and Technology Trends, 2(01), 10–19.
12. Wen. D., Wei, Z., Zhou, Y., Li, G., Zhang, X., & Han, W. (2018). Deep learning methods to process fmri data and their application in the diagnosis of cognitive impairment: A brief overview and our opinion. Frontiers in Neuroinformatics, 12, 23.
13. Heck, C. N., King Stephens, D., Massey, A. D., Nair, D. R., Jobst, B. C., Barkley, G. L. … … .. & Morrell, M. J. (2014). Two year seizure reduction in adults with medically intractable partial onset epilepsy treated with responsive neurostimulation: Final results of the RNS System Pivotal trial. Epilepsia, 55(3), 432–441.
14. Mao, Z., Su, Y., Xu, G., Wang, X., Huang, Y., Yue, W., & Xiong, N. (2019). Spatio-temporal deep learning method for ADHD FMRI classification. Information Sciences, 499, 1–11.
15. Christensen, D. V., Dittmann, R., Linares-Barranco, B., Sebastian, A., Le Gallo, M., Redaelli, A., … … & Pryds, N. (2022). 2022 roadmap on neuromorphic computing and engineering. Neuromorphic Computing and Engineering, 2(2), 022501.
16. Nazir, L., Haq, I. U., Khan, M. M., Qureshi. M. B., Ullah, H., & Butt, S. (2022). Efficient pre-processing and segmentation for lung cancer detection using fused CT images. Electronics, 11(1), 34.
17. Yedurkar, D. P., Metkar, S., Al-Turjman, F., Yardi, N., & Stephan, T. (2023). An IoT-based novel hybrid seizure detection approach for epileptic monitoring, IEEE Transactions on Industrial Informatics, 20(2), 1–13, 10.1109/tii.2023.3274913
18. Punitha, S., Stephan, T., Kannan, R., Mahmud, M., Kaiser, M. S., & Belhaouari, S. B. (2023). Detecting COVID-19 from lung computed tomography images: A swarm optimized artificial neural network approach. IEEE Access, 11, 12378–12393. 10.1109/ACCESS.2023.3236812

Part 3

Disease prediction and public health

Chapter 9

Improving prediction accuracy for neo-adjuvant chemotherapy response in breast cancer through 3D image segmentation and deep learning techniques

K V Ranjitha and T P Pushphavathi

Ramaiah University of Applied Sciences, Faculty of Engineering and Technology, Department of Computer Science and Engineering, Bangalore

9.1 INTRODUCTION

Image processing is a promising technology utilized in a variety of areas, such as medical and educational processes. Noise reduction in the image is a key focus for preserving image quality. Image quality reduces due to possession or diffusion of the image [1]. The image can be damaged by image noise. Noise degradation in the quality of an image, for which an image needs to be de-noise to restore its quality, refers only to the image's plane itself. In this type as well as a technique of Image processing is entirely based on pixel manipulation in images [2] and the frequency field analysis, which is quite time-consuming concerning the function or signals of mathematics.

"Image noise means an undesirable signal. It is an unwanted result of the image capture which enhances data from an extraneous, spurious. It is an unplanned change in color and image brightness and is usually an aspect of electronic noise."

Breast cancer is the most common tumor. In recent years, a vast amount of breast health inspections have been obtained that have required many medical imaging techniques, including tumor detection and segmentation to be developed [3]. These activities are intended to distinguish tumors from normal breast tissue, which may provide useful data analysis. Mammography and MRI are common approaches for detection as well as analysis of breast cancer. Early-stage diagnosis of breast cancer is more focused on mammography. The study of mammograms by the availability of a sufficiently broad data set has been successfully applied with deep learning techniques [4].

To determine improvements in the cancers' heterogeneity for the improved early forecast of the maximum "pathologic broad response (PCR)" and "recurrence-free survival (RFS)" following "neo-adjuvant chemotherapy (NAC)", "DCE-MR" images are analyzed of 132 females with nearby progressive breast cancer from experiments. To characterize heterogeneous changes inside tumor, image registration, tumor defects and changes in the DCE-MRI, kinetic features have been determined. The PCR and RFS respectively were carried out by 5-fold cross-validation, LR as well as Cox regression. Increased predictors like FTV and histopathology, as well as demographic factors, have tested the characterizations derived from images [5].

To look at the organ and structure confidentiality of the body, the Magnetic Resonance Imaging (MRI) practices an influential magnet and radio waves. Healthcare providers use MRI examination, from torn ligaments to cancers, to detect several diseases. The brain and spinal cord MRIs [6] are really important for research. Images from structural MRIs are used for the detection of diseases as they display a definite topological distribution of the brain. The reduction of grey matter and improvements in other time lobe systems is the main

DOI: 10.1201/9781003369059-12

reference point for the diagnosis of hippocampal atrophy. MRI has excellent spatial resolution and is exceptionally reliable in the classification of gray and white matter. Identity of anatomical alteration in the brain from RIMs requires the brain alignment to restrict itself to normal models, to distinguish gray and white tissue and brain fluid, and to detect atrophy regions based on the estimated volume of gray matter.

9.1.1 Image de-noising

Is used to eliminate noise from a damaged image to reestablish a true image. Although noise, edge, and shape are high-frequency machineries, the denotation of the images is difficult to discern and will eventually be missed by such information. Overall, it is an important challenge today to retrieve useful information in the process of noise reduction from noise images to achieve quality images. De-noising of photographs is a classic problem that has been studied for a long time. But it's still a challenging and unfinished task. The key explanation is that image de-noising is an inverse issue from a statistical point of view and is not a special solution. In the last few decades, great progress in image de-noising has been achieved [7].

Corrupted images are caused by several noises; some of them include [8] "Impulse Noise", "Photo electronic", "Gaussian", "Anisotropic noise", "Uniform or Quantization noise", and "Poisson noise".

Noise removal is a classic problem that is not yet fully resolved. This problem is thus constantly examined by researchers. Poisson noise depends on the signal, and additive noise removal approaches are not effective to remove this kind of noise.

In the medical field, digital modes, e.g., X-ray, Ultrasound, MRI, etc., are of great importance. These techniques do suffer from image noise that affects image quality considering their value. X-ray image formation is usually dependent on data on photon counters that obey Poisson's method and noise in X-ray images that are often distributed by Poisson [9]. This noise is therefore called Poisson noise and is recognized as shot noise. But proper diagnosis needs to eliminate the noise from medical x-ray images. This Poisson noise is known as signal-dependent noise, which varies concerning signal in magnitude. Even then, in low power regions of an image, this noise affects more because the signal power at low-intensity levels is smaller than the noise level. While noise is more powerful, it is also more signal power at high-intensity levels. So, the relatively low-level noise loss is less than the low intensity.

9.1.2 Feature extraction

Is the most important phase of image classification. It helps to remove the ideal feature of an image. Feature extraction methods or techniques are used for the classification and recognition of images. The image classification is used to differentiate between the local characteristics of the image. These characteristics are analyzed with different core components of the imaging data such as color intensity, image edges, texture, etc. [10]. The reliability of the functional extraction approach significantly increases an image's further processing. These functionalities may be used for the detection and retrieval of images. The function extraction technique is used to derive characteristics from a vast number of image data while preserving as much information as possible. Efficiency and effectiveness in the selection and extraction of functions are today a big problem. Color, texture, and type can all be eliminated as vector features using various techniques. The feature extraction techniques are classified in Figure 9.1.

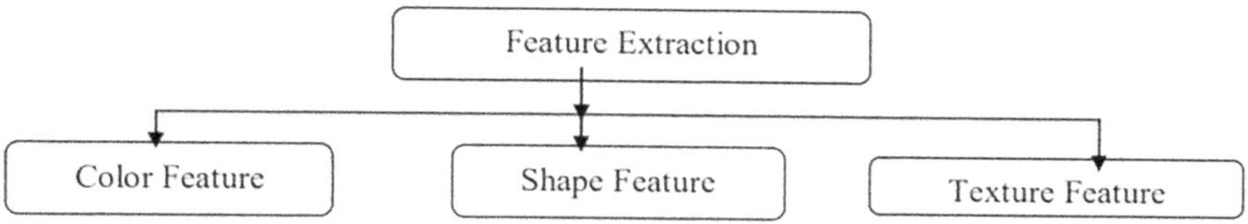

Figure 9.1 Classification of FE method.

9.1.3 Cancer

Is an ailment which is characterized by the progress of uncontrollable cell division, which can invade and destroy normal body cells. Safe cells in the bodies divide and swap in measured fashion throughout life. Cancer [11] starts when a cell is different to increase out of control. About 100 categories of cancer include breast, skin, lung, colon cancer, prostate, and lymphoma. More than 100 different forms of cancer exist. Symptoms vary depending on the type.

One of the leading causes of death in recent years is breast cancer [12]. Most studies have been conducted with different image analysis as well as classification techniques for diagnosis and detection of breast cancer. The disease remains nonetheless deadliest. Prevention becomes impossible because the cause of breast cancer remains obscure. Early breast cancer detection is the only way that breast cancer can be cured. At the beginning of the illness, primary prevention becomes multifaceted when causes are virtually unidentified. It is possible to incorporate such typical signatures as masses and microcalcifications on mammograms in the creation of early diagnostic methods, which are essential for improving people's quality of life. The most important tool for screening and early detection, which are crucial to improving the prognosis of breast cancer, is X-ray mammography. As usually low contrast masses and benign glandular tissue appear as well as very repetitive, many computers aided diagnostic systems have been built to support radiologists and internists in diagnosing them [13]. The most precise and fastest method to find breast cancer is by using CAD on a mammogram. Exact discovery will effectually decrease the death rate of mamma cancer. Early symptoms of prospective breast cancer are masses and micro calcification clusters. Users can help predict breast cancer in one's early life.

MRI is a gold standard imaging tool for assessing the "Neo-adjuvant chemotherapy (NAC)" response in breast cancer as it benefits both; morphology analysis as well as the provision of functional information obtainable by injection. These characteristics were known to be unique to MRI before the recent advent of contrast-enhanced mammography as an auspicious form of breast imaging [14].

An important measure for evaluating treatment response and the likelihood of overall survival for women with locally advanced breast cancer may be longitudinal patterns of tumor response during NAC. The dynamic contrast-enhanced MRI (DCE-MRI) is a component of the NAC protocol because it provides the opportunity to test variations in improvement models representing functional tumor characteristics as potential early indicators of patient response in addition to evaluating structural improvements in tumor size and form. [15–17]. To end this although much improvement has been created, the majority of methods noticed till date remain significant, either by dependent on aggregate tumor composition and structural steps or by overlooking specifics of the longitudinal phenotype of the image [18].

This paper's main contribution is split into two phases; Image segmentation is done on the MRI images collected from the ISPY TRIAL Breast MRI database. Segmentation phase takes place which is the detection of "Region of Interest (ROI Extraction)." The novelty of the work is based on the CNN method and U-NET model for image segmentation. Classification is done for the extracted features to make a diagnosis. Different feature extractions methods are explained. The Research study also explains the Segmentation model and Classification of breast images using Convolution Neural Network.

The review paper organization is done as follows. Literature Review is explained in Section 9.2. Section 9.3 provides more information on the methodology utilized for image segmentation and classification for mammography tumor identification and diagnosis. Convolution Neural Network Classification is described in Section 9.4 along with an introduction to the dataset and discussion of it. The Challenges are explained in Section 9.5. The conclusion is in Section 9.6.

9.2 LITERATURE REVIEW

Saeed Kermani et al. proposed the Gaussian mixture model (GMM) for color segmentation. Gaussian components in this system are ideal in the RGB color space for pixel values. The common iterative EM algorithm is used to estimate model parameters. Clusters are well-organized after segmentation to increase their average temperature. Two validity indices, Calinski–Harabasz and Davies–Bouldin, will be utilized to determine the ideal no. of clusters. Outcomes indicated an increase for a low number of clusters for the Davies–Bouldin index. Often this will lead to an improper pixel classifying, such that the index of Calinski–Harabasz is preferred. The proposed approach has high efficiency in separating temperature regions that can be used in screening applications as their outcomes and in the individual estimation of expert radiologists [19].

Jordina Torrents-Barrena et al. For the first time, state-of-the-art fetal brain, lungs, liver, spine, placenta and entire fetus segmentation, and classification approaches of MRI and (2D/3D) ultrasound are studied. A total of 123 works were examined and deliberated. Potential uses in clinical settings of the surveyed approaches are explored. Computer fetal surgical study fields are highlighted which are feasible and not previously discussed [20].

Yan Fang et al. proposed an innovative approach to the medical application depended on CNN approaches and image quality assessment (IQA) algorithms, which is a classification of breast cancer. First, they utilized CNN architecture to determine the pixel count in the lesions with the highest pooling layer. Broad pixel density and large-quality ranges are then allocated, indicating more texture as well as grayscale characteristics. Finally, using the obtained quality scores, they created a multi-SVM-based image kernel to classify breast cancer. Their suggested approach exceeds one image classification method based on identification, like pixel grayscale and gradient [21].

Gabriele Piantadosi et al. This work accurately separates breast parenchyma from the air as well as other tissues, like the chest wall, using a series of deep CNN's using 3D MR data. The novelty is the multiplanar mixture of U-Net CNN's utilizing an effective project fusing approach, in addition to implementing cutting-edge radionics techniques, allowing multi-protocol implementations. For 109 DCE-MRI instructions with histopathological defined lesions with 2 diverse acquisition protocols, the proposed approach is validated in two different sets of data. On both datasets, the median dice-like index is 96.60% (±0.30%) and 95.78% (±0.51%), correspondingly, $p < 0.05$ and 100% neoplastic lesion coverage [22].

Roberto Lo Gullo et al. The visual analysis of the multiparametric MRI tumor of a patient is inadequate to predict the NAC response of this patient. ML and DL methods via a mixture of qualitative and quantitative MRI structures have been lately useful to predict response to treatment early in or after the start of NAC. This is a new area, but published data shows promising results so far. They describe ML and DL models built up to now and deliberate some of the clinical application challenges [23].

N. Shobha Rani et al. This study evaluated segmentation techniques for tumor or glioma identification on T2 weighted 3D MRI images using BraTs 2018 data sets. The methods used to compare this efficiency with the proposed approach include Pixel Wise Linear Binary Pattern (LBP), geographic development and Otsu thresholds. This work initially slices 3D MRI images which are normalized from left and right sides to about 10%, as these slices have no significant information (empty slices). Also, the improvement of tumor/glioma regions on regular slices is carried out by high-improvement processing of the convolution kernel in many trials through different kernel sizes with a high boost kernel convolution. Glioma regions which are improved by the use of the kernel receive local adaptive glioma-extraction techniques. The gliomas detected are compared to the effects of segmentation of the ground truth to create efficiency of the technique planned. Glioma is correctly identified in 80% of slices, including in cases of low-grade and high-grade glioma (HGG). Via evaluating findings, it has been noted that the suggested approach surpassed the 87.20% and 89.18% average Jaccard & Dice similarity for HGG, and 83.77% and 87.74% for LGG are found [24].

K. Padmapriya et al. BTC's neural network structures were explored in depth by carrying out experiments that leveraged transfer learning but without record extensions. In this analysis, they give a thorough analysis of the surveys and new BTC techniques in deep learning. Furthermore, this analysis explores the required basic data sets used in the entire BTC evaluation. In addition to reviewing the previous literature concerns, this review also lists several tracks for analysis, which may be occupied in the next item, especially for the customization of intelligent health care, in this area [25].

M.Z. Liu et al. Via I-SPY TRIAL MRI Breast dataset, CNN was applied to predict neoadjuvant chemotherapy response. The I-SPY TRIAL breast MRI database was transmitted to 131 patients in 9 hospitals for study. For 3D segmentation with a 3D slicer, first, postcontrast MRI images were used. CNN is loaded with 3/3 kernels & linear layers. There were 6 residual layers in the convolutional kernels, a total of 12 convolutional layers. A 0.5 probability drop-out and normalization of L2 are used. The Adam Optimizer was applied for training. For performance assessment, 5-fold cross-validation was applied. The diagnostic precision was 72.5% (SD±8.4) and 65.5% (SD±28.1) sensitivity, as well as 78.9% (SD±15.2) specificity, of the two categories of their CNN [26].

Jyoti Parashar et al. Utilized a Deep learning experience in the identification and preliminary research on breast cancer. Mammography images were used from DDSm and Mias in the procedure proposed. CNN hybridization is proposed by improving cumulative, class-oriented, and optimization of tree-based learning [27].

Yi-Cheng Zhu et al. Suggested the generic DCNN model for learning algorithms for thyroid, including breast cancer models with the same architectural parameters (TNet as well as BNet) as well as test the feasibility of such a generalized approach in clinical ultrasound scans. The capacity of the thyroid model is also discussed in terms of learning common features and how it classifies breast and thyroid lesions. The following research uses a historical dataset from October 2016 to December 2018 of 719 thyroid and 672 breast images taken from various machines. Test findings indicate that TNet and BNet are both based on the similar DCNN architecture with decent outcomes for classification (TNet's average accuracy was 86.5% while BNet's was 89%.) [28].

Tomoyuki Fujioka et al. Breast MRI image classification with many recent CNNs has been carried out. The CNNs have demonstrated identical diagnoses for the classification of breast MRI by human readers. The highest CNN was 96.0% specificities and 0.895 AUC for MRI breast classifying [29].

Marco Caballo et al. The feasibility of proposed theories for the segmentation of breast masses is examined from the standpoint of radiomic research. A DL network has been developed and verified for breast mass segmentation in breast CT imaging. In between annotations of several radiologists and the DL network, radiomic stability was examined. The majority of radiomic characteristics have been established as stable in many mass segmentations. Deep segmentation of breast lesions dependent on learning can replace manual annotation in radiomic studies [30].

Suvidha Tripathi et al. Using BiLSTMs to classification tumors required background data between patches in the same area. The method is sturdy as per the tumor area. This work suggested an endwise network to image classification. A shallow network without heavy training discovered patch scanning approach for the image extract patches. The best accuracy of 84% was achieved. They found that BiLSTMs had much better results in model patches in a network for the end-to-end image classification [31].

Vivek Kumar Singh et al. Presented an enhanced automatic segmentation of tumors based on a discussion from the proposed system and it mainly focuses on the adversarial learning system. First, atrous convolution (AC) is introduced to capture the context of position as well as scale (i.e., tumor position as well as tumor size) to handle diverse sizes and shapes. Second, channel attention and channel weighting mechanisms are proposed to facilitate tumor-relevant functions (without extra monitoring) and to minimize artifacts' impacts. Third, they recommend incorporating the L1-norm and the Structural Similarity Index Metric into an adversarial learning framework to gain knowledge about the local context in the vicinity of tumors. The effectiveness of the suggested model was tested using two BUS image datasets. The test results show that in competition with modern segmentation models about dice and IoU metrics, the proposed model shows competitive results [32].

M. Malathi et al. Explored the CAD breast system for adaptive fusion by way of deep features of the CNN. The investigation shows that the random forest algorithm has the highest accuracy (97.51%) and the lowest error rate of the CNN classifier (95.65%). DBN can detect breast image abnormalities. The work provides active segmentation of contours to distinguish the abnormal image which can be identified by the DBN. The algorithm used in process of low-dose MRI-CT is used to remove the properties of the point spreading feature and restoration. By sparse transformation, the performance and speed of the segmentation are improved [33].

Ghulam Murtaza et al. A multiclassification tree-based DL model for breast cancers. Model for the diagnosis of a 4-subtype breast tumor is used in the diagnosis. The model is computer-friendly and was developed on a typical desktop. The model produced better outcomes when compared to cutting-edge existing models [34].

Dhanalekshmi Prasas, Shilpa P.Metkar, Fadi, Thompson Stephan, Manjur Kolhar, and Chadi Altrjman et al. A novel approach is proposed for multichannel epilepsy seizure for Internet of Things (IoT) based framework. Wireless technology is utilized to note the EEG signal of the epileptic patients. SVM based classifier is used for classification of seizure and non-seizure patients using as the feature. The proposed approach showed a better performance with 98.83% sensitivity and 95.89% average detection rate. The model proposed better helps diagnose the epileptic behavior for various EEG signals which is useful for the neuro-experts to analyze different results from the regions of the brain [35].

Divya Biligere Shivanna, Thompson Stephan, Fad Al-Turjman, Manjur Kolhar and Sinem Alturjman et al. A Multistage Classification Scheme is proposed to resolve complex medical diagnosis for neural network-based systems. This method helps identify antibodies in the blood serum and it better classifies Hep-2 cells using ANN and SVM based models. The proposed model showed an accuracy of 84.9% for intermediate cells and 95.8% for positive cells considering the SVM based model. For ANN based model gave an accuracy of 88.4% for intermediate and 97.1% for positive cells. The proposed models better improved the efficiency, turned down the medical expenses and was easily accessible for any healthcare facilities thereby useful in risk management and in developing new products [36].

9.2.1 Discussion of literature-related findings

From Table 9.1. it has been determined that "CNN (Deep Learning Technique)" produces better outcomes for image segmentation and breast tumor classification. To improve EDA performance, a variety of filtering techniques are used to reduce noise and segment the images. The research work is carried out by making enhancements and by utilizing various filtering mechanisms like Weiner and median filters to remove noise in the images. Data Segmentation is done by identifying the "Region-of-Interest (ROI)" in the breast tumor image. Classification of the extracted features to make the diagnosis is carried out by using a novel CNN model and also some enhancements are made in the CNN model to achieve better performance. Data Augmentations, regularizations are carried out to yield better efficiency and accurate performance.

9.3 BREAST CANCER DIAGNOSIS METHODS BASED ON DEEP LEARNING

9.3.1 U-NET model

Image Segmentation (IS) popularly known as Semantic Segmentation was studied and applied from 1980s. The main task of Image Segmentation is, given a RGB or grey scale image each of the logical segments in the image are colored with a unique color. IS can vastly and brilliantly be used in Medical Imaging like brain MRI's, other types of cancer diagnosis etc., IS also classifies each pixel in an image into one of the 2 or more classes. Pixel level Segmentation is a type of IS where a class label is created for every pixel.

The model or architecture of a U-NET [42] mainly comprises of five operators.

The U-NET architecture is shown in Figure 9.2. An Input-Image of size 572 × 572 × 1 is considered, since it is a grey scale image the depth is 1. Next, a conv 3 × 3 is performed with no padding and using ReLU activation an image size of 570 × 570 is got with 64 such kernels. Again, conv 3 × 3 is performed with ReLU, no padding and 568 × 568 × 64 tensor is seen as the output.

Next, max pool 2 × 2 is performed with stride 2; now the size of the image becomes half since pooling with a stride size of 2 is done on the images and thus, a 284 × 284 image is seen in the output. The steps are repeated by performing two more convolutions. Again, a max pool 2 × 2 with stride 2 is presented; size of the image becomes half so we get 140 × 140 image. Since the number of convolutions increase, the depth of the image is doubled. The same down sampling is repeated again.

Next, up-conv is performed on the image size of 28 × 28 × 1024 and copy and crop from a 64 × 64 × 512 image is done. Now an image size of 56 × 56 × [512 + 152] is seen, where the first 512 is from up-conv and the other 512 from copy and crop. In up-conv or up-sampling the size of rows and columns is duplicated to increase the size of image. With copy and crop, from an image size of 64 × 64, a 56 × 56 is considered by cropping and then the same is copied and given as an input to the next layer. By performing these operations, the

Table 9.1 Existing related work

Author and Ref.	*Methods Used*	*Research Findings*	*Limitations of the study*	*Dataset*
"Yan Fang, Jing Zhao, Lingzhi Hu, Xiaoping Ying, Yanfang Pan, Xiaoping Wang" [21].	In order to categorize breast cancer, CNN-based methods and "Image Quality Assessment (IQA)" algorithms are employed. The pixels in the lesions are counted using CNN architecture.	The best number is 0.82 when it comes to the accuracy of early breast cancer diagnosis. The effects on early breast cancer diagnosis are indicated by the AUC of stacking self-coding, which yields a value of 0.85.	The AUC values may vary due to varied modal data, and the quality of the data may have an impact on how breast cancer is differentiated.	"Mammogram images".
"Roberto Lo Gullo, Sarah Eskreis-Winkler, Elizabeth A. Morris, Katja Pinker" [23].	To predict response to early treatment during or after the beginning of NAC, machine learning and deep learning techniques like Linear SVM, Logistic Regression, and Linear Classifiers are utilized. Many of the problems with clinical application are also resolved by these models.	The NAC prediction accuracy for the CNN algorithms used was 88%. Early response treatment and prognostication were made possible by the machine learning classifiers, such as linear SVM and logistic regression, which displayed an AUC value of 0.86.	The reliability and reproducibility should be enhanced by the quantitative MRI techniques. Large datasets must be trained on deep learning models in order to prevent overfitting. To ensure the diagnostic accuracy of the created machine learning models, more standardized validation techniques are needed.	"Mammogram MRI Images".
"Yi-Cheng Zhu, Alaa AlZoubbi, Sabah Jassim, Quan Jiang, Yuan Zhang, Yong-Bing Wang, Yian Du Ye, Hongbo DU" [28].	To train the models for both thyroid and breast cancer, a general DCNN architecture with transfer learning is suggested. 672 breast scans and 719 thyroid images total are gathered from US machines.	With an accuracy rate of 86.5% for the thyroid network and 89% for the breast network, the test results showed good classification findings. The "TNet" model's performance was improved by using it to classify breast lesions, which yielded a sensitivity and specificity of 86.6% and 87.1%, respectively.	The data sample needed to be increased because the augmentation methods' data samples were insufficient to train CNN models. The radiologists' incorrect classification of the US images for malignant thyroid and breast tumors could lead to incorrect outcomes.	719 thyroid and 672 breast images collected from various US equipment.
"Tomoyuki Fujioka, Yuka Kikuchi, Jun Oyama, Mio Mori, Kazunori Kubota, Leona Katsuta, Koichiro Kimura, Emi Yamaga, Goshi Oda, Tsuyoshi Nakagawa, Yoshio Kitazume" [29].	106 normal and malignant breast MRI scans were obtained for training and testing purposes. The CNN models were used to determine the likelihood of cancer.	The best mean AUC was 0.840, according to CNN models. InceptionResNetV2 was discovered to be the ideal model. This model had an AUC of 0.895, a sensitivity of 78.7%, and a specificity.	The cut-off values in CNN models can occasionally differ between human readers and CNN, changing the model's sensitivity and specificity. Additionally, the CNN models frequently misread the MRI findings and the pathological characteristics of masses, producing erroneous results.	106 normal and malignant breast MRI pictures were taken into consideration.

"Marco Caballo, Domenico R. Pangallo, Ritse M.Mann, Ioannis Sechopoulos" [30].	A deep learning network was created to segment 2D breasts. Using "Intra-class correlation (ICC)" and "multivariate analysis of variance (MANOVA)" approaches, the feature stability and diagnostic performance between malignant and benign lesions were distinguished.	With an ICC rate > 0.75, the DL-based approaches produced a compliance rate of 0.085 0.66 and discovered that over 90% of all radiomic characteristics were stable. As a result, the segmentation of breast CT images using DL techniques was successful or shown high segmentation performance.	Due to capacity-based problems caused by the DL models' complexity, it is challenging to locate designated datasets. The problem with mass classification algorithms is their look and shape while taking into account different model parameters and non-optimal features.	Patient ages ranged from 50 to 86 years old, and 69 mammography breast images totaling 93 mass-like lesions were gathered.
'Igbe Tobore, Jingzhen Li, Liu Yuhang and Zedong Nie" [37].	Cancer cells are identified using segmentation and bulk detection using convolution neural networks. The model's effectiveness in using the training samples is assessed using XGBOOST.	The best mean AUC was 0.840, according to CNN models. InceptionResNetV2 was discovered to be the ideal model. This model had an AUC of 0.895, a sensitivity of 78.7%, and a specificity.	Due to capacity-based problems caused by the DL models' complexity, it is challenging to locate designated datasets. The problem with mass classification algorithms is their look and shape while taking into account different model parameters and non-optimal features.	The "Digital Mammography Data Base (DDSm)" and "DDSM-Mias" images were used to create the dataset.
"Mohd Usama, Belal Ahmad, Jiafu Wan, M. Shamim Hossain, Mohammed F.Alhamid and M.Anwar Hossain" [38].	CNN's 8-Layer network is intended as its foundation. Batch normalization, dropout, and a deep neural network called the "BD-CNN" are all utilized to enhance prediction. The underlying CNN Network is changed to Rank-based stochastic pooling approach. It was suggested that GCN could categorize the data and detect and predict cancer.	For the "base-CNN", "BD-CNN", and "BDR-CNN" networks, the findings are noted. When GCN is added, performance rate improves. As a result, the GCN-based classifiers produce reliable findings. Additionally, with n*=5, the performance is increased, demonstrating that the "BDR-CNN-GCN" network produces the best outcomes.	Despite the great accuracy that the "BDR-CNN-GCN" network achieves, it is unable to comprehend heterogeneous data, such as patient history and heart rate. The network produces workable results when using small datasets, but more optimization is needed to enhance detection while using larger datasets.	Breast mini-MIAS dataset (containing 322 mammographic images).
"Mohammad Jamshidi, Ali Lalbakhsh, Jakub Talla, Wahab Mohyuddin" [39].	Early detection of breast cancer involves the use of machine learning models like SVM, KNN, Random Forest, Naive Bayes, and Logistic Regression. In order to address CAD-related problems, DCNN is employed in the analysis for categorizing breast abnormalities.	The ANN offers high resolution multi-image modalities for breast cancer classification and prediction. The best breast cancer classification network was created using ML models, yielding accuracy of 97.74%. For various article datasets, the deep learning model delivers the best accuracy between 100% and 74.92%.	The Edge Detection approach, which is used to identify breast cancer, is not effective with contrast images, indistinct edges, or edges with many edges. The histogram threshold method exhibits inefficient working with the color spectrum and performs badly with discernible peaks. Due to its memory usage and processing time, the region-based deep learning method is also quite expensive.	Datasets from the "DDSM (Digital Database for Screening Mammography)", "WBC (Breast Cancer Wisconsin)", and "MIAS (Mammographic Image Analysis Society)" organizations.

(Continued)

Table 9.1 (Continued) Existing related work

Author and Ref.	*Methods Used*	*Research Findings*	*Limitations of the study*	*Dataset*
"Yifan Xianga, Lanqin Zhaoa, Zhenzhen Liua, Xiaohang Wua, Jingjing Chena, Erping Longa, Duoru Lina, Yi Zhuab, Chuan Chenab, Zhuoling Lina, Haotian Lina" [40].	Analyzing mammograms makes use of deep learning algorithms. Classification also uses the Adaptive De-Convolution Network with Max Pooling. The performance of breast mammography analysis is enhanced by the combination of these CNN and customized characteristics.	Performance is improved by combining CNN functionality with custom features. Additionally, System Architecture Evolution performs best when classifying features. Better performance is attained by faster RCNNs by excelling at feature extraction and classification.	Even while deep learning techniques work well, they require a lot of computations, therefore only a small number of systems might perform poorly with fewer computations. Additionally, mammography analysis is not yet done using YOLO methods, which reduces the effectiveness of finding breast cancer.	"MIAS Mini Mammographic Database (mini-MIAS)", "Digital Database for Screening Mammography (DDSM)", "Mammographic Image Database for Automated Analysis (MIDAS)" and "Breast Cancer Digital Repository (BCDR)" datasets are used.
"Behzad Soleimani Neysiani, Nasim Soltani, Reza Mofidi, Mohammad Hossein Nadimi-Shahraki" [41].	In feature extraction, Naive Bayes is employed. As part of the classification process to determine the type of mass from extracted features, decision tree classifier, K-NN, SVM, and linear regression algorithms are implemented.	Deep learning is a method. The area under curve (ROC) score for ResNEt-50 is 0.96, indicating improved cancer detection performance. The average ROC curve performance, taking into account various CAD techniques, is calculated to be 0.[illegible].	The GARM algorithm does not increase the accuracy of similar item identification recommendations. Due to the algorithm's slow processing speed and lengthy verification process, an indexing mechanism could be utilized to improve the algorithm's efficiency.	"Mammogram Images".

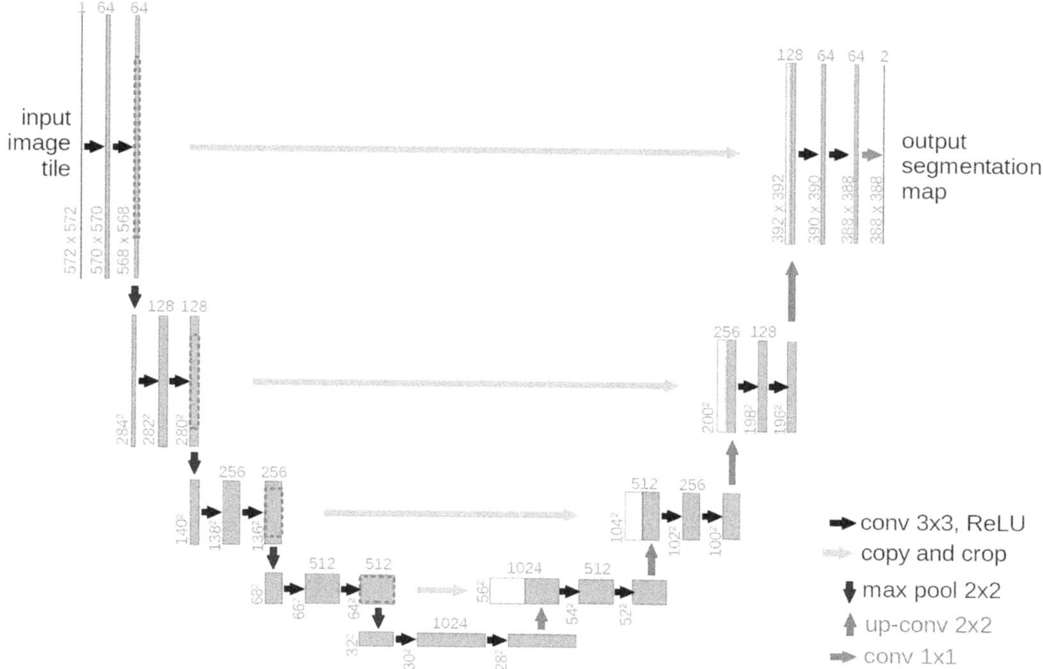

Figure 9.2 U-NET architecture.

information is taken from the previous layers which is sort of like skip connections. In this U-NET model loss can be computed using cross entropy [43]. Data Augmentation also is recommended for the U-NET model where instead of just using the raw image itself, shift, rotate, shear, zoom can be performed on an image to get better model accuracy.

The U-Net model achieves best mass segmentation and the performance rate is improved when used on the mammographic datasets. It also performs well when the training data for segmentation is limited considering the medical images [44]. The U-Net model incorporates the residual network to improve the model performance and yields less noisy boundaries in the images to the radiologists thereby playing a vital role in the breast cancer diagnosis.

9.3.2 Convolution Neural Network

Convolution Neural Network (ConvNets) were specifically designed for visual tasks like MNIST dataset. ConvNets were also designed for object recognition tasks. Most of the developments in CNN happened at the intersection of Computer Vision and Deep Learning [45]. The research on ConvNets were done on the cat's brain and some of the key findings from the research were, there are few neurons in the Visual Cortex (part of the brain responsible for visual tasks) that fire when presented with lines of horizontal, vertical or at any specific angle. V1 is the primary visual cortex which detects the edges. There are also edge detector neurons which can detect motion, depth, color, shapes, faces and these could be V2, V3, V4, and so on. There is a nice hierarchical structure amongst V1, V2, V3 ... where at the lower levels, edges could be detected, going above the color, and still above shape of the object could be detected. And finally, the object itself could be detected at the higher level.

The architecture is got from the biological inspiration of the images present in mammalian or human brains like the V1, V2, V3 we design convolution layer ... There could also be multiple edge detectors which might needs multiple kernels so learning the Kernel matrices from an input image I is important in convolutional layer [46]. Multiple kernels like k1 can be utilized which could do horizontal edge detection, k2 which might do vertical edge detection and k3 can do an edge detection for 45 horizontal edge and so on. So different kernels could read different weight matrices.

So, a convolutional layer has multiple kernels all of the same size (k x k). Padding and strides should be taken care; the input image could be a 3D RGB image with 3 channels. The length and width of the output image depends on padding p and strides s, kernel k. The depth(d) depends on m, the number of kernels. Kernels, p and s are the hyperparameters. Two stages in the convolution layer are considered, where in Stage 1 the input is considered to Convol with Kernel k.

Input (n × n × c) * Kernel1 (k × k × 3) → n × n × 1.
As part of Stage 2 element wise, ReLU is done to get the final output image.

The CNN architecture is best used in breast cancer classification and diagnosis as it outperforms feature extraction, thereby enhancing the malignancy detection in breast masses [47]. The network is used to pixelate the images and to classify each of the pixels in an image. Gradient boosting is applied to make predictions and then the predicted class is got by the probability score. The CNN model has specific design which uses fully connected layers to extract the features from the input and then classifies it to see if the cancer is malignant or benign. The validations are done using 10-fold cross validation. The CNN model can include different methods like Pooling, Augmentation to train the model datasets efficiently, which is explained in the next section.

9.3.2.1 CNN training: Optimization

For Multi Layered Perceptron, back propagation can be applied if they are differentiable. For both Convolution Layer and Max Pooling, both need to be differentiable. For Convolution Layer, the Conv operator and ReLU must be differentiable. In ConvNet, the relationship between an input pixel and output pixel can be determined using dot product and since element wise multiplication followed by addition is done, they are differentiable [48]. When we do Max Pooling, from a range of pixel values the maximum values are taken into account, considering the padding and strides. So whatever maximum value is obtained, the model should be able to back propagate. When the maximum value is given back, we pass it only to the maximum unit. Thus, Max Pooling also is differentiable.

For the max value → derivative = 1
For non max value → derivative = 0

Since Convolution Layer and Max Pooling are differentiable, back propagation can be applied and thereby different techniques can be used, like SGD, Adagrad, Adam, and dropouts in deep CNN.

ResNet50 models also can be used as a part of breast image recognition, which takes a deep CNN layer as the output adding to the input tensor. ResNet model uses convolution layer and batch normalization with pooling layers added in between the residual layers.

9.3.2.2 *Max pooling*

Max Pooling is a very popular method in modern convNets. Pooling is like a layer that we can add after applying two layers of convolution in an image. Pooling makes our model invariant to location, scaling and rotation. If suppose in the Convolutional Neural Network the face needs to be detected to check if it is present in the image, the location invariance does not bother where the face is. Scale invariant detects if the face is small or big. Rotation invariant tells if the face is straight or tilted. Max Pooling takes the maximum value in the image pixels. The maximum value taken depends on the padding and strides considered. A Max Pooling based CNN is designed to detect the cancer in breast images. Max Pooling says the edge can be present anywhere and the value is high in that region or in that area of pixels, and thus it is said to be invariant of the location and other parameters [49].

9.3.2.3 *Data augmentation*

Data Augmentation is very popular for image datasets. When the CNN models want to be robust to things like rotation, scale, cropping of images, etc., this technique can be employed. When an image wants to be flipped, or perform horizontal shift, vertical shift, rotation, or zoom, shear(stretch) data augmentation is used. Consider a dataset D with input image Xi and Yi as the output, augment the image dataset as D' = {Xij, yi}. Here, for every input image, the images are augmented in the dataset, keeping the original image. Lot of invariances can be seen like shift invariance. Invariance could mean the input to output mapping does not change if it changes slightly. Fifty or 60 random color augmentations can be performed to better analyze the microscopic images. Rotation invariances, zoom, shear, noise invariances can be seen. Data augmentation increases the size of the dataset to 10 times the original one, thereby preventing overfitting when using less data. It can be used in these types of invariances to keep the model robust [50]. The Keras ImageDataGenerator can be instantiated to get batches of different tensor images with Data augmentation.

9.3.3 Activation functions in neural network

Activation functions (fij's) like sigmoid and tanh are most popularly used in Neural Networks [51]. Function unit fij is considered with x1, x2, x3 ... to be the inputs with weights W1, W2, W3. The input that goes to fij is the weighted sum of xi Wi, and it is Z.
σ is the sigmoid unit. fij = σ

$$\sigma(Z) = \frac{e^z}{1 + e^z} \quad \text{and} \quad \frac{\partial \sigma}{\partial z} = \sigma(z)(1 - \sigma(z))$$

The activation function needs to be differentiable, and it needs to be easy and fast to differentiate. The derivate of sigmoid function is represented as the sigmoid function itself. The sigmoid function (z) can be used both in forward propagation as well as in computing derivatives for back propagation to update the weights [52]. Sigmoid function fits nicely into the framework of logistic regression.

Tanh function is similar to sigmoid activation. The derivative of tanh is represented as the tanh function itself.

$$\frac{dtanh}{dz} = 1 - \tan h^2(z) \text{ where } \tanh(z) = a = \frac{e^z - e^{-z}}{e^z + e^{-z}}$$

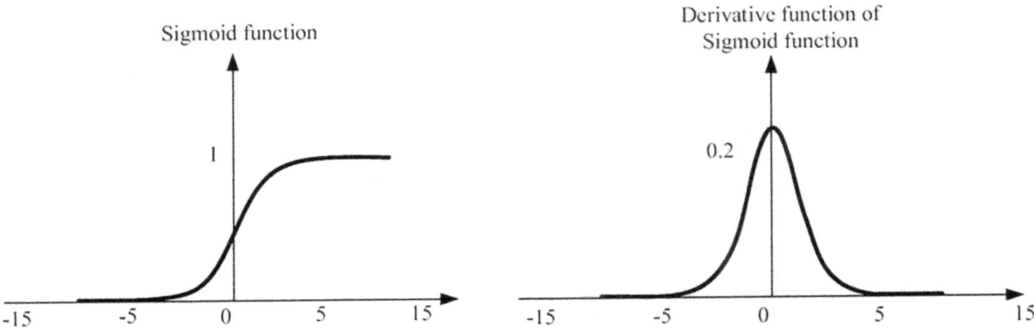

Figure 9.3 Sigmoid activation function and its derivative.

The major differences of tanh and sigmoid activation is; in sigmoid function the value lies between 0 and 1, as shown in Figure 9.3, whereas in tanh it lies between −1 to 1, as shown in Figure 9.4.

And the derivative of tanh, wrt z, lies between 0 and 1, and the maximum value it can take is 1 and minimum value −1. Classically, sigmoid and tanh activation were mostly used in Neural Networks because they were differentiable, and both the derivatives of tanh and sigmoid are represented in terms of themselves[53].

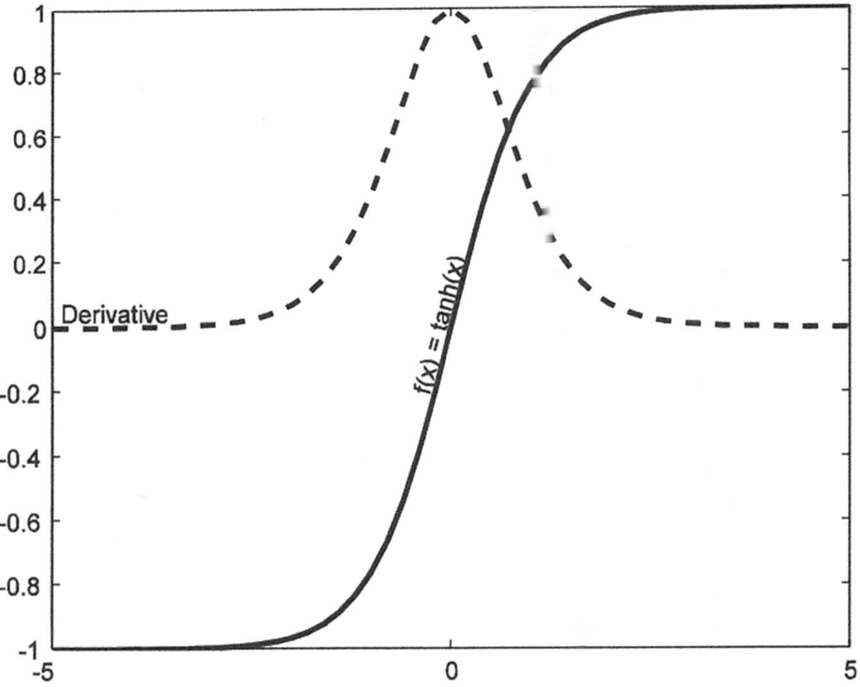

Figure 9.4 tanh activation function and its derivative.

9.3.4 Dropout and regularization

In a Deep Neural Network, the biggest problem is overfitting, where there are many layers that have too many weights to train [54]. So, overfitting has to be avoided and L1, L2 regularization is used. Dropout technique is extremely simple and elegant. In Random Forest method, a subset of columns is sampled where many trees are built. The trees trained in Random Forest are fully grown. Two important things are intuitively considered in Random Forest where we first take a random subset of features and train each of the base learners using randomization for regularization. The core idea in Random Forest is using randomization of features to create regularization.

In Dropout, at any point or iteration whenever forward or backward propagation is considered, subsets of inputs or hidden layers are randomly taken and the connections are removed. The dropout rate lies between 0 < = p < = 1, if p = 0.2 dropout is 20%, which implies 20% of the neurons are inactive or dropped out. Dropout is very similar to having a random subset of features in Random Forest. A Dropout Neural Network model is shown in Figure 9.5. At training time, activation unit or an input is present with a probability p. At test time, all activation units or inputs are always present, all of the weights are multiplied with p. So, at test time a fully connected Neural Network is seen. Dropout and Regularization can be used in predicting invasive cancer with a regularization rate of 25% to prevent overfitting. The breast image is then flattened and given to the next dense layer.

9.3.5 ReLU activation

Vanishing gradient descent is one of the big problems in classical neural networks, especially when sigmoid or tanh activation is used; also the convergence slows down. It is not possible to train the deep neural networks [55]. And thus, ReLU are the best activation function when using medical images in cancer diagnoses.

$$f_{ReLU}(z) = z^{+} = \max(0, z) = \{0 \ if \ z \leq 0, \ z \ otherwise\}$$

For any activation function, computing the derivative is important. The ReLU function f(z) is not differentiable at zero. Since the derivative of ReLU $\frac{dReLU}{dz} \in \{0, 1\}$ exploding gradient

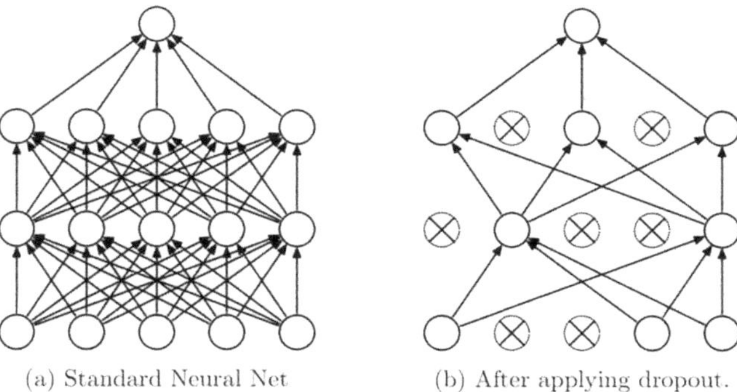

Figure 9.5 Shows a Dropout Neural Network model. (a): A standard Neural network with 2 hidden layers. (b): A network applying dropout to the network.

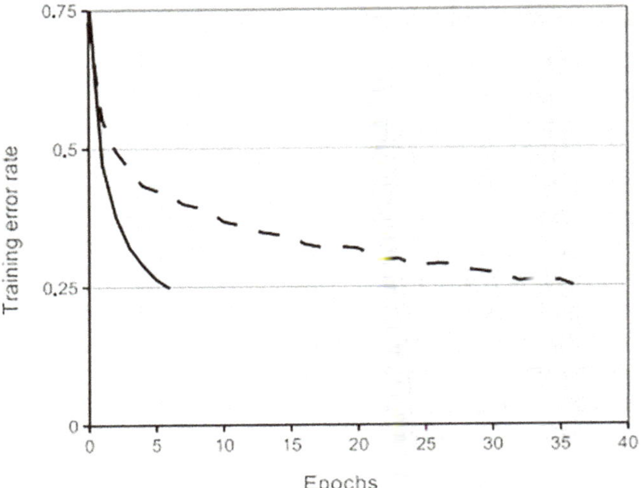

Figure 9.6 Shows a four-layer convolution neural network with ReLU.

problem and also the problem of vanishing gradient is not encountered. But since the derivate has the value of 0, the problem of dead activations is seen.

A four-layer Convolution Neural Network with ReLU is shown in Figure 9.6 x-axis is the number of epochs; y-axis is the error. As the number of epochs increases, error should reduce. The solid line represents a model built using ReLU. Dashed line is of the result got using tanh function [56]. After 5 epochs, for tanh an error equal to 0.4 is seen, but ReLU has much low error of 0.28. This shows that ReLU converges toward the solution faster than tanh, and it is because ReLU does not have the problem of vanishing gradients.

ReLU is not differentiable at 0. So soft plus function can be used as a smooth approximation to ReLU. Soft plus function is defined as.

$$f(x) = \log(1 + \exp(x))$$

The soft plus function with ReLU is explained in Figure 9.7.

And the derivative of soft plus function is defined as:

$$f'(x) = \frac{\exp(x)}{(1 + \exp(x))}$$

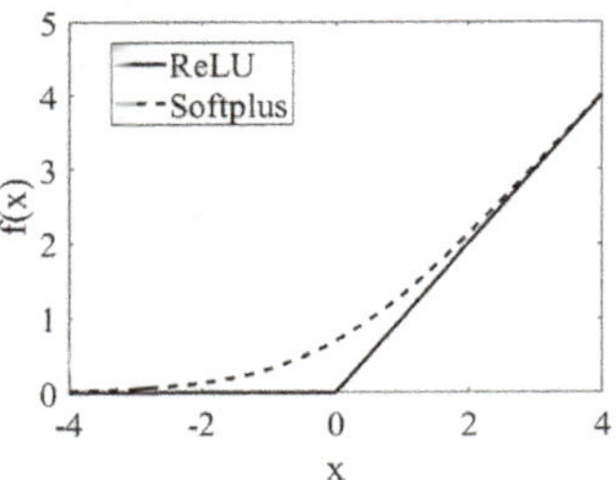

Figure 9.7 Soft plus function and Rectifier (ReLU) activation.

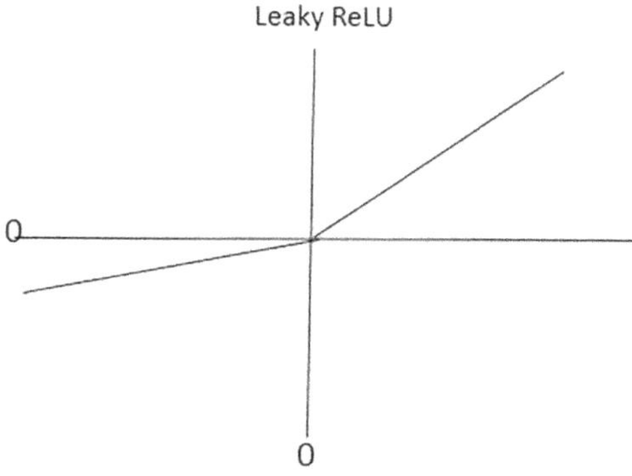

Figure 9.8 Leaky ReLU activation.

Leaky ReLU can be used as a variant to ReLU. A lot of gradients are multiplied in chain rule. Even if one of them becomes 0, the whole derivative becomes 0 and the update function does not change much, and this creates a problem. When weights are negative, z becomes negative, f(z) and $\frac{df}{dz}$ becomes 0 or negative and this leads to dead activations. If too many activations become dead the model performance deteriorates. A simple fix for this is Leaky ReLU. Leaky ReLU activation is shown in Figure 9.8.

Leaky ReLU is f(x) = ax where a = 0.01, and

$$\frac{df_{LR}}{dz} = \{1\ if\ z\ is + ve,\ \ a\ if\ z\ is - ve\}\}$$

With a small 'a' of 0.01, we could get rid of dead activations.

ReLU activation speeds up convergence. And it is easy to compute f(z), $\frac{df}{dz}$ and exp (). But we could run into the problem of dead activation which could be resolved using Leaky ReLU.

9.3.6 Feature extraction methods

Pre-processing of the image data or cleaning the data is considered to first step where the unwanted noise is eliminated. In this study various filters like gaussian, wiener, and the combination of these filters are used, thereby removing the noise effectively and in-turn helping in understanding the cancer dataset better for segmentation to be done as a next step. The MRI images taken from the dataset are preprocessed using these filters, and the visualized images are shown in Figure 9.9(a) and (b).

Featurization is important in any ML or DL model predictions. Featurization is converting some type of data into numerical vectors. Feature Engineering modifies the data such that it works well with ML models [57]. For text data we have Bag of Words, TF-IDF, and avg W2V. For categorical data, one-hot encoding, mean-response for data, is done. For time series, data is first converted into numerical vectors and then ML techniques are applied. For image data like X-rays and MRI scans, the data is first converted into numerical data and then ML or DL techniques are applied.

After the Pre-Processing step, the images are broken down into different segments for simplicity of the data. Different thresholding methods are used to enhance the brightness in

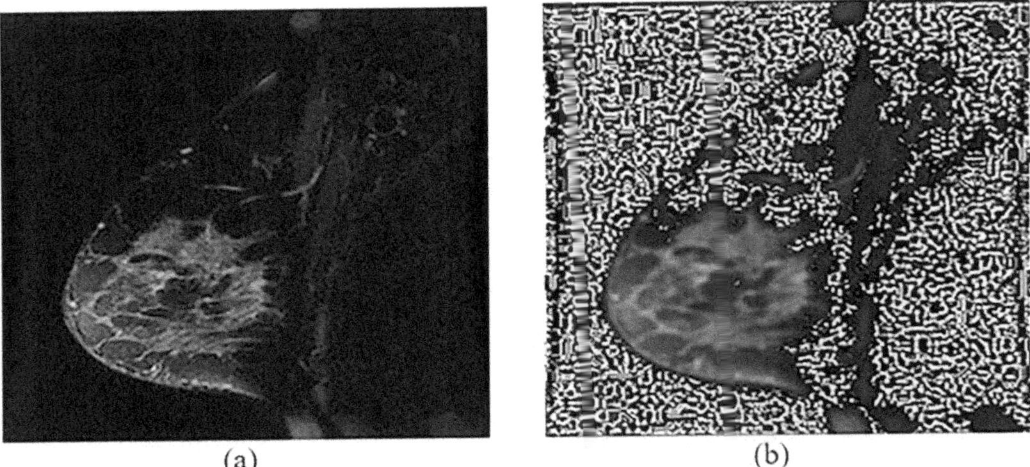

Figure 9.9 **(a)** Represents the original MRI image. **(b)** Represents the Pre-Processed image.

the image. Different feature extraction techniques can be used like GLCM (Gray Level Co-Occurrence Matrix) for better texture analysis. Different feature textures like mean, variance, contrast, homogeneity, standard deviation is obtained from the analysis. This method helps better understand the spatial relationship between the image pixels considering the gray intensity and angle. The pre-processed image with segmented and feature extracted MRI images are visualized in Figure 9.10(a)–(e).

Moving window is the simplest featurization of time series. The window width is defined and the features are used [58]. Deep Learning methods automatically learn correct featurizations when there is a lot of data. Fourier Decomposition method is used to represent Time-Series data. When a composite wave is used, and if there are "repeating" patterns, then it is decomposed into the sum of multiple sine waves. The Time-Waveform is converted into frequency domain specific to the one using Fourier transform, and these frequencies and amplitude are used to represent a feature vector. Fourier representations are very important when using repeating waveforms. Deep Learning features are the best features, where it automatically learns the best featurizations for your data. Deep Learning techniques are used mostly in Medical Image or Time Series data [59].

CNN, a deep learning method, is the best way to featurize image data. For X-ray or MRI scans, lots of data or images are given, and in each image histograms like color histogram and edge histogram can be used in image recognition and detection. Color histograms take all the red or blue or green values for each pixel with (nxm) data points and then plot a histogram. Edge histogram can be used to detect edges of specific angles and for every region edge-value or edge angle there is, and then the histogram is plotted.

Scale Invariant Feature Transforms (SIFT) is useful in detecting objects in an image [60]. SIFT detects key points in an image and creates a 128-dim vector for each key points. SIFT is popular in image search. SIFT is scale invariant or rotational invariant because the features do not change much, even if the image is big or small, or even if the image is a little tilted [61].

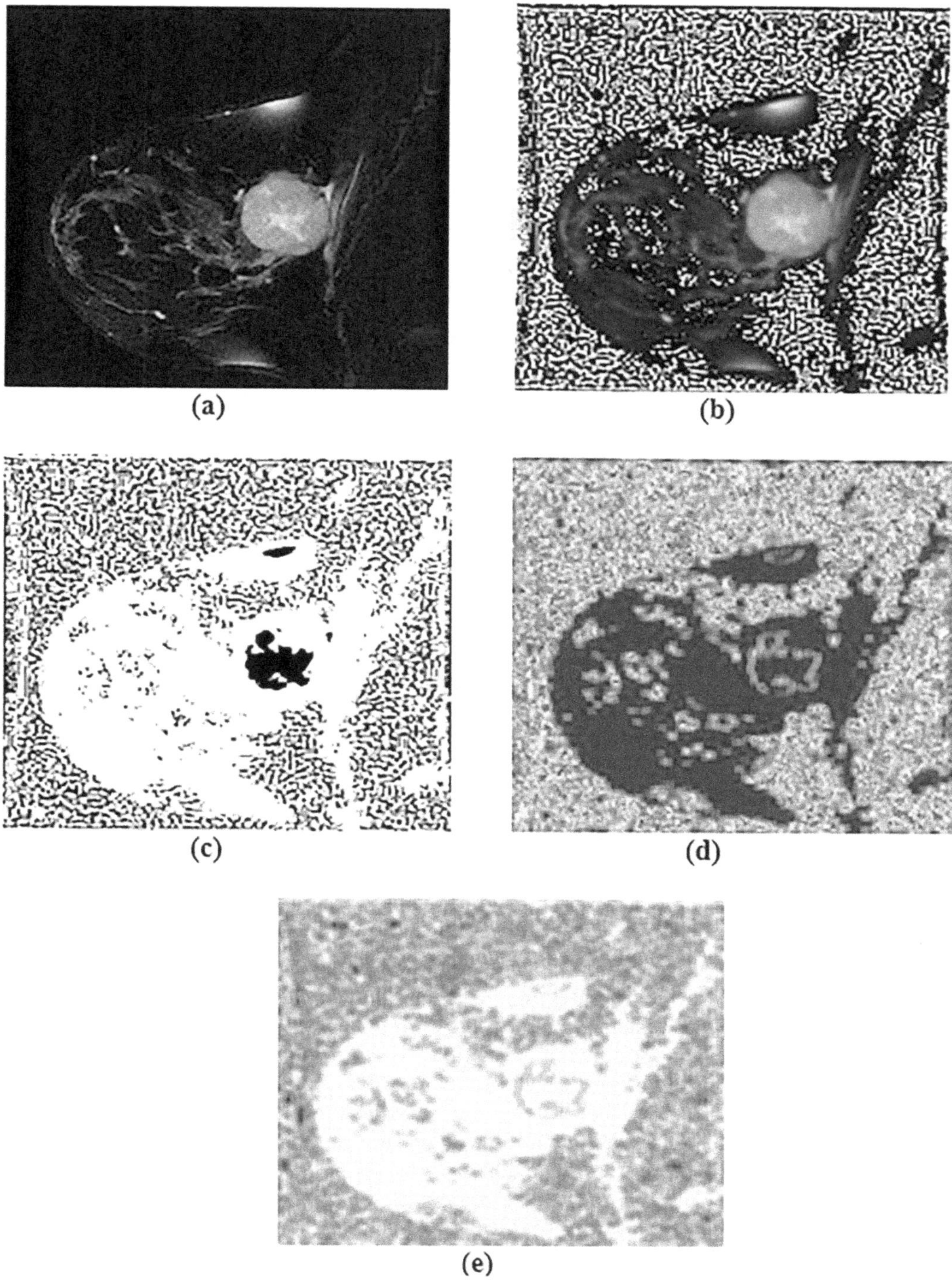

Figure 9.10 (a) Represents the original breast MRI image. (b) Represents the Pre-Processed image. (c) Represents the segmented output image. (d) Shows the texture feature 'Contrast' extracted from the segmented image. (e) Represents the texture feature 'Homogeneity' extracted from the segmented output image.

9.4 DISCUSSIONS

9.4.1 Dataset description

Imaging and genetic analyses were used in the "ISPY 2 (Inve tigation of Serial Studies to Predict Your Therapeutic Response)" study. Using the Trial Breast MRI Database, 131 cases from nine institutions were gathered [62]. Data from MRIs was gathered. "ISPY2" was created to assess the effectiveness of new breast cancer patients receiving neoadjuvant chemotherapy (NAC). "The local institutional review boards" and the "American College of Radiology" both authorized the process, and the database was "HIPAA-compliant." A better treatment plan can be found using the I-SPY2 based on molecular features. High probability regimens are more efficient. If a regimen has a low chance, it is dropped.

The dataset collected are MRI images of patients with breast cancer. The size of the dataset images is considered to be around 2 to 3GB. Different parameters were taken into account for the patient clinical data which included the "Age" of the Patients, Patient race. Also, the Pre-Treatment patient demographics like the 'Estrogen Receptor Status' with positive or negative results, "Progesterone Receptor Status", or "Her2 IHC" results for missing community.

Women who have breast cancer with no distant metastases and a tumor size greater than 2.5 cm are eligible to participate in the experiment. The collection consists of histopathologic output data, parametric maps for I-SPY2 patients, and DCE MRI data, which is a compilation of original acquired pictures. Various imaging metrics and prediction models for the treatment of breast cancer can be developed, tested, and compared using this imaging data. This database set includes 719 patients. The first subset of publicly published imaging data from the "I-SPY 2 TRIAL", "I-SPY2 Imaging Cohort 1," consists of 985 individuals in addition to 266 patients from the "ACRIN-6698/ISPY2" TCIA collection. The performance of the prediction models is assessed on a subset of 384 patients with a median age of 49 years old in the study to see whether multi-MRI feature prediction models outperform models using single features [63]. Each MRI scan assessment included important calculations for four features, including functional tumor volume longest diameter, sphericity, and contralateral background parenchymal enhancement.

9.4.2 Convolution neural network in breast cancer classification

Convolution Neural Networks from the segmented images are extracted, and neural networks are heavily utilized in categorization [64]. The process of classification comes after diagnosis. Figure 9.11 displays the CNN architecture as a whole. Convolutions of varying degrees, maximum pooling, and completely connected layers are performed by CNN. Image features are initially sent to the network as an input, and element-wise multiplication and addition are then carried out between the input and the variables of the neuron, followed by the use of the convolution operator as a kernel in each layer [65]. The error rate and loss function are then calculated using the output results from the network. Additionally, the chain rule is used to determine each variable's gradient. The novel CNN architecture takes an input image size of 256 × 256. Different filter sizes of 3 × 3, 4 × 4 are employed along with striding (1 × 1), average pooling size of 7 × 7 and max pool layer size of 3 × 3 with padding. A dropout of 50% is implemented by making the neurons inactive thereby reducing overfitting. Different metrics like accuracy and loss are calculated as a part of classification.

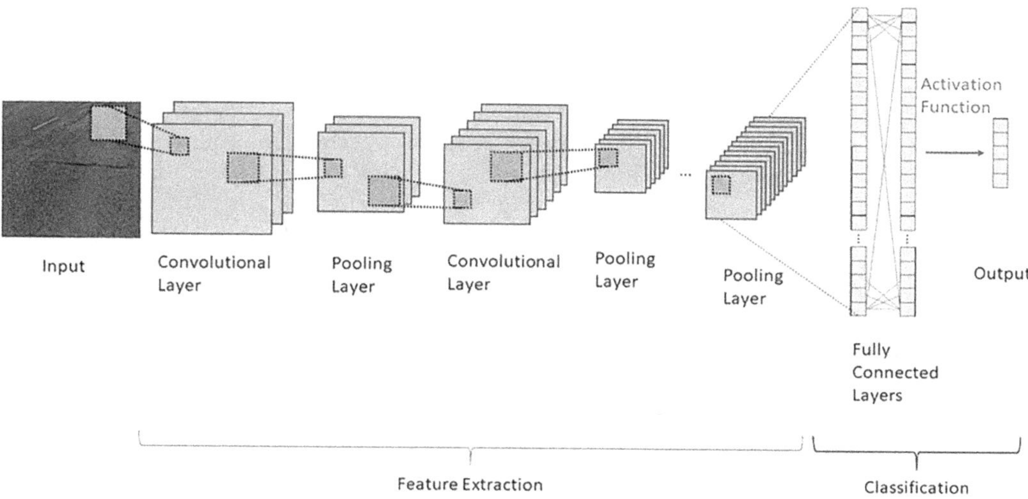

Figure 9.11 Overview of Convolution Neural Network Architecture.

For extracting local features from mammography pictures, CNN is employed. The back propagation technique is utilized to produce the best results for the weights among the network connections [66]. Rectified Linear Unit, or ReLU, is employed as an activation mechanism. The kernel or filter matrices are multiplied by the input pictures to produce the feature maps. By moving the filter left to right or up and down with varying stride sizes, as well as with enough padding, feature maps are created, and high features like edges are removed [67]. Max Pooling reduces the size of the output neurons by using the feature maps' maximum value of the matrix. Finally, by categorizing the existence of tumors in the output feature picture, CNN was able to extract the optimal features in the mammogram images.

9.5 CHALLENGES

- Poisson based signal noise are not useful in eliminating noise, and hence the data used needs to deal with noisy and inconsistent databases, thereby preserving the edges of ultrasound images.
- Feature extraction techniques do not function well since they rely on human extracting essential characteristics. Thus, different slicing and segmentation methods needs to be developed which could extract the best features.
- Training time is high in this research study which in turn deteriorates the performance.
- The overall Accuracy rate needs to be improved compared to the research done using the Convolution Neural Network with another best optimizer algorithm.
- Overfitting and Underfitting leads to poor predictions on the given data sets. Thus, a novel model can be proposed which enhances conceptual knowledge of a CNN as well as offer real guidance on how to prevent model over-fitting as well as under-fitting if a CNN is utilized for tasks of image recognition.
- The data sample used in augmentation methods is not sufficient in training CNN models. Adam Optimizer works well in dealing this issue.
- Gray-Level Co-occurrence Matrix and different SIFT based techniques can be proposed as a future study to extract different features from the collected raw images.

9.6 CONCLUSIONS

The study introduces a novel approach that uses a segmented tumor technique to predict chemotherapy response and classify breast tumors with high accuracy using CNN. The study suggests future research to explore various pre-processing techniques and feature extraction methods to improve the model's performance, such as content-based image retrieval approaches and Gray-Level Co-occurrence Matrix. A novel CNN with different filter sizes can also be proposed to address overfitting/underfitting problems and improve tumor detection speed.

ACKNOWLEDGMENTS

The authors sincerely thank the anonymous reviewers and associate editor for valuable and constructive comments to enhance the quality and organization of the manuscript.

REFERENCES

1. Rahul Singh et al.: "A brief review on image de-noising techniques", In Proceedings Springer in Visual Computing for Industry, Biomedicine and Art, vol no. 04, pp. 336–344, no. 01 (April 2015).
2. Jyotsna Patil, and Sunita Jadhav: "A comparative study of image de-noising techniques", In Proceedings International Journal of Innovative Research in Science, Engineering and Technology, vol no. 2, pp. 787–794, no. 3 (March 2013).
3. M. Kaufmann, G. von Minckwitz, E.P. Mamounas, D. Cameron, L.A. Carey, M. Cristofanilli, C. Denkert, W. Eiermann, M. Gnant, and J.R. Harris, et al.: "Recommendations from an international consensus conference on the current status and future of neoadjuvant systemic therapy in primary breast cancer", In Proceedings Annals of Surgical, vol no. 19, pp. 1508–1516 (December 2012).
4. A. Hamidinekoo, E. Denton, A. Rampun, K. Honnor, and R. Zwiggelaar: "Deep learning in mammography and breast histology, an overview and future trends", In Proceedings Elsevier Medical Image Analysis, vol no. 47, pp. 45–67 (March 2018).
5. Nariman Jahani et al.: "Prediction of treatment response to neo-adjuvant chemotherapy for breast cancer via early changes in tumor heterogeneity captured by DCE-MRI registration", In Proceedings Scientific Reports, vol no. 9, no. 1 (August 2019).
6. Sami Andberg, Parvathy Sudhir Pillai, and Tze-Yun Leong: "Magnetic resonance imaging (MRI) image processing Workbench for Alzheimer's disease classification", In Proceedings Indian Journal of Medical Informatics, pp. 1–5 (January 2015).
7. L. Fan, F. Zhang, H. Fan et al.: "A Brief review of image de-noising techniques", In Proceedings Visual Computing for Arts 2, vol no. 7, pp. 1–2, (2019).
8. Ashish Semwal, Akshay Chamoli, and Ankit Semwal, "A SURVEY: On image de-noising and its various techniques", In Proceedings International Research Journal of Engineering and Technology (IRJET), vol no. 04, no. 07, pp. 1512–1515 (July 2017).
9. Kirti V. Thakur, Omkar H. Damodare, and Ashok M. Sapkal, "Poisson noise reducing bilateral filter", In Proceedings Procedia Computer Science 7th International Conference on Communication, Computing and Virtualization, vol no. 79, pp. 861–865, ISSN 1877-0509 (2016).
10. Rajkumar Goel, Vineet Kumar, Saurabh Srivastava, and A. K. Sinha: "A review of feature extraction techniques for image analysis", In Proceedings International Journal of Advanced Research in Computer and Communication Engineering, vol no. 6, Special Issue 2, pp. 153–155 (February 2017).

11. Saif Ali, Aneeqa Tanveer, Azhar Hussain, and Saif ur Rehman: "Identification of cancer disease using image processing approaches", In Proceedings International Journal of Intelligent Information Systems, vol no. 9, no. 2, pp. 6–15 (2020).
12. Prannoy Giri, and K. Saravanakumar: "Breast cancer detection using image processing techniques", In Proceedings Oriental Journal of Computer Science and Technology, vol no. 10, pp. 391–399 (2017).
13. Rafael Guzman-Cabrera, José Rafael Guzmán-Sepúlveda, Miguel Torres-Cisneros, D. May-Arrioja, José Ruiz-Pinales, Oscar Ibarra-Manzano, Juan Avina-Cervantes, and Adrian Gonzalez-Parada: "Digital image processing technique for breast cancer detection", In Proceedings International Journal of Thermo physics, vol. 34, no. 8, pp. 1519–1531 (October 2013).
14. R.M. Kamal, S.M. Saad, A.F.I. Moustafa et al.: "Predicting response to neo-adjuvant chemotherapy and assessment of residual disease in breast cancer using contrast-enhanced spectral mammography: a combined qualitative and quantitative approach", In Proceedings Egypt Journal Radiology Nuclear Medical Analysis, vol. 51, no. 161, pp. 1–14 (2020).
15. A. Fangberget et al.: "Neo-adjuvant chemotherapy in breast cancer-response evaluation and prediction of response to treatment using dynamic contrast-enhanced and diffusion-weighted MR imaging", In Proceedings Springer European Radiology, vol no. 21, pp. 1188–1199 (2011).
16. N. M. Hylton et al.: "Locally advanced breast cancer: MR imaging for prediction of response to neo-adjuvant chemotherapy— Results from ACRIN 6657/I-SPY TRIAL", In Proceedings Journal Radiology, vol no. 263, no. 3, pp. 663–672 (2012).
17. J. R. Teruel et al.: "Dynamic contrast-enhanced MRI texture analysis for pretreatment prediction of clinical and pathological response to neo-adjuvant chemotherapy in patients with locally advanced breast cancer", In Proceedings Journal NMR in Biomedicine, vol no. 27, pp. 887–896 (August 2014).
18. J. Wu et al.: "Intratumoral spatial heterogeneity at perfusion MR imaging predicts recurrence-free survival in locally advanced breast cancer treated with neoadjuvant chemotherapy", In Proceedings Journal in Radiology, vol no. 172462, pp. 1–10 (2018).
19. Saeed Kermani, Nasser Samadzadehaghdam, and Mahnaz EtehadTavakol: "Automatic color segmentation of breast infrared images using a Gaussian mixture model", Optik, vol no. 126, no. 21, pp. 3288–3294, ISSN 0030-4026 (2015), 10.1016/j.ijleo.2015.08.007.
20. Jordina Torrents-Barrena, Gemma Piella, Narcís Masoller, Eduard Gratacós, Elisenda Eixarch, Mario Ceresa, and Miguel Ángel González Ballester: "Segmentation and classification in MRI and US fetal imaging: Recent trends and future prospects, medical image analysis", vol no. 51, pp. 61–88, ISSN 1361-8415 (2019), 10.1016/j.media.2018.10.003.
21. Yan Fang, Jing Zhao, Lingzhi Hu, Xiaoping Ying, Yanfang Pan, and Xiaoping Wang: "Image classification toward breast cancer using deeply-learned quality features", In Proceedings Journal of Visual Communication and Image Representation, vol no. 64, 102609, ISSN, pp. 1047–3203 (2019), 10.1016/j.jvcir.2019.102609.
22. Gabriele Piantadosi, Mario Sansone, Roberta Fusco, and Carlo Sansone: "Multi-planar 3D breast segmentation in MRI via deep convolutional neural networks", In Proceedings Artificial Intelligence in Medicine, vol no. 103, 101781, ISSN 0933-3657 (2020), 10.1016/j.artmed.2019.101781.
23. Roberto Lo Gullo, Sarah Eskreis-Winkler, Elizabeth A. Morris, and Katja Pinker: "Machine learning with multiparametric magnetic resonance imaging of the breast for early prediction of response to neoadjuvant chemotherapy", In Proceedings The Breast, vol no. 49, pp. 115–122, ISSN 0960-9776 (2020), 10.1016/j.breast.2019.11.009.
24. N. Shobha Rani, Karthik U, and Ranjith S: "Extraction of Gliomas from 3D MRI images using convolution Kernel processing and adaptive thresholding", In Proceedings Procedia Computer Science, vol no. 167, pp. 273–284, ISSN 1877-0509 (2020), 10.1016/j.procs.2020.03.221.
25. K. Padmapriya, S. Divya, and P. Ezhumalai.: "A scrutiny on brain tumor classification using deep learning technique", In Proceedings Materials Today, ISSN 2214-7853, pp. 1–5 (2021), 10.1016/j.matpr.2020.11.561.

26. Michael Z. Liua, Simukayi Mutasab, Peter Changc, Maham Siddiqueb, Sachin Jambawalikara, and Richard Ha: "A novel CNN algorithm for pathological complete response prediction using an I-SPY TRIAL breast MRI database", In Proceedings Magnetic Resonance Imaging, vol no. 73, pp. 148–151 (2020).
27. Jyoti Parashar, Sumiti, and Munishwar Rai: "Breast cancer images classification by clustering of ROI and mapping of features by CNN with XGBOOST learning", In Proceedings Materials Today, pp. 2214–2219, ISSN 2214-7853 (2020) 10.1016/j.matpr.2020.09.650.
28. Yi-Cheng Zhu, Alaa AlZoubi, Sabah Jassim, Quan Jiang, Yuan Zhang, Yong-Bing Wang, Xian-De Ye, Hongbo DU: "A generic deep learning framework to classify thyroid and breast lesions in ultrasound images", Ultrasonics, vol no. 110, 106300, pp. 1–26, ISSN 0041-624X (2021), 10.1016/j.ultras.2020.106300.
29. Tomoyuki Fujioka, Yuka Yashima, Jun Oyama, Mio Mori, Kazunori Kubota, Leona Katsuta, Koichiro Kimura, Emi Yamaga, Goshi Oda, Tsuyoshi Nakagawa, Yoshio Kitazume, and Ukihide Tateishi: "Deep-learning approach with convolutional neural network for classification of maximum intensity projections of dynamic contrast-enhanced breast magnetic resonance imaging", In Proceedings Magnetic Resonance Imaging, vol no. 75, pp. 1–8, ISSN 0730-725X (2021), 10.1016/j.mri.2020.10.003.
30. Marco Caballo, Domenico R. Pangallo, Ritse M. Mann, and Ioannis Sechopoulos: "Deep learning-based segmentation of breast masses in dedicated breast CT imaging: Radiomic feature stability between radiologists and artificial intelligence", In Proceedings Computers in Biology and Medicine, vol no. 118, 103629, ISSN, pp. 0010–4825 (2021), 10.1016/j.compbiomed.2020.103629.
31. Suvidha Tripathi, Satish Kumar Singh, and Hwee Kuan Lee: "An end-to-end breast tumour classification model using context-based patch modelling – A BiLSTM approach for image classification", In Proceedings Computerized Medical Imaging and Graphics, vol no. 87, 101838, pp. ISSN 0895-6111 (2021), 10.1016/j.compmedimag.2020.101838.
32. Vivek Kumar Singh, Mohamed Abdel-Nasser, Farhan Akram, Hatem A. Rashwan, Md. Mostafa Kamal Sarker, Nidhi Pandey, Santiago Romani, and Domenec Puig: "Breast tumor segmentation in ultrasound images using contextual-information-aware deep adversarial learning framework", In Proceedings Expert Systems with Applications, vol no. 162, 113870, pp. ISSN 0957-4174 (2020), 10.1016/j.eswa.2020.113870.
33. M. Malathi, P. Sinthia, Fareen Farzana, and G. Aloy Anuja Mary: "Breast cancer detection using active contour and classification by deep belief network", In Proceedings Materials Today, 2721–2724, ISSN 2214-7853 (2021), 10.1016/j.matpr.2020.11.551.
34. Ghulam Murtaza, Ainuddin Wahid Abdul Wahab, Ghulam Raza, and Liyana Shuib: "A tree-based multiclassification of breast tumor histopathology images through deep learning", In Proceedings Computerized Medical Imaging and Graphics, vol no. 101870, pp. 1–17, ISSN 0895-6111 (2021), 10.1016/j.compmedimag.2021.101870.
35. Dhanalekshmi Prasad, Shilpa P. Metkar, Fadi Al-Turjman, Thompson Stephan, Manjur Kolhar, and Chadi Altrjman: "A novel approach for multichannel epileptic seizure classification based on Internet of Things framework using critical spectral verge feature derived from flower pollination algorithm", In Proceedings MDPI Sensors journal, vol no. 22, no. 23, pp. 1–18 (2022).
36. Divya Biligere Shivanna, Thompson Stephan, Fadi Al-Turjman, Manjur Kolhar, and Sinem Alturjman: "IoMT-based automated diagnosis of autoimmune diseases using multistage classification scheme for sustainable smart cities", In Proceedings MDPI Sustainability Journal, vol no. 14, no. 21, pp. 1–15 (2022).
37. Igbe Tobore, Jingzhen Li, Liu Yuhang, and Zedong Nie: "Breast cancer images classification by clustering of ROI and mapping of features by CNN with XGBOOST learning", In Proceedings Materials Today (November 2020), pp. 422–430.
38. Mohd Usama, Belal Ahmad, Jiafu Wan, M. Shamim Hossain, Mohammed F. Alhamid, and M. Anwar Hossain: "Improved breast cancer classification through combining graph convolution network and convolution neural network", In Proceedings Information Processing and Management, vol no. 58, pp. 1–25 (January 2021).

39. Mohammad Jamshidi, Ali Lalbakhsh, Jakub Talla, Wahab Mohyuddin: "A brief survey on breast cancer diagnostic with deep learning schemes using multi-image modalities", In Proceedings IEEE Access, vol no. 100, pp. 165780–165810 (June 2020).
40. Yifan Xianga, Lanqin Zhaoa, Zhenzhen Liua, Xiaohang Wua, Jingjing Chena, Erping Longa, Duoru Lina, Yi Zhuab, Chuan Chenab, Zhuoling Lina, and Haotian Lina: "A study on convolution neural network for breast cancer detection", In Proceedings Second International Conference on Advanced Computational and Communication Paradigms (October 2018), pp. 1–7.
41. Behzad Soleimani Neysiani, Nasim Soltani, Reza Mofidi, and Mohammad Hossein Nadimi-Shahraki: "Methods used in computer-aided diagnosis for breast cancer detection using mammograms: A review", In Proceedings Journal of Healthcare Engineering (March 2020), pp. 1–21.
42. Olaf Ronneberger, Philipp Fischer, and Thomas Brox: "U-Net: Convolutional networks for biomedical image segmentation", In Proceedings arXiv Informatik University of Freiburg, Germany (2015), pp. 1–8.
43. Penghui Li, Lijun Zhang, Jinlong Qiao, and Xiangguo Wang: "A semantic segmentation method based on improved U-net network", In Proceedings 4th International Conference on Advanced Electronic Materials, Computers and Software Engineering (March 2021), pp. 1–7.
44. Heyi Li, Dongdong Chen, Bill Nailon, Mike Davies, and Dave Laurenson: "Improved breast mass segmentation in mammograms with conditional residual U-net", In Proceedings Medical Image Computing and Computer Assisted Interventions Conference (August 2018), pp. 1–8.
45. Xiuzhen Cai, Xia Li, Navid Razmjooy, and Noradin Ghadimi: "Breast cancer diagnosis by convolutional neural network and advanced thermal exchange optimization algorithm", In Proceedings Computational and Mathematical Methods in Medicine, vol no. 21, pp. 1–13 (2021).
46. Wessam M. Salama, and Moustafa H. Aly: "Deep learning in mammography images segmentation and classification: Automated CNN approach", In Proceedings Alexandria Engineering Journal Elsevier, vol no. 60, pp. 4701–4709 (2021).
47. Hiba Chougrad, and Zouaki Hamid: "Deep convolutional neural networks for breast cancer screening", In Proceedings Computer Methods and Programs in Biomedicine Elsevier Journal, vol no. 157, pp. 19–30 (April 2018).
48. Priyanka, and Sanjeev Kumar: "A review paper on breast cancer detection using deep learning", In Proceedings IOP Conference Series: Materials Science and Engineering, vol no.10, pp. 757–899 (2020).
49. Saad Awadh Alanazi, M. M. Kamruzzaman, Md Nazrirul Islam Sarker, Madallah Alruwaili, Yousef Alhwaiti, Nasser Alshammari, and Muhammad Hameed Siddiqi: "Boosting breast cancer detection using convolution neural network", In Proceedings Journal of Healthcare Engineering, vol no. 21, pp. 1–11 (April 2021).
50. Hiba Chougrad, and Zouaki Hamid: "Deep convolutional neural networks for breast cancer screening", In Proceedings Computer Methods and Programs in Biomedicine Elsevier Journal, vol no. 157, pp. 19–30 (April 2018).
51. Chigozie Enyinna Nwankpa, Winifred Ijomah, Anthony Gachagan, and Stephen Marshall: "Activation functions: Comparison of trends in practice and research for deep learning", In Proceedings 2nd International Conference on Computational Sciences and Technologies, pp. 17–19 (December 2020).
52. Jianli Feng, and Shengnan Lu: "Performance analysis of various activation functions in artificial neural networks", In Proceedings International Journal of Physics Conference Series, vol no. 1237, pp. 1–7 (2019).
53. Shiv Ram Dubey, Satish Kumar Singh, and Bidyut Baran Chaudhuri: "Activation functions in deep learning: A comprehensive survey and benchmark", In Proceedings Neurocomputing Elsevier Journal, vol no. 503, pp. 92–108 (September 2022).
54. Nitish Srivastava, Geoffrey Hinton, Alex Krizhevsky, Ilya Sutskever, and Ruslan Salakhutdinov: "Dropout: A simple way to prevent neural networks from overfitting", In Proceedings Journal of Machine Learning Research, vol no. 15, pp. 1929–1958 (2014).

55. Alex Krizhevsky, Ilya Sutskever, and Geoffrey Hinton: "ImageNet classification with deep convolutional neural networks", In Proceedings Communications of ACM, vol no. 60, pp. 84–90 (June 2017).
56. Puja Gupta, and Shruti Garg: "Breast cancer prediction using varying parameters of machine learning models", In Proceedings Third International Conference on Computing and Network Communications (CoCoNet' 19), vol no. 171, pp. 593–601 (2020).
57. Xiang Yu, Qinghua Zhou, Shuihua Wang, and Yu-Dong Zhang: "A systematic survey of deep learning in breast cancer", In Proceedings International Journal of Intelligence Systems, vol no. 10, pp. 152–216 (August 2021).
58. Lihua Lei, and William Fithian: "AdaPT: an interactive procedure for multiple testing with side information", In Proceedings Journal of the Royal Statistical Society, vol no. 80, pp. 649–679 (2018).
59. Angela Oberhofer, Abel J. Bronkhorst, Carsten Uhlig, Vida Ungerer, and Stefan Holdenrieder: "Tracing the origin of cell-free DNA molecules through tissue-specific epigenetic signatures", In Proceedings National Library of Medicine diagnostics, vol no. 12, pp. 1–26 (July 2022).
60. T. P. Shiji, S. Remya, and V. Thomas: "Computer aided segmentation of breast ultrasound images using scale invariant feature transform (SIFT) and bag of features", In Proceedings 7th International Conference on Advances in Computing and Communications, vol no. 115, pp. 518–525 (2017).
61. Yu-Yao Wang, Zheng-Ming Li, Long Wang, and Min Wang: "A scale invariant feature transform based method", In Proceedings Journal of Information Hiding and Multimedia Signal Processing, vol no. 4, pp. 2073–4212 (April 2013).
62. Natsuko Onishi, Wen Li, Jessica Gibbs, Lisa J. Wilmes, Alex Nguyen, Ella F. Jones, Vignesh Arasu, John Kornak, and Bonnie N. Joe: "Impact of MRI protocol adherence on prediction of pathological complete response in the I-SPY 2 neoadjuvant breast cancer trial", In Proceedings Tomography MDPI, vol no. 6, no. 2, pp. 77–85 (June 2020).
63. Natsuko Onishi, Wen Li, David C. Newitt, Roy J. Harnish, Fredrik Strand, Alex Anh-Tu Nguyen, Vignesh Amal Arasu, Jessica Gibbs, and Ella F. Jones: "Breast MRI during neoadjuvant chemotherapy; lack of background parenchymal enhancement suppression and inferior treatment response", In Proceedings Radiology Breast Imaging, vol no. 301, pp. 295–308 (2021).
64. Alexander Rakhlin, Alexey Shvets, Vladimir Iglovikov, and Alexander A. Kalinin: "Deep convolutional neural networks for breast cancer histology image analysis", In Proceedings International Conference Image Analysis and Recognition, pp. 737–744 (2018).
65. Majid Nawaz, Adel A. Sewissy, Taysir Hassan, and A. Soliman: "Multi-class breast cancer classification using deep learning convolutional neural network", In Proceedings International Journal of Advanced Computer Science and Applications, vol no. 9, pp. 316–322 (2018).
66. F.A. Spanhol, L.S. Oliveira, C. Petitjean, C., and L. Heutte: "Breast cancer histopathological image classification using convolutional neural networks", In Proceedings International Joint Conference on Neural Networks, pp. 2560–2567 (2016).
67. Z. Han, B. Wei, and Y. Zheng: "Breast cancer multi-classification from histopathological images with structured deep learning model", In Proceedings Scientific Reports, vol no. 7, pp. 4172 (2017).

Chapter 10

A machine learning predictive framework for diabetes management using blood parameters

A Poonguzhali[1], *P Ramkumar*[2], *Reji Thomas*[2], *S Tamil Selvan*[3], *and Angel Latha Mary*[4]

[1]Department of Electronics and Communication Engineering, Sri Sairam College of Engineering, Anekal, Bangalore, Karnataka, India
[2]Department of Computer Science and Engineering, Sri Sairam College of Engineering, Anekal, Bangalore, Karnataka, India
[3]Department of Computer Science and Engineering, Saveetha School of Engineering, Chennai, Tamil Nadu, India
[4]Department of Computer Science and Engineering, SNS College of Technology, Coimbatore, Tamil Nadu, India

10.1 INTRODUCTION

Diabetes type 1 is a chronic condition wherein the body's immune system inflicts damage upon the beta cells responsible for insulin production, subsequently affecting insulin secretion by the pancreas. An estimated 415 million individuals worldwide suffer from the non-communicable metabolic disorder known as diabetes mellitus. Diabetes mellitus constitutes the most prevalent manifestation of this condition. The pancreas releases insulin, a peptide hormone that aids in assimilating glucose from ingested carbohydrates, a process termed glycogenolysis [1]. Diabetes mellitus, commonly referred to as Diabetes, arises from inadequate production of the hormone insulin by the body [2], resulting in the onset of diabetes. The ailment encompasses three subtypes: type 1, type 2, and gestational diabetes. Notably, type 1 diabetes holds the highest incidence.

Diabetes type 2, as well as diabetes associated with pregnancy, further underscore the chronic nature of this ailment. In type 1 diabetes, the immune system's attack on beta cells impairs insulin production, thereby influencing insulin secretion. Consequently, type 1 diabetes remains the predominant form of the disease. Type 2 diabetes progresses as insulin utilization becomes restricted, leading to elevated blood sugar levels. Gestational diabetes, affecting about one in every hundred pregnant women, entails elevated blood glucose levels during pregnancy that typically subside postpartum [3].

In 2016, the World Health Organization ranked diabetes as the seventh leading global cause of mortality. Impressively, the number of diabetes cases in the United States surged from 108 million in 1980 to 425 million in 2017. Projections indicate that type 1 diabetes will account for a mere 5 to 10% of all diabetes cases, while type 2 diabetes will encompass 80 to 90% [4]. Diagnosed diabetes cases in adults escalated from 4.7% in 1980 to 8.8% in 2017, reflecting a significant rise. Moreover, India is projected to have nearly one million Type II diabetes cases by 2030. Notably, an estimated 86 million individuals in the United States are considered to be in a pre-diabetic state. Furthermore, 20 to 40% of diabetics grapple with diabetes-related complications, including diabetic nephropathy. Diabetic retinopathy, affecting over 60% of type 2 diabetes patients, represents a leading cause of

DOI: 10.1201/9781003369059-13

vision impairment. Diabetic patients face a 68% higher mortality rate due to heart disease and stroke compared to the general population. In India, heart-related conditions contribute to over half of all diabetic patient fatalities.

Diabetes is intricately linked to a plethora of complications, each specific to the disorder. The repercussions of elevated blood glucose or diabetes extend to organs such as the heart, kidneys, eyes, peripheral nerves, and blood vessels, leading to coronary heart disease, ischemia-related issues, renal disorders, diabetic foot conditions, and nerve damage. Early-stage anticipation of these complications remains challenging, often only surfacing in advanced disease states, thereby heightening patient vulnerability. Notably, numerous biological parameters exhibit contrary trends before the manifestation of symptoms, underscoring the importance of early intervention. However, due to multifaceted factors, the early detection and prediction of diabetic complications pose challenges. The primary objective of this project is to anticipate diseases resulting from elevated blood sugar levels in diabetic patients [5]. To achieve this, blood parameters will be collected from diabetic patients and employed to construct a computer-aided diagnostic model. These combined efforts aim to enable early detection of complications, ultimately enhancing patient quality of life and alleviating financial burdens.

Data analysis involves scrutinizing, cleansing, transforming, and modeling substantial datasets, ultimately yielding data models. The primary goal of data analysis is to uncover hitherto unknown patterns and extract applicable insights. In the medical context, data analysis yields enhanced accuracy, reduced costs, and optimized human resource utilization. Data mining within healthcare settings presents a novel avenue for identifying recurring themes in patient data. This specific study revolves around forecasting the impact of diabetes on the heart and kidneys. Present prediction strategies for diabetes onset are viable only within constrained datasets.

Diabetes Mellitus, a chronic metabolic disorder, profoundly impacts global populations. Early diabetes detection proves pivotal for improved patient outcomes and reduced healthcare expenses. Data analysis techniques hold potential for early diabetes detection, accomplished by identifying patterns and trends in blood parameters. Patient records serve as a foundation for this endeavor. Within the medical landscape, data analysis yields enhanced accuracy, reduced costs, and streamlined human resource utilization. Data mining within healthcare settings presents a novel avenue for identifying recurring themes in patient data. This specific study revolves around forecasting the impact of diabetes on the heart and kidneys. Present prediction strategies for diabetes onset are viable only within constrained datasets.

This study intends to predict diabetes mellitus through data analysis, utilizing blood parameters and the K-Nearest Neighbors (KNN) classifier. The study involves collecting data from diagnosed diabetes patients and healthy individuals devoid of prior diabetes history. Noteworthy parameters include fasting blood sugar, hemoglobin A1c (HbA1c), serum creatinine, total cholesterol, triglycerides, and high-density lipoprotein (HDL) cholesterol. These parameters form the foundation for training the KNN classifier [6].

The KNN algorithm, a supervised machine learning tool, classifies data based on proximity to other data points. Notably, it operates without making assumptions about data distribution, embracing a non-parametric approach. To elucidate the study entails data collection from 768 patients, encompassing variables such as blood glucose, blood pressure, and body mass index (BMI), which are then partitioned into training and testing subsets.

This study demonstrates the potential of data analysis and machine learning algorithms, specifically KNN, in predicting diabetes mellitus. Such methodologies promise to transform early detection and management, ultimately fostering improved patient well-being.

However, the validation of results and algorithm optimization for clinical applications necessitate further research.

10.2 LITERATURE STUDY

Diabetes Mellitus (DM) stands as a persistent ailment affecting millions globally, underscoring the importance of timely detection and effective management to avert complications. In recent times, the utilization of data analysis and machine learning techniques has garnered increasing attention for the prediction and control of DM. The ensuing literature review delves into the application of data analysis in the realm of DM prediction.

Mujumdar et al. [7] introduced a method for predicting significant diabetic complications through concealed pattern recognition. Their approach postulates the emergence of issues such as diabetic retinopathy, diabetic kidney disease, and heart disease in type 2 diabetes patients. The study utilized a dataset furnished by type 2 diabetic patients, subjecting it to diverse algorithms for complications identification. Among these, the Random Forest algorithm emerged as the most adept in forecasting complications, showcasing potential as a healthcare decision-making tool. The feature which has been chosen to predict the disease is not effective as it provides low accuracy.

Farhana et al. [8] conducted a study aiming to prognosticate diabetes-related features. They mined patient records employing assorted data mining techniques, culminating in a fuzzy classifier model geared towards precise predictions concerning cardiac and renal complications. The findings revealed a substantial proportion of diabetes patients at heightened risk for both cardiac and renal issues. This kind of analysis encompassed data from 485 DM patients and 490 non-DM patients, employing the Random Forest algorithm for DM prediction. The results exhibited a satisfactory accuracy of 81.8% in patient classification. Analogous to the previous study, age, BMI, and fasting plasma glucose levels emerged as critical predictors of DM. The chosen attributes were not given the precise value for classifiers.

Ahamed et al. [9] introduced a method for Diabetes Mellitus Disease prediction using Machine Learning Classifiers, bolstered by Oversampling and Feature Augmentation. Their model hinged on Bayesian and KNN algorithms, primed to aid medical practitioners in diabetes-related predictions. The study scrutinized a diabetic patient database, evaluating multiple diabetes features for disease prognosis. The classifiers have not given a worth full results for early predcition.

Bhat et al. [10] delved into the Prevalence and Early Prediction of Diabetes Using Machine Learning. This comprehensive survey examined diverse data mining approaches employed in previous diabetes prediction and analysis endeavors. This diabetes disease leveraged the Support Vector Machine (SVM) algorithm to scrutinize data from 585 DM patients and 557 non-DM patients. Impressively, the SVM algorithm achieved a commendable accuracy of 92.6% in classifying patients. This study pinpointed age, Body Mass Index (BMI), and family history of DM as pivotal factors for DM prognosis. This kind of early prediction have not satisfied a fruitful classification of this disease.

Tasin et al. [11] proposed a methodology involving machine learning and explainable AI techniques for diabetes prediction. Their research culminated in a refined diagnostic approach, leveraging various methods to rectify missing values and enhance classification accuracy. The study, anchored by the Pima Indian Diabetes Dataset, showcased a remarkable 99% accuracy in classification. A diabetes data have been encompassed from 2,000 DM patients, employing the K-Nearest Neighbor (KNN) algorithm for DM prediction. This study documented an accuracy of 73.5% in patient classification, with fasting plasma glucose levels and HbA1c levels identified as pivotal indicators for DM prediction. In this method, the accuracy of the proposed system was not effective.

Khaleel et al. [12] addressed about Data Mining for Diabetes and the Development of Prediction Models Using Rapid Miner. It merge the data from diabetic and non-diabetic participants, harnessing Rapid Miner for vital data mining tasks encompassing preprocessing, outlier detection, normalization, and more. This approach culminated in an algorithm capable of accurately anticipating diabetes onset and associated complications. The precision of this method has certain drawbacks such as the accuracy is 83%.

Massari et al. [13] explored the micro vascular effects of diabetes via assorted data mining techniques. Their approach harnessed C5.0 and neural networks to elucidate associations between diabetes complications like diabetic retinopathy, diabetic nephropathy, and diabetic foot issues. Statistical analyses conducted on a comprehensive subject pool yielded significant insights, particularly highlighting creatinine as a pivotal factor in diabetic retinopathy prognosis.The data mining techniques used by the author is only applicable to select the data from homogeneous group of diseases.

Zbiciak et al. [14] briefed about the highlights that diabetes is a heterogeneous group of diseases characterized by chronically elevated blood glucose levels. It is divided into several categories, including type 1 diabetes, type 2 diabetes gestational diabetes, and diabetes due to other causes. Type 2 diabetes and type 1 diabetes account for the majority of diabetes cases. Biomarkers such as islet autoantibodies and genetic tests can help establish the subtype of diabetes. However, the current classification system inadequately captures the heterogeneity seen in patient presentations, disease course, response to therapy, and disease complications. Therefore, the paper aims to refine diabetes subtypes using data-driven approaches based on clinical phenotypes and genetic information. The researchers applied a clustering methodology to assign participants into five predefined diabetes subtypes based on age at diabetes diagnosis, BMI, HbA1c, fasting C-peptide levels, and the presence of glutamate decarboxylase antibodies at baseline. The effect of glargine (insulin) versus standard care on hyperglycemia was compared between subtypes using logistic regression models. The interaction between subtype and intervention was also assessed. Multiple hypothesis testing was performed to adjust for the analysis of retinopathy and cardiovascular diseases.

Yousef et al. [15] utilized data mining techniques for diabetes prediction. The classification method that assigns data items into target categories or classes based on their similarity to neighboring data points. The paper compares the accuracy of the data mining algorithm for classifying diabetes data. It addresses the major health challenge of diabetes by applying data mining methods to extract knowledge from healthcare data, such as sugar patient sets. The study highlights the importance of data records in healthcare, as they help doctors study different patterns in the dataset, contributing to the understanding and management of diabetes.

In summation, these studies underscore the potential of data analysis and machine learning algorithms in DM prediction and management, offering promising avenues for early detection, care, and complication prevention. However, further research is imperative to corroborate findings and fine-tune algorithms for real-world clinical implementation. Moreover, the integration of Internet of Things (IoT) devices holds promise for disease prediction [16,17], affording enhanced symptom identification and early-stage prognosis. The amalgamation of patient blood parameters within a comprehensive database, subsequently subjected to KNN classifier algorithm for pattern recognition, exemplifies a robust methodology for predictive analysis [18].

10.3 METHODOLOGY

The objective of this study was to assess the feasibility of predicting diabetic disorders through data analysis using a comprehensive set of blood parameters collected from diabetic patients. The measured parameters included age, fasting blood sugar (FBS), postprandial blood sugar (PPBS), HbA1c, average glucose, serum cholesterol, monocytes, albumin, and creatinine levels. To facilitate efficient data retrieval and processing of numerous continuous queries over an extended duration, we implemented a structured data storage system based on a conceptual framework, ultimately establishing a comprehensive data repository. These endeavors were undertaken to enhance the overall research efficiency. The data analysis process, primarily conducted using Python programming, centered on diagnosing diabetic diseases, with a specific focus on heart diseases and kidney complications associated with diabetes.

Figure 10.1 presents a procedural flowchart illustrating the methodology employed for assessing cardiovascular and renal risks in diabetic individuals. Initially, we established a comprehensive data repository comprising physiological data from approximately 140 cases, obtained with the requisite permissions from the relevant authorities. The collected data can be classified into two primary categories: continuous datasets and categorical datasets. The data used in this proposed work falls into the category of continuous datasets. Subsequently, following rigorous data analysis, we segregated the dataset into distinct subsets: the training dataset and the testing dataset. Seventy percent of the data were utilized for training, with the remaining 30% used for the testing. This approach ensures robust evaluation and prediction (Figure 10.2).

The recognition was achieved by developing an algorithm to forecast the dangers to both the heart and the kidneys. For the purpose of predicting diabetic kidney diseases, the K Neighbor classifier was utilized. A diagrammatic presentation of the steps involved in the procedures in the method that is used to forecast diabetic complications by using a KNN classifier can be seen in the figure [8]. This method is described in more detail later. The KNN classification algorithm is then applied to the data set that was previously saved in the database after first getting the relevant blood parameters from the patients and storing them in the database. Following that, a cutoff value for the criteria is agreed upon, and this decision is determined after interacting with professionals working in the field of health care.

In the table that is seen in figure [9], both the normal levels and the values that are considered to be abnormal for the various blood parameters that were used for this investigation are presented. The potential repercussions that could arise as a result of each distinct combination of blood parameter readings are also provided. These values represent the threshold that must be reached with an essential for the algorithm to be able to produce an accurate estimate of the complications that may arise. If it is identified that the patient has diabetes, the algorithm will mark this as an abnormality, and it won't be until later that the problems will be found that they will be discovered. The programme checks the additional parameters of cardiac and renal problems to make sure they are correct. The patient is

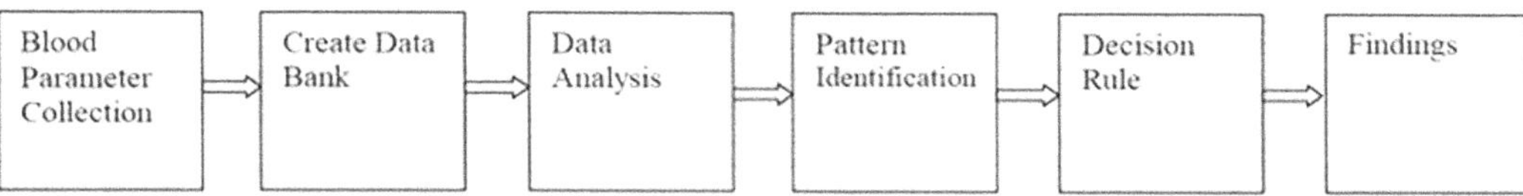

Figure 10.1 Flowchart of the methodology.

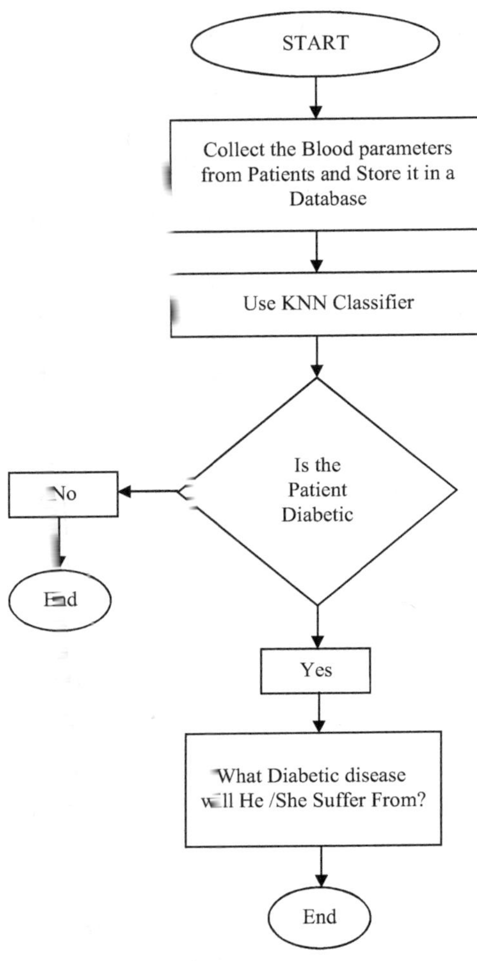

Figure 10.2 Data flow.

classified as having the corresponding diseases that they would be suffering from by the procedure if the principles of certain strictures are more than the inception measures or the usual level. For example, diabetics are classified as having the disease if the critical point or level is exceeded.

Table 10.1 outlines essential risk parameters for diabetes mellitus, offering normal, mid-range, and high values for key tests crucial in diabetes management. These parameters serve as a valuable reference for healthcare professionals and individuals with diabetes to gauge their risk and potential complications. Notably, HbA1C levels, indicating long-term blood sugar control, are associated with heart diseases and stroke when elevated. Serum creatinine levels, when exceeding 1.3 mg/dL, are indicative of diabetic kidney diseases. Low serum albumin levels, below 3.4 g/dL, may signal mild kidney disease. Elevated serum cholesterol levels, above 150 mg/dL, increase the risk of heart diseases and stroke. Moreover, heightened monocyte levels, surpassing 8%, are linked to arteriogenesis and heart diseases due to their role in inflammation and plaque formation in blood vessels. Monitoring and managing these parameters within recommended ranges are crucial for minimizing diabetes-related complications and maintaining overall health.

Table 10.1 Risk parameters of diabetes mellitus

Tests	*Normal values*	*Mid-range*	*High values*	*Complications*
HbA1C	4–6	7–9	10–13	Heart diseases, stroke
Serum creatinine	0.7–1.3 mg/dL	–	Greaterthan1.3	Diabetic kidney diseases
Serum albumin	3.4–5.4 g/dL	–	Lower than 3.4	Mild kidney disease
Serum cholesterol	Less than 150 mg/dL	–	Higher than 150 mg/dL	Heart diseases Or stroke
Monocytes	3–7%	–	Greaterthan8%	Arterogenisis (heart diseases)

10.3.1 Data analysis

Data mining is the systematic process of discovering previously undisclosed patterns within a given dataset, with the aim of extracting actionable insights. The proposed work involved the collection of blood data from diabetes patients to predict potential heart and kidney-related issues. Two primary research approaches, quantitative and qualitative, each with its own distinct methodology, are employed for data analysis. The acquired data undergoes a structured organization process before undergoing rigorous data cleansing procedures, leading to the establishment of a comprehensive data repository [19]. Subsequently, the information is subjected to meticulous data analysis techniques. To ensure the precision of our predictions and, consequently, the achievement of our intended outcomes, appropriate classifiers were used. The insights derived from this analysis play a pivotal role in shaping the decision-making processes.

10.4 RESULTS AND DISCUSSIONS

To substantiate the research, datasets were obtained from the UCI data repository. Illustrated in Figure 10.4, predictive analysis was conducted on the gathered dataset using the K-Nearest Neighbors (KNN) classifier. This analysis covered a total of 140 distinct cases, post data aggregation and storage in a designated database. The KNN algorithm carries out classification by utilizing newly acquired data points, making decisions rooted in similarity metrics. The dataset was partitioned into 20 subsets, with each subset containing data from five different subjects. Classification decisions relied on majority voting, where the consensus of nearest neighbors determined the classification outcome. The model's accuracy directly correlated with the number of neighbors considered in the analysis. The KNN classifier yielded a commendable accuracy level of 71.42%. Furthermore, the dataset was split into 20 sets, each including data from five distinct patients, as indicated in the accompanying figure. Optimal accuracy was observed at the fifth neighbor ($k = 5$). With input from medical professionals, threshold values for each parameter were established. These thresholds were subsequently incorporated into calculations to provide prognostic insights concerning diabetes-related complications. Key features such as Serum Creatinine, Cholesterol, Albumin, Glucose, PPBS, Age, and FBS, as outlined in Table 10.2, are integral to this research work.

Table 10.2 Pre-processed dataset used for analysis

Age	*FBS (mgs/dl)*	*PPBS (mgs/dl)*	*Avg.Glucose*	*Monocytes (%)*	*Serum cholesterol*	*Serum Creatnine*	*Albumin (g/dl)*
70	120	180	6.1	136	2	128	1
40	100	160	4.1	87	5	175	0.4
32	120	180	7.2	259	3	161	1.2
68	108	197	7.8	300	2	170	2.1
47	180	250	7.1	320	6	310	0.6
56	184	261	8.1	182	2	224	0.8

Table 10.2 presents a pre-processed dataset utilized for analysis. The table includes several health-related parameters for a group of individuals. It comprises their age in years, fasting blood sugar (FBS) levels in milligrams per deciliter (mg/dL), postprandial blood sugar (PPBS) levels, average glucose levels (mg/dL), the percentage of monocytes in their blood, serum cholesterol levels (mg/dL), serum creatinine levels, and albumin levels in grams per deciliter (g/dL). This dataset offers a comprehensive view of various health markers and can be used for diverse analyses, including exploring relationships between these parameters, identifying potential health trends or risk factors, or developing predictive models for specific health outcomes. Such analysis holds the potential to yield valuable insights into health conditions, aiding in informed decision-making regarding medical interventions or lifestyle adjustments.

In this datasets, the extracted features are involved for preprocessing task. After preprocessing, the values are feed to the classifier to estimate the mellitus status. In this chapter, the performance measurement of prediction accuracy is compared with Decision tree induction with all the considered parameters. The comparative analyzes depicted that K means algorithm have given high accuracy of predicting the diabetes mellitus, Table 10.3 presents a performance analysis of two classifiers, K-Nearest Neighbors (KNN) and Decision Tree Induction, based on key performance metrics expressed as percentages. KNN demonstrates superior performance across multiple metrics, including accuracy (71.42% vs. 69.3%), precision (70.21% vs. 67.36%), recall (70.38% vs. 69.4%), and F-Score (70.48% vs. 68.3%). These metrics are crucial in assessing the effectiveness of classification algorithms in tasks such as machine learning and data mining. The data in the table suggests that KNN may be the more favorable choice for the specific task under consideration, as it consistently outperforms Decision Tree Induction. However, the selection of the best classifier ultimately depends on the specific goals and requirements of the application in question.

The comparative analysis methods have produced the values based on the parameters that have been considered to carry out this work. The comparative analysis chart has been depicted in Figure 10.3.

Table 10.3 Performance analysis of classifiers

S.No	*Performance (%)*	*KNN*	*Decision Tree Induction*
1	Accuracy	71.42	69.3
2	Precision	70.21	67.36
3	Recall	70.38	69.4
4	F- Score	70.48	68.3

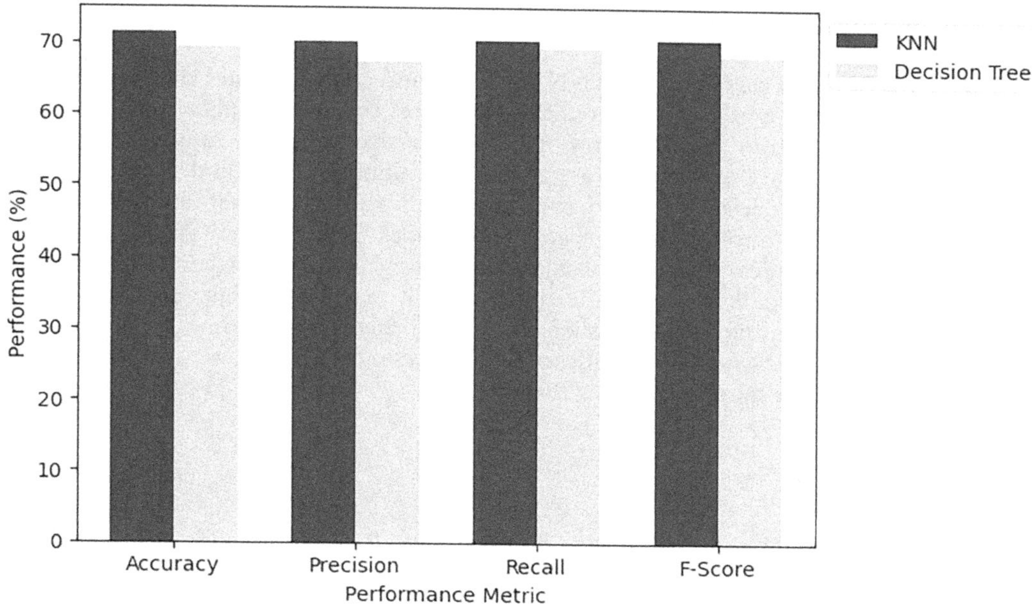

Figure 10.3 Performance analysis of classifier to predict the diabetes disease.

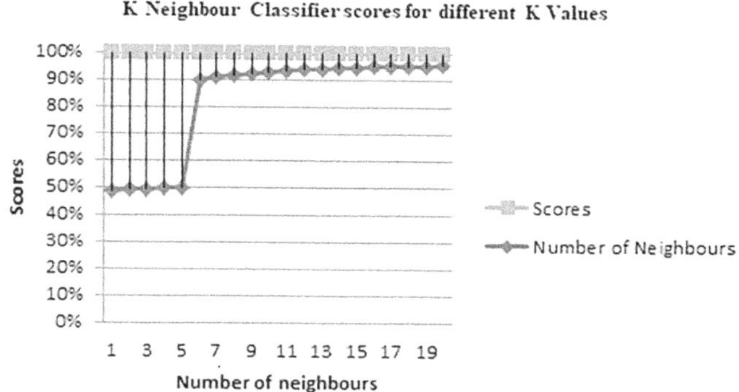

Figure 10.4 A graph illustrating the KNN classifier scores for a variety of K values.

The comparative analysis techniques employed in this study have yielded values based on carefully selected parameters. These findings are visually presented in Figure 10.3, where the x-axis represents performance metrics, and the y-axis illustrates classifier performance. Notably, the K-Nearest Neighbors (KNN) algorithm has demonstrated superior accuracy when compared to the Decision Tree Induction method, particularly concerning the chosen disease prediction parameters. Consequently, this chapter offers a graphical representation highlighting the effectiveness of the KNN classifier in achieving higher accuracy. Figure 10.4 delves into the diverse values of K employed for disease classification, further emphasizing the robust performance of the KNN approach across these parameters when contrasted with alternative classifiers.

10.5 CONCLUSION

Leveraging the K-Nearest Neighbors (KNN) classifier and comprehensive data analysis, the study underscores the potential of predicting diabetes-related complications. Extensive medical variables contributed to achieving an impressive accuracy rate of 71.42% in forecasting the occurrence of heart disease and kidney ailments. This model not only holds promise as a valuable decision support tool for healthcare practitioners but also has the potential to contribute to improved patient outcomes and reduced healthcare costs. Subsequent research endeavors may consider augmenting prediction accuracy through the utilization of larger datasets and the inclusion of additional relevant parameters. Furthermore, incorporating variables such as lifestyle factors and family genetic history could further enhance classification and prediction accuracy for diabetic mellitus disease, extending the scope for more precise outcomes.

REFERENCES

1. Han, L., Luo, S., Yu, J., Pan, L., & Chen, S. (20 8). Rule extraction from support vector machines using ensemble learning approach: an application for diagnosis of diabetes. IEEE J. Biomed. Health Inform., 19, 728–734. doi: 10.1109/JBHI.2014.2325615
2. Bengio, Y., & Grandvalet, Y. (2005). Bias in Estimating the Variance of K-Fold Cross-Validation. New York, NY: Springer, 75–95. doi: 10.1007/0-387-24555-3
3. Su, Z. D., Huang, Y., Zhang, Z. Y., Zhao, Y. W., Wang, D., Chen, W., et al. (2018). iLoc-lncRNA: predict the subcellular location of lncRNAs by incorporating octamer composition into general PseKNC. Bioinformatics, 34(24), 4196–4204. doi: 10.1093/bioinformatics/bty508 [Epub ahead of print].
4. Liao, Z., Ju, Y., & Zou, Q. (2020). Prediction of G protein-coupled receptors with SVM-Prot features and random forest. Scientifica, 2016, 8309253. doi: 10.1155/2016/8309253
5. Tang, W., Wan, S., Yang, Z., Teschendorff, A. E., & Zou, Q. (2019). Tumor origin detection with tissue-specific miRNA and DNA methylation markers. Bioinformatics, 34, 398–406. doi: 10.1093/bioinformatics/btx622
6. Liao, Z. J., Wan, S., He, Y., & Zou, Q. (2018). Classification of small GTPases with hybrid protein features and advanced machine learning techniques. Curr. Bioinform., 13, 492–500. doi: 10.2174/1574893612666171121162552
7. Mujumdar, A., & Vaidehi, V. (2019). Diabetes prediction using machine learning algorithms. Procedia Comput. Sci., 165, 292–299. doi: 10.1016/j.procs.2020.01.047
8. Farhana, B., Munidhanalakshmi, K., & Mohana, R. M. 2021). Predict diabetes mellitus using machine learning algorithms. J. Phys., 2089(1), 012002. doi: 10.1088/1742-6596/2089/1/012002
9. Ahamed, B. S., Arya, M. S., & Nancy, A. O. (2022). Diabetes mellitus disease prediction using machine learning classifiers with oversampling and feature augmentation. Adv. Human-Comput. Interaction, 2022, 1–14. doi: 10.1155/2022/92 0560
10. Bhat, S. S., Selvam, V., Ansari, G. A., Ansari, M. N., & Rahman, M. H. (2022). Prevalence and early prediction of diabetes using machine learning in North Kashmir: a case study of District Bandipora. Comput. Intell. Neurosci., 2022, 1–12. doi: 10.1155/2022/2789760
11. Tasin, I., Nabil, T. U., Islam, S., & Khan, R. (2022). Diabetes prediction using machine learning and explainable AI techniques. Healthcare Technol. Lett., 10(1–2), 1–10. doi: 10.1049/htl2.12039
12. Khaleel, F. A., & Al-Bakry, A. M. (2023). Diagnosis of diabetes using machine learning algorithms. Materials Today: Proceedings, 80, 3200–3203. doi: 10.1016/j.matpr.2021.07.196

13. Massari, H. E., Sabouri, Z., Mhammedi, S., & Gherabi, N. (2022). Diabetes prediction using machine learning algorithms and ontology. J. ICT Standardisation, 10(02), 319–338. doi: 10.13052/jicts2245-800x.10212
14. Zbiciak, A., & Markiewicz, T. (2023). A new extraordinary means of appeal in the Polish criminal procedure: the basic principles of a fair trial and a complaint against a cassatory judgment. *Access to Just. E. Eur.*, 25.
15. Yousef, M. Z., Yasky, A. F., Al Shammari, R., & Ferwana, M. S. (2022 Jul 22). Early prediction of diabetes by applying data mining techniques: A retrospective cohort study. Medicine (Baltimore), 101(29), e29588. doi: 10.1097/MD.0000000000029588
16. Chithaluru, P., Al-Turjman, F., Kumar, M., & Stephan, T. (2023). Computational-intelligence-inspired adaptive opportunistic clustering approach for industrial IoT networks. IEEE Internet Things J., 10(9), 7884–7892. doi: 10.1109/JIOT.2022.3231605
17. Rajendran, M., Stephan, P., Stephan, T., Agarwal, S., & Kim, H. (2022). Cognitive IoT vision system using weighted guided Harris Corner feature detector for visually impaired people. Sustainability, 14(15), 9063. 10.3390/su14159063 Appendix: Taylor & Francis-Author Discount
18. Lin, C., Chen, W., Qiu, C., Wu, Y., Krishnan, S., & Zou, Q. (2020). LibD3C: ensemble classifiers with a clustering and dynamic selection strategy. Neurocomputing, 123, 424–435. doi: 10.1016/j.neucom.2013.08.004
19. Habibi, S., Ahmadi, M., & Alizadeh, S. (2019). Type 2 diabetes mellitus screening and risk factors using decision tree: results of data mining. Glob. J. Health Sci., 7, 304–310. doi: 10.553 9/gjhs.v7n5p304

Chapter 11

A combined neuro-fuzzy and Naive Bayes approach for swine flu disease prediction

P Santhi[1], *M Sathya Sundaram*[2], *and P Pandiaraja*[3]

[1]TIFAC-CORE in Cyber Security, Amrita School of Engineering, Amrita Vishwa Vidyapeetham, Coimbatore, Tamil Nadu, India

[2]Department of Computer Science and Engineering, Paavai Engineering College, Namakkal, Tamilnadu, India

[3]Department of Computer Science and Engineering, M Kumarasamy College of Engineering, Karur, Tamilnadu, India

11.1 INTRODUCTION

Swine flu is a micro organism disease. It is caused by fungi and viruses. This disease can be spread, directly or indirectly, from one person to another, which is known as a communicable disease. Swine flu, Hepatitis A, HIV/AIDS, TB, etc., are some forms of communicable diseases. Swine flu is caused by Influenza viruses. It has five subtypes: H1N1, H1N2, H2N3, H3N1, and H3N2. Previously, those who had direct contact with pigs were affected by this flu. Since 2009, it has spread very fast; a new strain of H1N1 is labeled as a pandemic by WHO. It is communicated by people's interaction with non-living objects infested by viruses and is transported to the nose and the eyes. It encode 11 different proteins (NA, HA, PB1, PB2, PB1-F2, PB, PA, M1, M2, NS2 and NS1). The RBC are grouped together and connect the viruses to the infected cells. The virus particles are moved to the infected cells and the NA helps to grow the host cells [1].

Influenza and RNA viruses can be divided based on the protein consumption A, B, and C. Influenza A can be further subdivided into HA and NA depending on the protein surface. To identify the origin of pandemic swine flu virus strains, this author applied SVM and decision tree machine learning techniques. This existing work uses the sequences of nucleotides and protein for decision tree and SVM classifiers. The decision tree is trained using three host groups. They built different HMM profiles for finding the Influenza virus host. They developed a prediction tool using LAMP technology to detect a swine flu origin [2].

Influenza-A H1N1 virus leads to problems including pneumonia, lung infection, and other breathing problems. Sometimes it could be life-threatening problems. In the year 2017, as per the media reports, more than 22,000 cases have been reported across India. It can be easily curable if it is diagnosed in the earlier stage. The epidemic of Influenza-A H1N1 was classified as A, B, and C Viruses. 'A'-Category will be categorized by the patients with mild fever, cough or sore throat, headache, body ache, vomiting, and diarrhea. Here the patients are separated in the home and are not allowed to mingle with others. 'B'-Category will contain high grade fever and severe sore threat and effect pregnant woman, child < 5 years, adults > 65 years, and patients with lung diseases, cancer, kidney disorders, HIV/AIDS, diabetes, etc,. A deep learning approach is used to extract the spatial and temporal features [3]. 'C'-Category will also have symptoms such as chest pain, breathlessness, fall in BP, and nails with blood bluish staining [4].

DOI: 10.1201/9781003369059-14

Influenza virus communication is powerfully modified by weather conditions like humidity and temperature. Influenza is strongly circulated during winter time, and is detected around two or three months. In this work, the researcher has tested viral spread between the host by considering the ambient temperature and relative humidity. They detected that transmission was active between 5 to 30 degrees Celsius. They also considered another important parameter for transmission as RH. When the RH factor is very low, the virus was constantly stable [5].

The people above 65 and the children below 5 are at high risk. Children with asthma and COPD are at high risk. Women who are pregnant would be suggested for limited tests. The swine flu could be found by use of chest x-ray, routine blood tests, and the CBC test. The symptoms of swine flu are fever, cough, runny nose, sore throat, body ache, chills, and fatigue. If it is in serious stage, skin would be a gray or bluish color, and patients would have difficulty breathing and abdominal pain, etc.

The previous study helps to identify attributes such as proteins, weather conditions, age, sex, suffering from respiratory diseases, changes in skin color, platelet count, complete blood cell count, hemoglobin tests, etc., to reduce the risk factors and the death rate. It is very difficult to collect information at the initial stage. Proper mining of data could help in controlling the diseases and improve the effectiveness in treatment.

Due to the growth of the internet, many people ask for help regarding their health issues. We can predict the disease using big data analytics with enormous data available on tweets, survey reports, news, search query data, etc. Based on the results, more awareness will be provided and the death rate will be reduced.

11.1.1 Research data

The data was collected from social media, databases available from the government, tweets, search query data, etc., and protein sequences can be retrieved from the database using GenBank. The multiple sequence alignment and phylogenetic trees for emergent pandemic virus strains were computed using the HKY + gamma model of evolution with six gene segments (PB2, PB1, PA, HA, NP, NS). Concentric circle-based clustering and multi class classification is also used for image clustering and also for the classification [6].

In swine flu, a major factor is climate and weather conditions. This disease is also caused by the monsoon patterns in certain areas. Another weather factor at play here is the difference between maximum and minimum temperatures at a place [7]. The data were collected from different geographical conditions [8]. Some healthcare systems are developed for diagnosing the swine flu. Shikimic acid is used to treat the swine flu. This acid is produced from the fermentation process [9,10]. Swine flu is detected using the concepts of neural networks and map reduced concepts [11,12].

The big data was collected through the web crawler using the python selenium library from twitter. The communicable diseases were recorded daily. It includes age, sex, respiratory conditions, etc [9]. Search engines and social networking can show the trajectory of different diseases. It also includes patient data in electronic patient records, clinical data from clinical decision support systems, machine generated data from monitoring vital signs, human generated data from paper documents, etc. [13,14].

The map reduced based LSTM approach is also used for the purpose of classification [15]. The proposed approach in this article demonstrates the use of IoT-based techniques for seizure detection in epilepsy monitoring. This work can be cited as a future direction to explore the integration of IoT devices and data analytics techniques for real-time monitoring and prediction of swine flu. By incorporating IoT sensors and data analysis methods similar to the ones used in this article, the authors can enhance the data collection process and improve the accuracy of the swine flu prediction system [16]. This article investigates the impacts of COVID-19 on renewable energy transitions and air quality using machine learning analysis. The authors of the chapter can cite this work to highlight the potential for applying machine learning techniques to analyze the impact of swine flu on various aspects such as public health, healthcare infrastructure, and environmental factors. By incorporating similar analysis methods, the authors can provide a comprehensive assessment of the consequences and potential mitigation strategies associated with swine flu outbreaks [17].

11.2 METHODS AND IMPLEMENTATION

Large amounts of data are created from a variety of sources every day. Big data in healthcare is unbelievable not only because of its volume but also due to the variety of data types and the velocity at which it must be managed [18–20]. The data collected may be structured, unstructured and semi structured etc. The collected data may contain missing values, inconsistent data, superfluous data, and also noisy data. Data should be preprocessed to change them, so that it contains only the essential attributes for our predication.

The data related to swine flu is collected from the Genbank https://www.ncbi.nlm.nih.gov/genomes/FLU/SwineFlu.html [21]. This database contains the virus sequence collected in the years 2009 to 2010. This database is has eight attributes with 934 data. The attributes are PB2, PA, PB1, NP, HA, NA, NS, and MP. This virus sequence is related to the Influenza A (H1N1) virus. The database contains various types of virus sequences. So, the data preprocessing is used to improve the quality of this research. In this work, data preprocessing techniques are used to generate quality data. The main tasks in data preprocessing are data normalization and data reduction. Min-Max normalization is concentrated for the normalization to convert the different values into normalized values. Before Min-Max normalization, standard scalar method is applied to convert the various virus sequence into numeric form. Feature Selection is an important task for the classifier, which selects a highly impact feature from the dataset [22,23]. Any classifier mainly depends on the highly impacted features for producing the higher result with better performance. This chapter using the Neuro-Fuzzy logic for feature selection, which is the combination of both fuzzy and Artificial Neural Networks (ANN). After the feature selection, the high impact features are given to the classifier as an input, and finally it produces the classification output. Here the Naive Bayes classifier is used for the classification of swine flu data [24].

11.2.1 Feature selection using neuro-fuzzy system

The dataset contains 'M' features or attributes to perform the classification. In practice, some of these features are not relevant for our classification and it may be uncorrelated with the class labels. These features could not be able to produce the better classifier and sometimes it will degrade the performance of it. So avoid these kinds of situations; the feature selection is used for eliminating the irrelevant and avoiding the features having a low impact on the process. Here, the Neuro-Fuzzy approach is used for the purpose of selecting the features without decreasing the quality of the input dataset. In this system, the fuzzy controller is trained using the NN concepts of either back propagation or by a genetic algorithm. The main reason behind this combination is to increase the efficiency of the fuzzy controller. This system is constructed using either Mamdani approach or Takagi and Sugeno's approach [11].

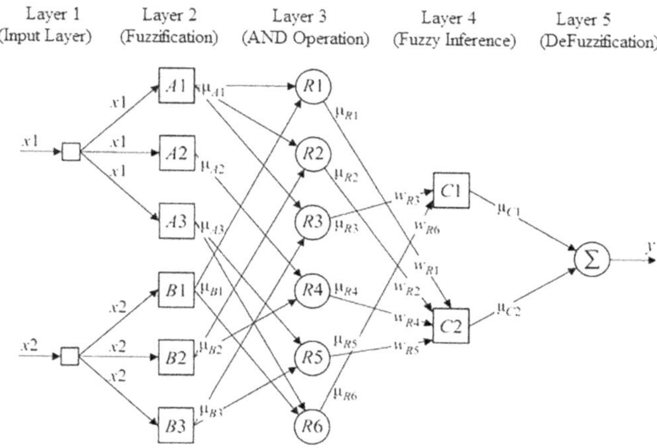

Figure 11.1 Architecture of neuro-fuzzy system using Mamdani approach.

Here the Neuro-Fuzzy is constructed using Mamdani approach. Figure 11.1 shows the architecture for Mamdani approach, in which it contains five layers: Layer 1 is an Input Layer, Layer 2 consists of fuzzification, AND operation is in Layer 3, and Fuzzy inference and defuzzification are the layers 4 and 5.

The input layer does not have any specific task. Here, it will perform the linear transformation, and the same input is passed to the process of fuzzification. Fuzzification is a process of converting the raw input into the fuzzy value through Membership Function (MF). A membership function is a building block of the fuzzy system, which contains the various shapes triangular, trapezoidal, Gaussian, etc. A membership function can be in any shape, but it is has a membership value between 0 and 1. The number of membership functions influences the computational time [8]. In most of the research, we can use the triangular shape for its simplicity and less computation time. If the problem is more complex, then other types of shapes will be in consideration, ones that find the fittest shape for the given problem [12]. This chapter concentrates on the Gaussian Membership function to generate the membership value. Figure 11.2 shows the example of Gaussian MF.

The Gaussian MF is represented as Gaussian of x: c, s. μ (x, c, s, m) is as follows:

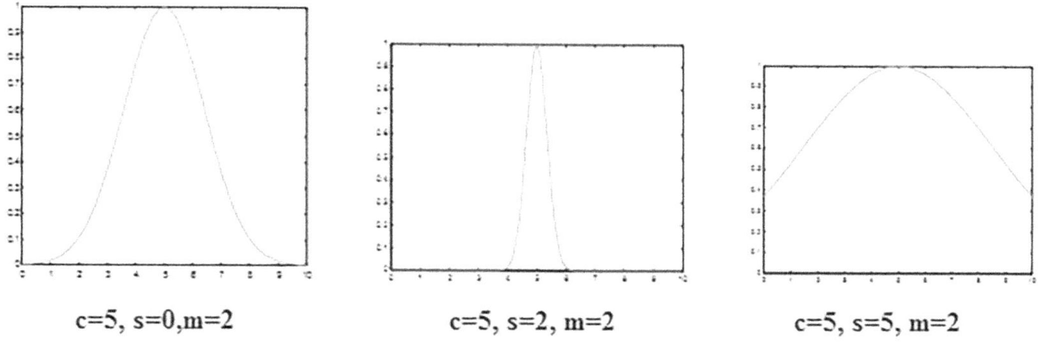

Figure 11.2 Different shapes in Gaussian membership function.

$$\mu(x, c, s, m) = exp\left[\left(-\frac{1}{2}\right)\left|\frac{(x-c)}{s}\right|^{m}\right] \tag{11.1}$$

Where,

c, s, and m indicate the mean, standard deviation, and fuzzification factor. The value of mean 'c' is calculated using:

$$c = \frac{(x1 + x2 + x3 + \ldots\ldots + xn)}{n} \tag{11.2}$$

$$S = \sqrt{\frac{(x-c)^2}{n}} \tag{11.3}$$

Where, x – Set of numbers, c – Mean, Value n – Total number of data

11.2.2 Naive Bayes classifier

Pattern recognition is used for automatic detection of uniformities of data through computer algorithms and with the use of these uniformities data can be categorized into different classes. The classes can be created by using the Naive Bayes classifier algorithm. The parameters used to categorize into different classes are phylogenetic segments, age, RH factors, temperature, Area, WBC count, and sex. Three different classes are created based on different parameters.

In this work, the whole dataset was divided into training, validation, and test data subsets. The Naive Bayes classifier was used to predict the probability based on Bayes' theorem. Each training data can easily update the probability distribution, calculating both the prior probabilities and conditional probabilities. Prior probability of diseases may occur on the basis of phylogenetic segments, age, Rh factors, and temperature. A Naive Bayes classification was trained using the features extracted from the training data and also included pattern matching rules.

Let A = $\{a_1, a_2, \ldots \ldots a_n\}$ be a set of pre computed features to show whether or not the particular categories belongs to one class. The main properties of the Naive Bayes classifier is class conditional independence. This property is represented as follows:

$$P\left(\frac{A}{B}\right) = \frac{P\left(\frac{B}{A}\right)P(A)}{P(B)} \tag{11.4}$$

Where, P(A/B) and P(B/A) – Posterior Probability P(A) and P(B) – Proir Probability,

The posterior probability of P(A/B) and P(B/A) is calculated using Eqs. (11.5) and (11.6).

$$P\left(\frac{A}{B}\right) = \frac{P(A \cap B)}{P(B)} \tag{11.5}$$

$$P\left(\frac{B}{A}\right) = \frac{P(B \cap A)}{P(A)} \tag{11.6}$$

11.3 RESULTS AND DISCUSSION

The dataset consists of eight features: Genotype, Subtype, PB2, PB1, PA, HA, NP, and NA. Table 11.1 shows the output of Fuzzification. In Gaussian distribution, X-axis denotes the mean value and Y- axis denotes the standard deviation. The different membership function is generated using fuzzification. Overall performance of the classifier system mainly depends on the membership function. By using this Gaussian distribution or Normal distribution, the irrelevant feature is replaced and the selected membership value is passed into the fuzzy inference system to generate the 'N' number of rules used for the prediction. Here, Gaussian distribution is constructed using Mean 'c' and Standard deviation 's' of each feature of the swine flu dataset.

The fuzzification output is passed to the Neural Networks to select the best features. The following figure shows the Neuro-Fuzzy system for the swine flu dataset, in which the features PB1 and HA are eliminated by using Gaussian Membership Function. Because these two attributes are not correlated to other attributes, they have been eliminated at zthe time of fuzzy inference, and finally, the best features are selected using the Back Propagation NN approach. Figure 11.3 shows the NN model with the features PB1 and HA having 0.010186 error rates. If these attributes are removed, then the performance of the Neuro-Fuzzy System has been increased when compared to previous models.

In the Neuro-Fuzzy system, the uncorrelated features are removed in the fuzzy inference. Fuzzy inference is a rule generation process, in which IF-THEN rules are generated for the swine flu dataset using fuzzification with the logic operation of "AND." This system has generated 48 inferences for eight inputs. Here the error rate of the Neuro-Fuzzy system is 0.010186 is shown in Figure 11.4. After the fuzzy inference, 48 inferences are reduced into 36 inferences for the six inputs. Here the error rate of the system is reduced and the performance has been increased.

The selected features using Neuro-Fuzzy is given to the Naive Bayes classifier. It is one of the most powerful and applicable for all types of datasets, like small sized to large sized datasets. The given dataset consists of 58 different tuples; these tuples are divided into 35 train datasets and 23 test datasets. The Naive Bayes classifier works based on the posterior, and also, the prior probability is called class conditional independence. Here, the Naive Bayes classifier produced 98.76% accuracy in prediction of the swine flu dataset. It was improved only because of the Neuro-Fuzzy feature selection method.

11.4 PERFORMANCE ANALYSIS

The various kinds of feature selection method are combined with the Naive Bayes classifier, and the accuracy is calculated for the input dataset. This accuracy result is shown in Figure 11.5. Here, the Neuro-Fuzzy System is analyzed against the feature selection of filter method, wrapper method, and fuzzy logic with the Naive Bayes classifier, in which the previously mentioned methods have an accuracy rate of 85.54, 88.76, 90.32, and 98.76. The Neuro-Fuzzy system has more accuracy when compared to the filter, wrapper, and fuzzy logic method. Figure 11.5 shows the accuracy rate of these methods.

This chapter uses the precision, recall, and F1 Score for calculating the performance of these algorithms. Precision is the ratio of correctly classified samples and the sum of both true positive and false positive. It is calculated using the formula 7. Formula 8 and 9 show the calculation of recall and F1 Score. Recall is the ratio between true positive and the sum of

Table 11.1 Membership function generation using Gaussian distribution

Number of Features	*Mean (c)*	*Standard Deviation (s)*	*Gaussian Distribution*
Genotype	0.827	0.920	
Subtype	1.155	1.411	
PB2	1.206	1.435	
PB1	3.982	3.521	

(Continued)

Table 11.1 (Continued) Membership function generation using Gaussian distribution

Number of Features	*Mean (c)*	*Standard Deviation (s)*	*Gaussian Distribution*
PA	0.5	0.903	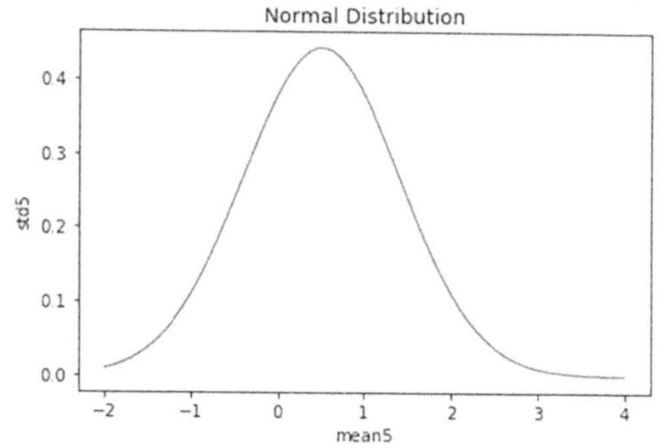
HA	3.172	3.027	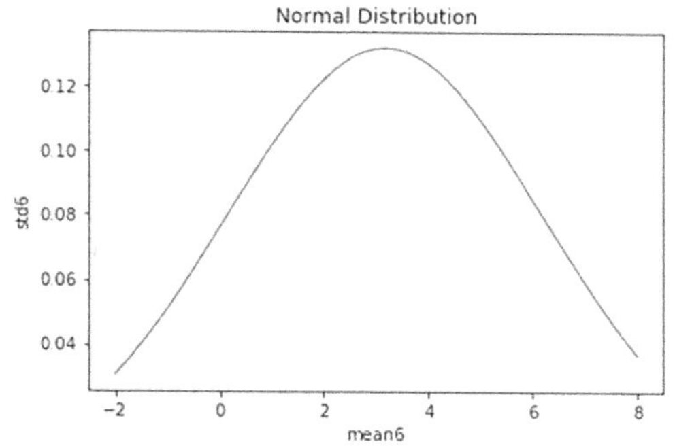
NP	0.862	1.0670	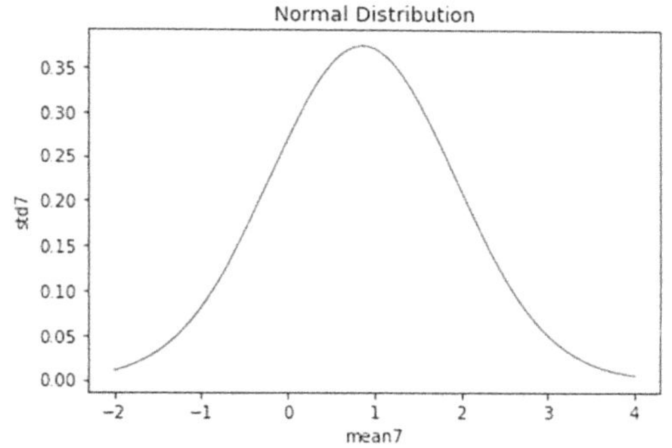
NA	0.448	0.729	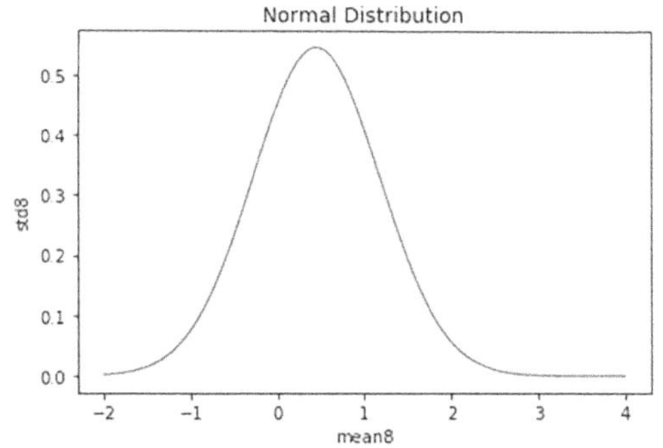

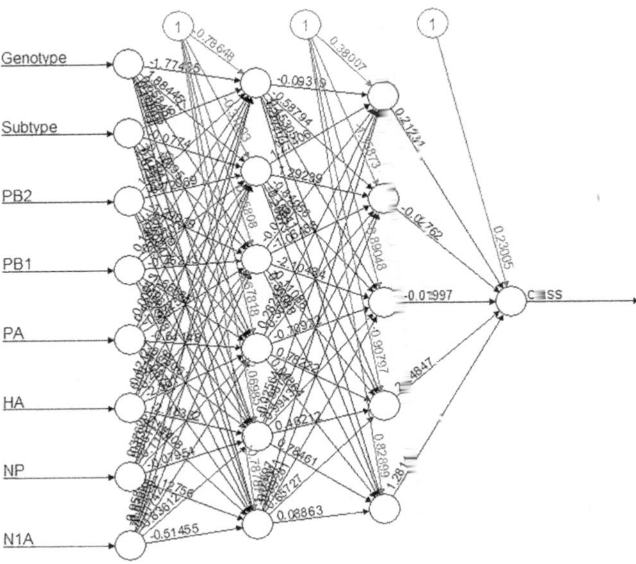

Figure 11.3 Neuro-fuzzy system with the error rate of 0.010186

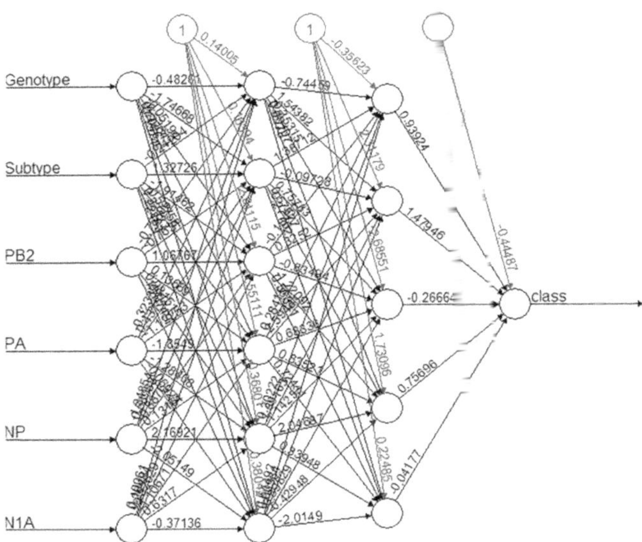

Figure 11.4 Neuro-fuzzy system with the error rate of 0.008506.

both true positive and false negative. F1 score is the ratio between the product of precision and recall and the sum of precision and recall. Performance analysis of these algorithms is shown in Table 11.2. Here, the proposed algorithm has a better performance when compared to other algorithms.

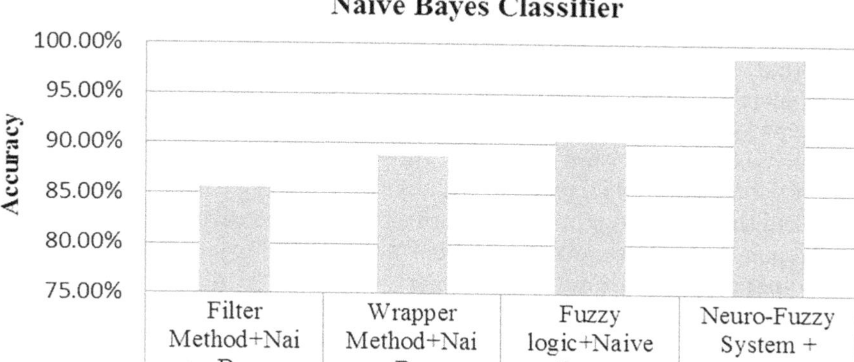

Figure 11.5 Accuracy of classification system.

Table 11.2 Performance analysis

Methods Used	*Precision (%)*	*Recall (%)*	*F1 Score (%)*
Filter +Naive Bayes Classifier	84.87	81.67	83.24
Wrapper +Naive Bayes Classifier	85.56	83.54	84.54
Fuzzy logic +Naive Bayes Classifier	88.67	84.42	86.49
Neuro Fuzzy +Naive Bayes Classifier (Proposed)	92.45	88.76	90.57

$$\text{Precision} = \frac{\text{True Positive}}{\text{True Positive} + \text{False Positive}} \tag{11.7}$$

$$\text{Recall} = \frac{\text{True Positive}}{\text{True Positive} + \text{False Negative}} \tag{11.8}$$

$$\text{F1 Score} = \frac{2 \text{ X Precision X Recall}}{\text{Precision} + \text{Recall}} \tag{11.9}$$

11.5 CONCLUSION

Swine Flu is a communicable disease caused by the pig. This disease affects the respiratory system and is caused by the influenza viruses. Because of this, many people have lost their lives. So, the prediction of swine flu would have a major impact in mortality rate reduction. In the past, most researchers have proposed many algorithms for feature selection to improve the accuracy of the prediction system. But these algorithms have rates up to 90.32%. This chapter is focused on the feature selection algorithm. Here, the performance of Fuzzy logic has been improved using the approach of Neural Networks, and the fuzzy is trained using a back propagation based NN algorithm called the Neuro-Fuzzy system. After that, the selected high impact features are given into the Naive Bayes classifier for prediction in which it produces an accuracy of 98.76%. The combined Neuro-Fuzzy and Naive Bayes approach can significantly improve the accuracy of swine flu prediction. This research improved clinical decision making and gives better performance in outcomes of public health. If the size of the data is increased, then it will degrade the performance of this proposed system. To avoid this limitation, in the future this research should be extended to use the deep learning approach in decision making, and IoT should be integrated with this approach to make the automated deep learning system.

REFERENCES

1. Jilani, T. N., Jamil, R. T., Siddiqui, A. H., H1N1 Influenza (Swine Flu), Book series, 2019.
2. Attaluri, P. K., Zheng, X., Chen, Z., Lu, G., "Applying machine learning techniques to classify H1N1 viral strains occurring in 2009 flu pandemic", The 6th Annual Biotechnology and Bioinformatics Symposium (BIOT-2009), 21–27, Oct, 2009.
3. Kanna, P. R., Santhi, P., "Unified deep learning approach for efficient intrusion detection system using integrated spatial–temporal features" Knowledge-Based Systems, 226, 1–2, 2021.
4. Mukherjee, S., Sen, S., Nakate, P. C., Moitra, S., "Management of swine flu (H1N1 flu) outbreak and its treatment guidelines", Journal of Community Acquired Infection, 2(3), 71–78, 2015.
5. Lowen, A. C., Steel, J., "Roles of humidity and temperature in shaping influenza seasonality", Journal of Virology, 88(14), 1–12, 2014. doi: 10.1128/JVI.03544-13
6. Santhi, P., Bhaskaran, V. M., "Improving the efficiency of image clustering using modified non Euclidean distance measures in data mining", International Journal of Computers Communications & Control, 9(1), 56–61, February, 2014.
7. Thakkar, B. A., Hasan, M. I., Desai, M. A., "Health care decision support system for swine flu prediction using Naive Bayes classifier", 2010 International Conference on Advances in Recent Technologies in Communication and Computing, Kottayam, India, 101–105, 2010.
8. Nelson, M. I., Souza, C. K., Trovão, N. S., Diaz, A., Mena, I., Rovira, A., Vincent, A. L., Torremorell, M., Marthaler, D., Culhane, M. R., "Human-Origin Influenza A(H3N2) reassortant viruses in swine, Southeast Mexico", Emerging Infectious Diseases, 25(4), 691–700, 2019 Apr.
9. Saxena, R. K., Tripathi, P., Rawat, G., "Pandemism of swine flu and its prospective drug therapy", European Journal of Clinical Microbiology & Infectious Diseases, 31, 3265–3279, 2012.
10. Kshatriya, R. M., Khara, N. V., Ganjiwale, J., Lote, S. D., Patel, S. N., Paliwal, R. P., "Lessons learnt from the Indian H1N1 (swine flu) epidemic: Predictors of outcome based on epidemiological and clinical profile", Journal of Family Medicine and Primary Care, 7(6), 1506–1509, Nov./Dec. 2018.
11. Miraclin Joyce Pamila, P. J. C., Senthamil Selvi, R., Santhi, P., Nithya, T. M., "Ensemble classifier based big data classification with hybrid optimal feature selection", Advances in Engineering Software, 173, 1–21, 2022.
12. Santhi, P., Lavanya, S., "Prediction of diabetes using neural networks", International Journal of Advanced Science and Technology, 29(7 Special Issue), 1160–1168, 2020.
13. Nogales, A., Martinez-Sobrido, L., Chiem, K., Topham, D. J., DeDiego, M. L., "Functional evolution of the 2009 pandemic H1N1 influenza virus NS1 and PA in humans", Journal of Virology, 92(19), Oct. 2018.

14. Baudon, E., Chu, D. K. W., Tung, D. D., Thi Nga, P., Vu Mai Phuong, H., Le Khanh Hang, N., Thanh, L. T., Thuy, N. T., Khanh, N. C., Mai, L. Q., Khong, N. V., Cowling, B. J., Peyre, M., Peiris, M., "Swine influenza viruses in Northern Vietnam in 2013-2014", Emerging Microbes & Infections, 7(1), 123, Jul. 2018.
15. Kanna, P. R., Santhi, P., "Hybrid intrusion detection using MapReduce based black widow optimized convolutional long short-term memory neural networks", Expert Systems with Applications, 194, 116545, 2022.
16. Yedurkar, D. P., Metkar, S., Al-Turjman, F., Yardi, N., Stephan, T., "An IoT-based novel hybrid seizure detection approach for epileptic monitoring," IEEE Transactions on Industrial Informatics, 20(2), 1420–1431, Feb. 2024. doi: 10.1109/TII.2023.3274913
17. Stephan, T., Al-Turjman, F., Ravishankar, M., Stephan, P., "Machine learning analysis on the impacts of COVID-19 on India's renewable energy transitions and air quality," Environmental Science and Pollution Research, 29(52), 79443–79465, Nov. 2022. doi: 10.1007/s11356-022-20997-2.
18. Ginsberg, J., Mohebbi, M. H., Patel, R. S. et al., "Detecting influenza epidemics using search engine query data", Nature, 457, U1012–U1101, 2009
19. Liang, Y., Kelemen, A., "Big data science and its applications in health and medical research: challenges and opportunities", Journal of Biometrics and Biostatistics, 7, 1–9, 2016. doi: 10.41 72/2155-6180.1000307
20. Liu, Y., Logan, B., Liu, N., Xu, Z., Tang, J., Wang, Y., "Deep Reinforcement Learning for Dynamic Treatment Regimes on Medical Registry Data", 2017 IEEE International Conference on Healthcare Informatics (ICHI), Park City, UT, USA, 380–385, 2017.
21. NCBI Influenza Virus Sequence Database: https://www.ncbi.nlm.nih.gov/genomes/FLU/SwineFlu.html, 2010.
22. Czekalski, P., "Evolution-fuzzy rule based system with parameterized consequences", International Journal of Applied Mathematics and Computer Science, 16(3), 373–385, 2006.
23. Keerthi, S., Santhi, P., "Precise multi-class classification of brain tumor via optimization based relevance vector machine", Intelligent Automation & Soft Computing, 36(1), 1173–1188, 2023.
24. Kosko, B., Mitaim, S., "What is the best shape for a fuzzy set in function approximation?" Proceedings of the 5th IEEE International Conference on Fuzzy Systems (FUZZ-96); September 1996, pp. 1237–1243.

Chapter 12

Enhancing decision-making in maternal public healthcare using a knowledge discovery-based predictive analytics framework

Shelly Gupta[1], *Jyoti Agarwal*[2], *and Disha Mohini Pathak*[3]

[1]Department of Computer Science and Engineering (Artificial Intelligence), KIET Group of Institutions, Ghaziabad, Uttar Pradesh, India

[2]Department of Computer Science and Engineering, Graphic Era Deemed to be University, Dehradun, Uttarakhand, India

[3]Department of Computer Science, ABES Engineering College, Ghaziabad, Uttar Pradesh, India

12.1 INTRODUCTION

The better women's health status is a symbol of strong healthcare system, so it is very important for a nation to sustain its maternal health status. The status of women's health can be determined in terms of MMR, which is the ratio of women deaths over 100,000 live births in a year. In 2005, WHO also stated that dilapidated women's health condition is the main reason for high MMR globally [1]. In India, the ruined status of women's health is a huge point of concern. To avoid this situation, there is a need to optimize the benefits of health services to the entire population by providing the accessibility of effective care at a population level [2,3]. Considering the previously mentioned concept of qualitative care, the developed countries have shown a high reduction in MMR, but the status for the same is still aching in many developing countries [4]. According to WHO, India is the 22% contributor to the total maternal deaths globally, as every year out of 536,000 global maternal deaths, almost 117,000 maternal deaths happen in India [5].

The Indian government is now very careful toward the status of women's health in the nation. It has launched the National Rural Health Mission (NRHM) in 2005 in order to provide qualitative, affordable, and accessible care at the population level. The Ministry of Health and Family Welfare (MoHFW) has started many schemes and projects like Janani Suraksha Yojana (JSY, in 2005), Accredited Social Health Activist (ASHA, in 2005), Janani Shishu Suraksha Karyakaram (JSSK, in 2011), Pradhan Mantri Surakshit Matritva Abhiyan (PMSMA, in 2016), and Labour Room Quality Improvement Initiative (LaQshya, in 2017), with an objective to reduce the national MMR by providing the qualitative and comprehensive antenatal care to all pregnant women nationwide. According to [6], the MMR rate in India reduced from 212 in 2007 to 178 maternal deaths per 100,000 live births in 2012, but the goal to achieve less than 100 is still a dream [7,8].

To work on this problem statement, data analytics on public healthcare data can play a reasonable role in identifying and highlighting the main factors and trends responsible for maternal deaths during delivery and just after delivery. This chapter is concerned with the challenges relevant to the usage of public maternal healthcare data and how the knowledge discovery process can make use of it for building a predictive model which can help healthcare practitioners in making decisions [9,10] at different levels, i.e., strategic, tactical,

DOI: 10.1201/9781003369059-15

and operational [11] in the public healthcare sector. Machine learning methods play a vital in the knowledge discovery process to generate knowledge and information. At the tactical level, the suggested framework is justified in that it would assist the state administration in making decisions regarding the distribution of priority and non-priority districts in accordance with NRHM requirements.

12.2 PUBLIC HEALTHCARE SYSTEM IN INDIA

Normally, the country supports public healthcare via nationwide healthcare systems. It is a setup to support the healthcare needs of a community or population funded and provided by the government or government approved committees. Public healthcare assures the healthy living of the society by providing the efficient healthcare services [12]. Public health is apprehensive towards the total health of the population rather than personal health, and it demands a joint effort to achieve this by addressing population-wide prevention, treatment, and care [13]. These inhabitants might be modest as like a village, or large as like a country. The public health and healthcare are important concerns for developing countries like India to gain access to healthcare that contributes to population health. From the elementary to the higher level [14] in India, the public sector or government provides healthcare at no cost through national healthcare systems as general health services. These are the main duties that the federal, state, and local governments all share [15]. Also, the private industry dominates the delivery of clinical services [16], but this study does not consider this fact. Primary, secondary, and tertiary care make up India's three-tiered healthcare system, which offers national healthcare services [17]. The primary tier includes three healthcare units which all are included at health care delivery system, i.e., Sub Centres (SCs), Primary Health Centres (PHCs) and Community Health Centres (CHCs). The secondary tier includes Sub District Hospitals (SDHs) and District Hospitals. The tertiary tier includes like medical college hospitals, AIIMS, PGI institutions [18].

12.2.1 Sub centres (SCs)

The Sub Centres is the very first refer unit between the village population and the health works. As per the national standards a SC population coverage is 3,000 hilly areas and 5,000 for plain areas. One male health professional and an Auxiliary Nurse Midwife (ANM) oversee a Sub Centre (SC).

12.2.2 Primary health centres (PHCs)

The Primary Health Centres are the rural populations' initial point of contact with the doctor. As per the national standards a SC population coverage is 20,000 for hilly areas and 30,000 for plain areas. There are four to six beds available at each PHC to provide the basic healthcare necessities. There is a PHC for six SCs. It features one male and one female health assistant to manage the basic healthcare needs.

12.2.3 Community health centres (CHCs)

The CHC is a referral unit for four PHCs. As per the national standards a SC population coverage is 80,000 for hilly areas and 120,000 for plain areas. There is a facility of 20 beds at each CHC. Every CHC has one physician, one pediatrician, one gynecologist, one surgeon, and 21 paramedical staff members to provide healthcare services. It also includes the laboratory facility for medical testing, one operation theatre Labour room, and X-ray machine.

The Indian healthcare management system is also at three levels: national, state, and district [19,20].

12.2.4 National level

The federal government oversees developing public healthcare policies and initiatives under the direction of the Ministry of Health and Family Welfare (MoHFW). The three main departments of this organization are the Department of Health Research, the AYUSH (Ayurveda Yoga-Naturopathy Unani Siddha and Homeopathy) Department, and the Department of Health and Family Welfare. They contribute to India's national healthcare management system.

12.2.5 State level

The Indian constitution takes the healthcare as a subject at state level. The healthcare delivery system is unique for every state. Both governmental and commercial service providers are integrated in this system. But the major funding coming from the state is 80% of the total, which is mostly available at public level. At state level the state government is responsible for formulating health policies and to activate the central policies independently. This is done under the direction of the state level ministry of health and family welfare.

12.2.6 District level

The district level in healthcare system is like a communication channel between the state level bodies and peripheral level units, i.e., PHCs/SCs. The designated officer is the Chief Medical Officer responsible to manage the work flow at the district level independently under the guidance of state level bodies in the system.

This management hierarchy leads to the decision making at three different levels: strategic, tactical, and operational [21], as shown in Figure 12.1. The strategic decisions are mainly taken by the central government at national level. The tactical decisions are taken by state government while the operational decisions are carried out at the district level. India is a

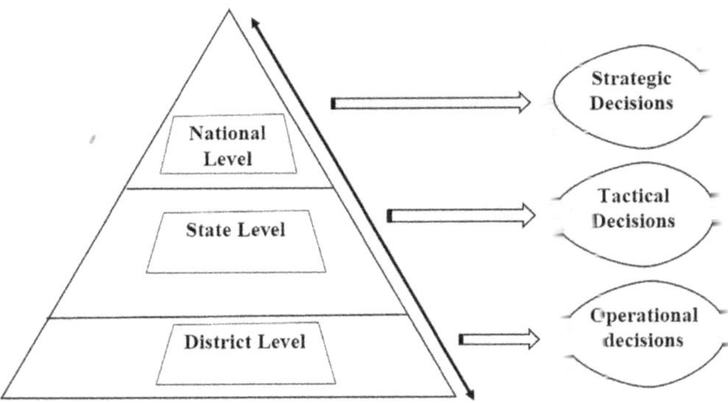

Figure 12.1 Healthcare management system hierarchy.

developing country that started off health programs at the national level but failed to make the effect on mass health issues and depletion in national maternal mortality and infant mortality rates [22].

The core of any administrative system is decision making, which is heavily reliant on the current information [23]. The ability of health administrators to make informed policy decisions would be enhanced by the establishment of a suitable method or procedure [24]. As a result, at all levels of system decision making, the integration of public healthcare data and analysis is crucial for healthcare planners [25].

12.3 KNOWLEDGE DISCOVERY FOR DECISION MAKING

The National Rural Health Mission platform was created by the Government of India (GoI) in 2005 to offer data on public health in rural areas [22], which is abundant in public healthcare data and growing daily. It is to mention that the usability of this public healthcare data in the Indian healthcare sector is quite low. The statistics report published by the Directorate General of Health Services, Central Bureau of Health Intelligence, and the Ministry of Health and Family Welfare provides government administrative data [26]. This statistical analysis does not provide optimal decision making at different decision levels, and its very unfortunate to see that such reasonably good data is rarely been used for policy and decision making.

A new generation of models and tools was sized to provide analytical solutions for the extraction of the valuable particulars or knowledge from this ever-increasing volume of data. Like in [27] A. Kamat et al. have implemented the classification algorithms to predict the mode of a new delivery, i.e., either normal or caesarean for a pregnant women. They have used the maternal dataset of 671 instances of 10 attributes. The attributes are about the status of women's medical health like BMI, glucose fasting, BPD, fundal height, cervical length, etc. Based on algorithms and performance comparisons, they identified that Naive Bayes performed much better as compared to ID3 decision tree to predict about the type of delivery. In [28] B. N. Lakshmi et al. have applied the two selected classification algorithms, i.e., C 4.5 and Naive Bayes, to predict the gestational risk level in pregnant women to prevent the delivery complications in them. They have collected the dataset of 370 data instances of 12 attributes from Bangalore, Karnataka. They applied the filter method to identify the relevant features for classification purpose and included only six attributes of relevance in the study. They compared the performance of the generated models and on comparison based, and they suggested the C 4.5 provided better results in predicting the risk level in pregnant women. In [29] G. Sahle used decision tree-based approaches, such as the J48 and JRip algorithms, to determine the parameters involved for the estimation of maternal healthcare appointments after delivery in Ethiopia. He employed a dataset of 6558 Ethiopian demographic health survey records for his research. After applying these algorithms which both almost have shown equal and high accuracy and identified delivery place, health delivery assistance by professional, professional in prenatal care health and age as the major factors that are responsible to make the new mother to go for post-natal checkups. In [30] S. Sharmilan et al. was using the Naive Bayesian and Artificial Neural Network based techniques to forecast pregnancy issues in order to manage the MMR and IMR. The algorithms have shown 70–80% accuracy for the same purpose and to improve this accuracy a new hybrid method utilizing the best practice of both methods have been proposed and the accuracy to predict the same is increased to 86%. In [31] O. B. Alaba et al. has applied decision tree, multi-layer perceptron, and Naive Bayes classifier to develop predictive models regarding the maternal mortality rate reduction in Nigeria. They have used the dataset of 200 medical records collected from three different health facilities of Nigeria. Among the three methods used for predicting the safe delivery with live new mother the multi-layer perceptron has worked most efficiently. In [32] R. Mehta et al. carried out a study and evaluation on data mining techniques applied in the maternal healthcare sector for decision making and improving women's health for a nation. They looked at a few research that used predictive analytics techniques to find answers to health-care restrictions in the maternal-care area. The key research focused on predicting high-risk pregnancies, obstetric risk factors, and premature birth risk factors, among other things. They have analyzed that the data mining methods performed good over the datasets for said predictions. But still, the problem of high MMR is not resolved.

This led to the knowledge discovery in databases, which is accountable for constructing high level knowledge from low level data stored in organization repositories for framing regulations. In order to improve the performance of public healthcare system of India, the knowledge must be fetched from the available data which will lead to informed decision making. The procedure of analyzing data in order to identify hidden relevant information or knowledge is known as data mining [33].

Many researchers have discussed the importance of data mining methods in decision support in various domains. Like in [34] the authors have used machine learning methods to investigate the influence of COVID-19 on India's climate and renewable energy transitions and concluded that renewable energy sources are projected to rise in the post-COVID period, as the epidemic has prompted a positive transformation. Whereas in [35] the authors proposed a method to reduce the overall trip time by reducing the entire time delayed at stop signs. The model is built on a two-level architecture. To improve the popularity of metaheuristic approaches, an original approach that incorporates the desirable features of each BA as well as GA was suggested to optimize the traffic issue.

The KDD process model and predictive analytics are used in this study to offer a theoretical framework model for decision-making. In order to build prediction models from databases and identify relevant and valuable trends, data analysis is the primary sub-step of the KDD process model. With the use of the KDD methodology, previously unknown patterns and knowledge in maternal care datasets may be found and used to create cleaner and more efficient conclusions for successful healthcare supervision. The primary goal of incorporating decision making with the KDD model is to significantly boost decision support by using the KDD framework, which is especially useful when a large amount of factual data is provided for information extraction. The primary goal of this study is to support national and Uttar Pradesh's maternal health services in being delivered in the most timely, precise, elevated, and sensitive fashion possible because healthcare providers require access to the latest available information to use across decision-making systems. To accomplish this objective, KDD and data mining procedures can be applied to extract significant amounts of concealed, beneficial, useable information from data, which can then be utilized to construct strategic decision-making models based on data analysis. Although decision support systems built on knowledge discovery and data mining techniques may be used to enhance decision making in a range of contexts, their application in the healthcare sector might assist policymakers in developing better policies and treatments.

12.4 KDD AND DATA MINING

The knowledge discovery is the motivation for processing data. This can be done by storing data about a specific process and retrieving it later in order to utilize it meaningfully. Data mining approaches are used in the KDD method to discover patterns and insights. The process of converting low-level records into good knowledge is known as KDD process. As a result, knowledge discovery in databases is defined as the challenging process of discovering correct, original, beneficial, and subsequently comprehensible patterns in data. Data Mining and Knowledge Discovery in Databases (KDD) are terms that are frequently used synonymously. This quandary stems from the three different approaches i.e., clustering, association, and classification to data mining, but data mining is a significant aspect in the KDD process. The procedures of uncovering valuable insights from huge amounts of data in databases, data warehouses, or other information repositories is referred to as data mining. It employs ml algorithms, statistical, and visual analytics to explore and present information in a way that we can understand. The diversity of scientific fields of interest contributes to the vividness and rapid evolution of the data mining field of study. Data mining applications can evaluate the data using a few parameters. The KDD and DM processes are explained later.

The necessary stages in the KDD iterative procedure as shown in Figure 12.2 are explained in brief:

A. Selection
The data necessary for the analytics job are extracted from the database in this stage. The target dataset, that is going to be evaluated, is founded during the selection procedure.
B. Pre-processing
Due to the large size, ambiguity, and probable origin from numerous diverse sources, accessible datasets are extremely prone to noise, miss and inconsistency in data. So, in this stage, the target dataset chosen in selection stage is pre-processed in order to address the issue.
C. Transformation
Smoothing, summarization or agglomeration, generalizability, simplification, differencing, and feature building operations are carried out in this phase to convert or integrate data into suitable forms for extraction.
D. Data Mining
Techniques for data mining process are used in the KDD Process model to retrieve data patterns. In this stage of the KDD Process model, sophisticated methods are employed to uncover patterns in the data. The set of data is evaluated using data mining procedures according the task.
E. Interpretation
This stage entails pattern recognition and knowledge discovery. This critical step employs visualization methods to aid users in comprehending and interpreting the findings from data mining.

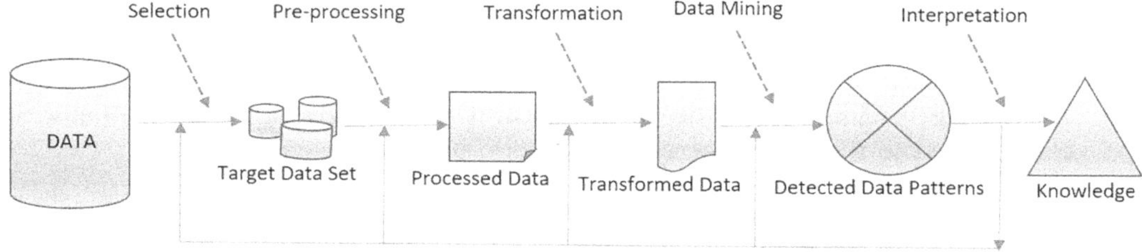

Figure 12.2 Various stages in KDD process model.

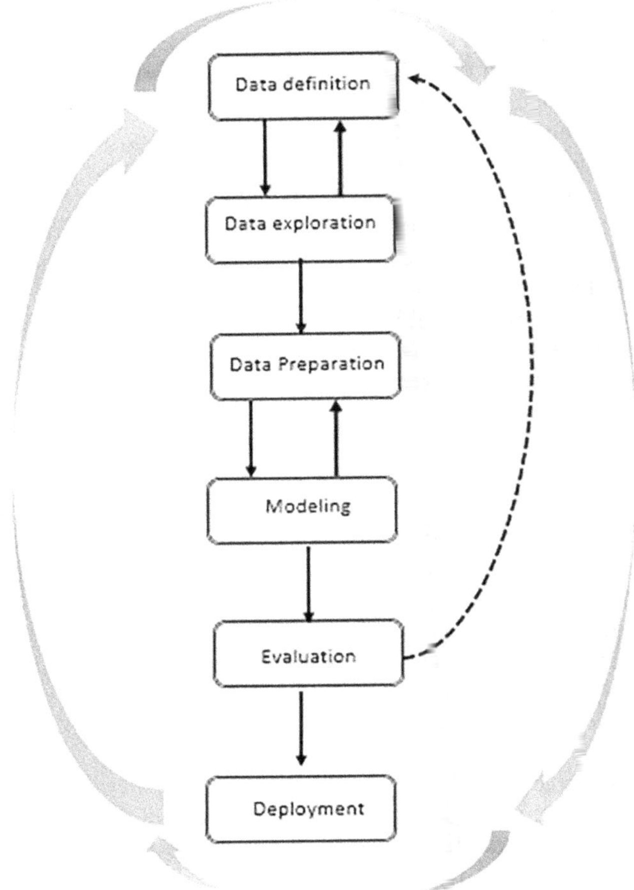

Figure 12.3 Data mining process steps.

The data mining process as shown in Figure 12.3 encompasses various steps are explained here:

A. Problem definition
   The first stage is to establish objectives. Depending on the intended purpose, the appropriate set of techniques may be used to analyze the data throughout to construct the related behavioral model.
B. Data exploration
   If the data accuracy is insufficient for an accurate model, advice on new data collecting and storage techniques might be provided. During analysis, each data must be consolidated so that it may be processed uniformly.
C. Data preparation
   The objective of this stage is to clean-up and convert the information in order to address lost and incorrect attributes that make all recognized genuine information comparable for further meaningful analysis.

D. Modelling
   A data mining method or collection of procedures is selected for evaluation according to the information and the intended outputs. These approaches encompass both traditional approaches like analytics, neighbourhood, and grouping, as well as upcoming approaches like incremental and iterative association and rule-based procedures. The technique is determined depending on the precise goal to be attained and the amount of information to be evaluated.
E. Evaluation and Deployment
   An investigation is conducted by utilizing the findings of such data mining technologies to derive extraordinary insight from the research and provide a sequence of suggestions for evaluation.

Because of the significance of KDD, the purpose of this research was to design a conceptual framework based on KDD for retrieving information in order to transform maternal health information from databases of healthcare into knowledge in a logical fashion for better healthcare administration. This proposed theoretical model will aid healthcare researchers to figure out and leverage new data and findings as patterns, correlations, guidelines, and connections from vast quantities of maternal health data that can be used to make decisions for the future. Furthermore, no research has been done in the research region on KDD and data mining approaches in the context of a variety of maternal health care aspects. As a conclusion, the current effort is the only one of its classes in the research field, and it has a high level of technical execution afterwards when the results analysis for changing trend, correlations, guidelines, and associations are communicated with various government agencies involved in the health sector of Uttar Pradesh state of India.

12.5 BACKGROUND

In this part, some noteworthy chapters that supported the current study are discussed. The notion for this conceptual framework model was inspired by a conceptual framework model called DM-PHCS [36] based on the CRISP-DM technique. The DM-PHCS model provided an illustration of data mining support for decision making at various levels of the Indian public healthcare system. In [37] the authors by incorporating and using big data (BD) analytics, tools, and methodologies built a BD driven safety decision-making (BD- SDM) framework to help people make safer judgments that are wiser and more fortunate. Also, a unified theoretical framework for data mining was created [38] by manufacturing composite functions for clustering, classification, and visualization. This framework is further shown utilising several real-world datasets and various data mining techniques. In [39] the researchers create a conceptual framework that can direct the management of data for better services in South African healthcare institutions. A framework was created based on the research findings, principally to direct and advance how data are saved, accessed, managed, and utilized to enhance quality healthcare. To construct a unique way for issue resolution, the authors [40] built a decision support system called DMDSS, which stands for data mining decision support system built on CRISP-DM. In [41], the constructed data mining framework may be used as the foundation for a subsequent optimization model that can be employed to distribute patients‘ visits as efficiently as feasible based on their current participation behaviour.

For better decision-making across a variety of areas, including health care, several academics have developed decision support systems using knowledge discovery and data mining approaches. These systems help officials develop improved policies and treatments.

The level of health consequences can be used to gauge how well primary healthcare is provided. Hence these health consequences and health indicators are interconnected.

Although maternal health care services databases are one of the most important components in the health sector, studies have shown that knowledge discovery using data mining methods is used less by investigators on databases relevant to public maternal healthcare databases. The Government of India's Ministry of Health and Family Welfare (MOHFW) launched an online National Rural Health Mission portal in 2005 and a Health Management Information System (HMIS) in 2008. They provide voluminous databases regarding various public healthcare related indicators like maternal health, child immunization, lab testing, family planning etc. But a limited research work related to application of knowledge discovery on this data for analysis has been done until now. Therefore, the application of KDD as a decision support system will aid in the creation of improved health policies and the provision of maternal health at all levels. The KDD and data mining specialists may design models and retrieve insights from the data on the HMIS portal to help the healthcare practitioners make the best decisions and create better health policies.

12.6 PROPOSED FRAMEWORK (KDPA-MH) MODEL

The main goal of creating the previously mentioned framework model is to promote the use of KDD and data mining methodologies in the decision-making process for handling and arranging maternal health pertinent and accessible data on the HMIS platform approved by the Ministry of Health and Family Welfare (MOFW-GOI). The KDD reference model [42] has been revised and is depicted in figure 12.4 in accordance with the recommendations of the proposed model, which is known as the Knowledge Discovery Based Predictive Analysis for Managing Maternal Health (KDPA-MH) framework KDPA-MH is initially used to develop several KDD models based on research of maternal health care data from prior years. The KDD process heavily relies on data mining hence this theoretical framework

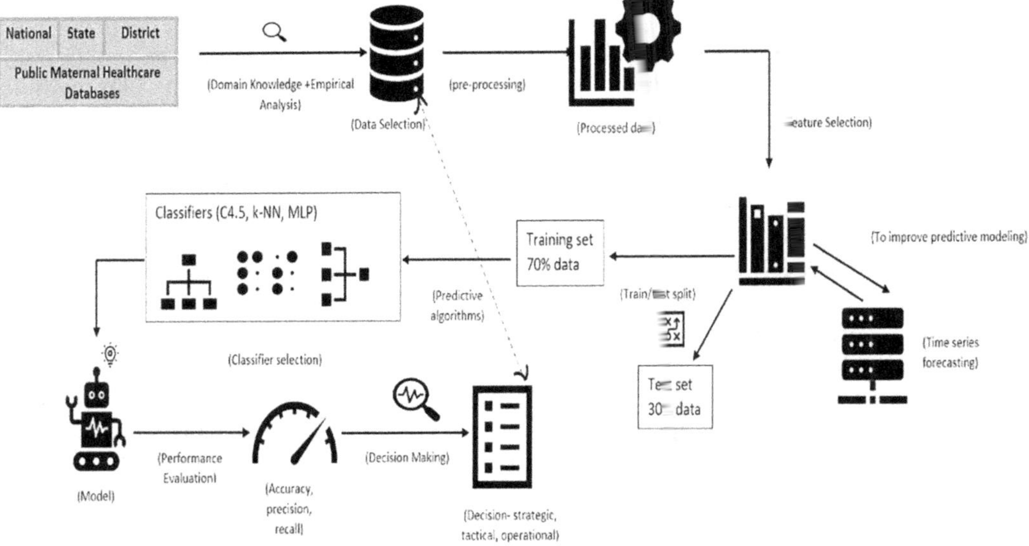

Figure 12.4 The proposed framework (KDPA-MH) model.

includes a variety of data mining methods like time series, classification, and others. The KDPA-MH builds the models using a range of data mining techniques in accordance with the publicly available maternal healthcare data, and then applies these models in the decision-making process. Health officials and specialists are then expected to participate in the final decision-making process, without delving too deeply into the model creation process. The various steps of the suggested conceptual framework model KDPA-MH are covered in detail below, and it adheres to the KDD research approach.

12.6.1 Empirical analysis for data selection

The empirical data analysis on public maternal healthcare data is to be done first in order to identify where the least reduction in maternal mortality rate of the nation exists. The first step before doing any data analysis task is to collect the dataset.

In [43] the maternal health data of the nation, specifically state-by-state, is collected via the NRHM-HMIS site in order to conduct the empirical investigation. It is secondary data. The data for various demographic variables was gathered from the Ministry of Health and Family Welfare of India's statistics report, Health, and Family Welfare Statistics [44] in India for the year (2012–2013). The data from the District Level Household Survey (DLHS-4) and the Annual Health Survey (AHS-4) for the years 2011–2013 are included.

According to the empirical data analysis of related to pregnancy accessible data from the census of 2011, it is noticed that the general maternal health condition of the country is not satisfactory. In this study, it is identified that the Kerala state has a great maternal health condition in contrast to the condition of maternal health in Uttar Pradesh, and the Bihar state is much more questionable and worrying. This leads to the conclusion that because these states have a higher number of women than other states. then increased efforts at the state level might result in a lower national MMR rate. Hence the Uttar Pradesh state is selected for further analysis to work toward the reduction in MMR rate.

12.6.2 Data preparation and feature selection

For good and sustainable data analysis, data preparation, and feature selection are essential. It is a data mining data pre-processing technique that simplifies the number of parameters for an analytical activity.

In [45] the decision tree based J48 classification method is employed to the native dataset of 20 variables, and the wrapper features subset selection method for selecting features is applied. The Classification Subcategory Optimizer for the J48 classification method has chosen the suitable parameters using the greedy strategy, i.e., best First, and decreased the overall data dimensionality from 20 to six variables. The accuracy increased from 67.69% to 72.3%, which is a significant increase that validates the relevance of selecting features for public maternal health care services data. According to the findings of this research, using proper feature selection techniques for categorization of maternal healthcare data with a particular goal value can assist health planners in identifying trends in desirable attributes.

12.6.3 Data mining: Time series and predictive modelling

Time Series Predictive Modelling is a key technique in the health sector for achieving the Millennium Development Goals (MDGs) for MMR in India. The suggested framework utilizes this to provide trend analysis and future values. And by assisting healthcare planners in making decisions, predictive analytics helps to enhance healthcare quality.

In [46] a model for time series forecasting in public maternal healthcare data is proposed. The time series forecasting is done for the selected features from the original data. The time series forecasting methods, i.e., ES, ANN, and LSTM, were utilized. Based on the comparative study, it is identified that the exponential smoothing procedures worked more bitterly than the other two proposed methods which is amazing because exponential smoothing methods are straightforward and acceptable to implement. The ES method is recommended for further prediction of future values and trends in the essential features of the specified domain.

In [47] a model for predictive modelling in public maternal healthcare data is proposed. The predictive modelling is done for the selected features category from the original data. Three types of classifiers were implemented for the purpose of the predictive modelling on state district level data. The C 4.5, MLP, and K-NN classification methods are applied on the three different categories of the public maternal healthcare databases. Based on a performance-based examination of the methodologies, the C4.5 decision tree method is found to be the best fit for the predictive task.

12.6.4 Decision making and knowledge representation

Healthcare stakeholders may use analytics to assist them make better decisions for the system. The analytics are used to make judgments and make forecasts at this stage. In [47] from the perspective of healthcare stakeholders, the predictive analytics enabled them to accurately determine the priority and non-priority distribution of districts based on three separate attribute categories of maternal health data in the Uttar Pradesh state of India.

12.7 CONCLUSION

KDPA-MH is essentially a knowledge discovery-based predictive analytic framework that promotes decision making by delivering evidence-based information. The relevant case study of the Uttar Pradesh state of India is shown in this chapter, utilizing this framework for priority and non-priority districts distribution as per NRHM standards at the state level. This more impactful distribution of districts will help the healthcare practitioners utilize the healthcare benefits more effectively to reduce the current MMR in the nation. As a result, healthcare professionals and administrators can utilize this proposed system at the tactical decision level. The proposed KDPA-MH framework can be utilized for predictive analysis, specifically for priority and non-priority districts distribution for any state of India, as it supports the Indian Healthcare system. Hence, the executives in the healthcare industry can use this integrative framework to make decisions for future initiatives across the decision-making stage with only a basic understanding of the KDD process.

12.8 FUTURE SCOPE

In order to improve decision-making at many levels, including national, state, and district, the current study suggests using a framework for knowledge discovery-based predictive analysis termed KDPA-MH. In the future, a platform built on the KDPA-MH framework will be developed to produce forecasts at the state and federal levels employing a variety of data mining techniques on maternal health data for better decision making. Also, state government stakeholders will produce a report of the current inquiry for technical research execution.

REFERENCES

1. World Health Organization (2005). World Health Report 2005: Make every mother and child count. Geneva: WHO. Available from: http://www.who.int/whr/2005/whr2005_en.pdf
2. S. M. Campbell, M. O. Roland and S. A. Buetow, "Defining quality of care," Soc. Sci. Med., vol. 51, no. 11, pp. 1611–1625, 2000. doi: 10.1016/S0277-9536(00)00057-5.
3. S. D. Iyengar, K. Iyengar and V. Gupta, "Maternal health: A case study of Rajasthan," J. Health Popul. Nutr., vol. 27, no. 2, pp. 271–292, 2009.
4. UNICEF Maternal Health Available from: http://www.unicef.org/health/index_maternalhealth.html
5. K. Hill, K. Thomas, C. AbouZahr, N. Walker, L. Say, M. Inoue and E. Suzuki, "Estimates of maternal mortality worldwide between 1990 and 2005: an assessment of available data," Lancet, vol. 370, no. 9595, pp. 1311–1319, 2007. doi: 10.1016/S0140-6736(07)61572-4.
6. UNICEF India – Maternal Health Available from: http://www.unicef.org/health/index_maternalhealth.html
7. K. S. Vora, D. V. Mavalankar, K. V. Ramani, M. Upadhyay, B. Sharma, S. Iyengar, et al., "Maternal health situation in India: a case study," J. Health Popul. Nutr., vol. 27, no. 2, pp. 184–201, 2009.
8. B. Randive, V. Diwan and A. de Costa, "India's conditional cash transfer programme (the JSY) to promote institutional birth: is there an association between institutional birth proportion and maternal mortality?" PLoS One, 8, 2013. 10.1371/journal.pone.0067452
9. A. Szeghegyi, "Investigation of decision-making process by the use of knowledge based system," Proceedings of 5th International Conference on Management, Enterprise and Benchmarking, pp. 209–222, 2007.
10. F. Janos, Introduction to Decision Making Methods. [Online] Available: http://academic.evergreen.edu/projects/bdei/documents/decisionmakingmethods.pdf.
11. L. M. Murtola, H. L. Laine and S. Salantera, "Information systems in hospitals: a review chapter from a nursing management perspective," Int. J. Netw. Virtual Organ., vol. 13, no. 1, 81–100, 2013.
12. Public Health Care. [Online]. Available: http://www.publichealthcareservice.com
13. From transition to transformation in public health, Local Government Association, London, 2012. [Online]. Available: https://lacors.webs.com/MariamPage/3%20Understanding%20the%20health%20role%20of%20local%20government.pdf
14. Chapter-VIII, Public Health Care System. [Online]. Available: https://niti.gov.in/planningcommission.gov.in/docs/aboutus/committee/strgrp/stgp_fmlywel/sgfw_ch8.pdf
15. Annual Report 2014-15. [Online]. Available: https://www.annualreports.com/HostedData/AnnualReportArchive/e/TSX-V_EIL_2015.pdf
16. S. Basu, J. Andrews, S. Kishore, R. Panjabi and D. Stuckler, "Comparative performance of private and public healthcare systems in low- and middle-income countries: A systematic review," PLoS Med., vol. 9, no. 6, 2012. doi: 10.1371/journal.pmed.1001244
17. A. Majumder and V. Upadhyay, "An analysis of the primary health care system in India with focus on reproductive health care services," Artha Beekshan, vol. 12, no. 4, pp. 29–38, 2004.
18. Rural health care system in India. [Online]. Available: http://www.nhm.gov.in/images/pdf/monitoring/rhs/rural-health-care-system-india-final-9-4-2012.pdf
19. India's Healthcare System - Overview and Quality Improvements, Swedish Agency for Growth Policy Analysis, Sweden, Stockholm, 2013. [Online]. Available: https://www.tillvaxtanalys.se/download/18.62dd45451715a00666f21a01/1586366220403/direct_response_2013_04.pdf
20. L. S. Vaz, Textbook of Public Health and Community Medicine, Ist ed., Rajvir Bhalwar, Department of Community Medicine, Armed Forces Medical College, Pune, 2009.
21. National Rural Health Mission Meeting people's health needs in rural areas Framework for Implementation 2005-2012 [Online]. Available: https://nhm.gov.in/WriteReadData/l892s/nrhm-framework-latest.pdf
22. C. Arpita 2013, Health care in India. [Online]. Available: http://www.marketexpress.in/2013/03/health-care-in-india.html

23. T. Lucey, Management Information Systems, 8th Edition, London: Letts Educational, 1997.
24. S. L. Goel, Management Techniques and Good Governance in Health Care System and Hospital Administration, Deep & Deep Publications, 2010.
25. The Governmental Public Health Infrastructure. [Online]. Available: http://www.nap.edu/read/10548/chapter/5
26. Health Information of India, Central Bureau of Health Intelligence, Ministry of Health and Family Welfare, Government of India.2012 [Online]. Available: http://cbhidghs.nic.in/introduction.asp
27. A. Kamat, V. Oswal and M. Datar, "Implementation of classification algorithms to predict mode of delivery," Int. J. Comput. Sci. Inform. Technol., vol. 6, no. 5, pp. 4531–4534, 2015.
28. B. N. Lakshmi, T. S. Indumathi and N. Ravi, "A comparative study of classification algorithms for predicting gestational risks in pregnant women," International Conference on Computers, Communications and Systems, pp. 42–46, 2015.
29. G. Sahle, "Ethiopic maternal care data mining: discovering the factors that affect postnatal care visit in Ethiopia," Health Inform. Sci. Syst. (Springer), vol. 4, 2016. doi: 10.1186/s13755-016-0017-2
30. S. Sharmilan and T. Chaminda, "Predictive data mining system to diagnose pregnancy complications," International Conference on Computational Modeling & Simulation (IC2MS), 2017.
31. O. B. Alaba, P. A. Idowu, O. A. Abass and I. O. Faniyi, ' Development of a predictive model for maternal mortality in Nigeria using data mining technique," 11th International Multi-Conference on ICT Applications (AICTTRA), pp. 25–32, 2017.
32. R. Mehta, N. Bhatt and A. Ganatra, "A survey on data mining technologies for decision support system of maternal care domain," Int. J. Comput. Appl., vol. 138, pp. 20–24, 2016.
33. X.-H. Li, J.-H. Zhao and B.-H. Li, "Investigation of fuzzy mathematical model for general evaluation of administrators in university," Proceedings of 2004 International Conference on Machine Learning and Cybernetics (IEEE Cat. No.04EX826), 2004, pp. 1977–1980, vol. 3, doi: 10.1109/ICMLC.2004.138210
34. T. Stephan, F. Al-Turjman, M. Ravishankar et al., "Machine learning analysis on the impacts of COVID-19 on India's renewable energy transitions and air quality", Environ. Sci. Pollut. Res., vol. 29, pp.79443–79465, 2022.
35. S. Srivastava, T. Stephan and S. K. Sahana, "An innovative hybrid biologically inspired method for traffic optimization problem," Int. J. Artif. Intell. Tools, vol. 31, no. 2, 2022. doi: 10.1142/s0218213022400048
36. A. Sharma and V. Mansotra, "Data mining based decision making: a conceptual model for public healthcare system," Proceedings of IEEE 3rd International Conference on Computing for Sustainable Global Development (INDIACom), pp. 1226–1230, 2016.
37. L. Huang, et al., "Big-data-driven safety decision-making: a conceptual framework and its influencing factors," Saf. Sci., vol. 109, pp. 46–56, 2018.
38. D. M. Khan, N. Mohamudally and D. K. R. Babajee, "A unified theoretical framework for data mining," Inf. Technol. Quant. Manag., vol 17, pp. 104–113, 2013.
39. T. Iyamu and K. Nunu, "Healthcare data management conceptual framework for service delivery," Educ. Inf. Technol., vol. 26, pp. 3513–3527, 2021. 10.1007/s10639-020-10413-y
40. K. Jindal, M. Sharma, B. K. Sharma, "Data mining to support decision process in decision support system," Int. J. Emerg. Technol. Adv. Eng., vol. 4, no. 1, pp. 41–46, 2014.
41. S. Abdallah, M. Malik and G. Ertek, "A data mining framework for the analysis of patient arrivals into healthcare centers," Proceedings of the 2017 International Conference on Information Technology, Singapore, pp. 52–61, December 27–29, 2017. ACM.
42. J. Han and M. Kamber, Data Mining: Concepts and Techniques, 2nd ed., San Francisco: Morgan Kauffmann Publishers, 2001.
43. S. Gupta, S. N. Singh and D. Kumar, "An empirical analysis of maternal health data: A case study of India," 2016 2nd International Conference on Next Generation Computing Technologies (NGCT), 2016, pp. 490–493, doi: 10.1109/NGCT.2016.7877465.

44. Health and Family Welfare Statistics in India 2015. [Online]. Available: https://nrhm-mis.nic.in/SitePages/Pub-FW-Statistics2015.aspx
45. S. Gupta, S. N. Singh and P. K. Jain, "Feature selection on public maternal healthcare dataset for classification," 3rd International Conference on Computing Informatics and Networks, vol. 167, pp. 573–583, Springer, 2021.
46. S. Gupta, S. N. Singh and P. K. Jain, "Time series forecasting to improve predictive modelling in public maternal healthcare data," Recent Patents Eng., vol. 14, no. 3, pp. 422–439, 2020.
47. S. Gupta, S. N. Singh and P. K. Jain, "Utilising predictive analytics for decision-making and improving healthcare services in public maternal healthcare database," Int. J. Reasoning-Based Intell. Syst., vol. 13, no. 2, pp. 85–91, 2021.

Part 4

Patient care and enhancements

Chapter 13

Enhancing patient care and treatment through explainable AI

A gap analysis

Shyni Carmel Mary S[1], *Dhyana Sharon Ross*[2], *Anbumani Bala*[3], *and Joe Arun*[4]

[1]Business Analytics, Loyola Institute of Business Administration (LIBA), Chennai, Tamil Nadu, India

[2]Healthcare and Human Resources Management, Loyola Institute of Business Administration (LIBA), Chennai, Tamil Nadu, India

[3]Medical Consultant Paediatrician & Child Psychiatrist, St Thomas Hospital, Chennai, Tamil Nadu, India

[4]Professor of Marketing, Loyola Institute of Business Administration (LIBA), Chennai, Tamil Nadu, India

13.1 INTRODUCTION

We started to wonder if human doctors might eventually be supplanted in the healthcare sector by AI tools because of recent advancements in AI technology. Practically speaking, Artificial intelligence (AI) tools are unlikely to replace human doctors, but they can improve outcomes and provide more accuracy in the healthcare context. The availability of healthcare data is a key factor supporting the emergence of AI solutions in the healthcare industry. Intelligence is a state of being, not just a technology but a collection of technologies [1]. Technology has always proven to be beneficial for humankind, especially for patients. One good example of technology, that helps in patients' treatment is the study [2] where with the use of technology, patients were able to detect early the epileptic episodes before its occurrence.

Healthcare is one of the most significant industries in the broader big data environment due to the productive society. Artificial intelligence (AI) is the power of technology-embedded algorithms to understand data to do automated activities without needing every single step of the procedure to be specifically coded by a human. AI's application in healthcare industry has the real prospect of either help or hurt patients. AI can support normal tasks for healthcare workers including doctors, nurses, and others. Preventive care, overall patient outcomes, and quality of life can all be improved by AI in healthcare and also it can develop more accurate diagnoses and treatment plans. AI and related technologies are spreading throughout industry and society, and they are beginning to be utilised for patient treatment in healthcare. The many facets of patient care, in addition to operating methods inside pharmaceuticals, payers, and service provider organizations, these technologies have the potential to revolutionis\ze. Numerous research has already indicated AI's capability of improvising crucial occupations in healthcare, such as ailment detection on par with or superior to that of humans [3]. By looking at information from the government, the healthcare sector, and other sources, AI can indeed be utilized in predict and track the emergence of serious diseases. AI can play a significant role in global public health activities to fight pandemics and epidemics.

DOI: 10.1201/9781003369059-17

13.1.1 AI and healthcare

AI could help in the healthcare industry by analysis of medical records, creating therapy programmes, predicting medical events, helping with monotonous tasks, conducting online discussions, support for clinical judgement, and drug administration, creating new drugs, helping people make healthier decisions, and more. More individualization is needed in healthcare. Also, it should be interactive, proactive, and precautionary and AI could considerably advance these objectives. We anticipate that the growth and maturation of AI will continue with potent tools for biomedicine based on an overview of the advances being accomplished [4].

13.1.2 AI relevance to healthcare

AI and related technologies are starting to be applied in healthcare. They are becoming more and more common in business and society. In reality, artificial intelligence is comprised of a wide variety of technologies. Despite the fact that most of these technologies can be used right away in the healthcare industry, the specific processes and tasks they support vary substantially. The last generation was dependent on the curation of medical specialists, but artificial intelligence is outpacing them. In order to uncover patterns in data that can explain complex interactions, AI research recently made use of machine learning techniques that are now in use. Applications of AI have been used in healthcare to improve how clinical researchers understand patient circumstances [5].

13.1.2.1 WHO on AI in patient care and treatment

WHO acknowledges that AI's application in medicine and public health offers enormous promise. The potential for AI to advance how health services are provided, including illness prevention, assessment, and intervention, has already transformed how healthcare services are provided in some higher-income nations. Although AI applications are becoming more potential in health and medicine, the use of AI outside of high-income nations may be constrained due to insufficient infrastructure. Applications can be categorized depending on the precise aims for using AI and the methods employed to accomplish those goals [6].

13.1.2.2 ICMR on AI in patient care and treatment

The use of AI in healthcare is having the capacity to provide answers to important problems in the field of medicine, including those relating to diagnostics, treatments, and preventive measures, predicting the prognosis of diseases, complicated data processing, and public health surveillance. This list is probably going to keep expanding in the future [7]. The need for healthcare is constantly growing, and countries are struggling with a lack of competent workers. AI developments have created new possibilities for addressing this shortfall. Among the topics that has seen substantial expansion in recent years is telemedicine and self-care through conversational chatbots and wearable monitoring technology. Additionally, this gives healthcare professionals a substitute for remote monitoring and early disease detection [7,8].

13.2 EXPECTATIONS PERCEPTION AND EXPERIENCE OF PATIENTS

What satisfies the needs of consumers is the quality of the services and what they accept as being provided. The level of service quality is defined as the extent to which services are customized to meet customer expectations. Perception, or more specifically, how services are presented, is

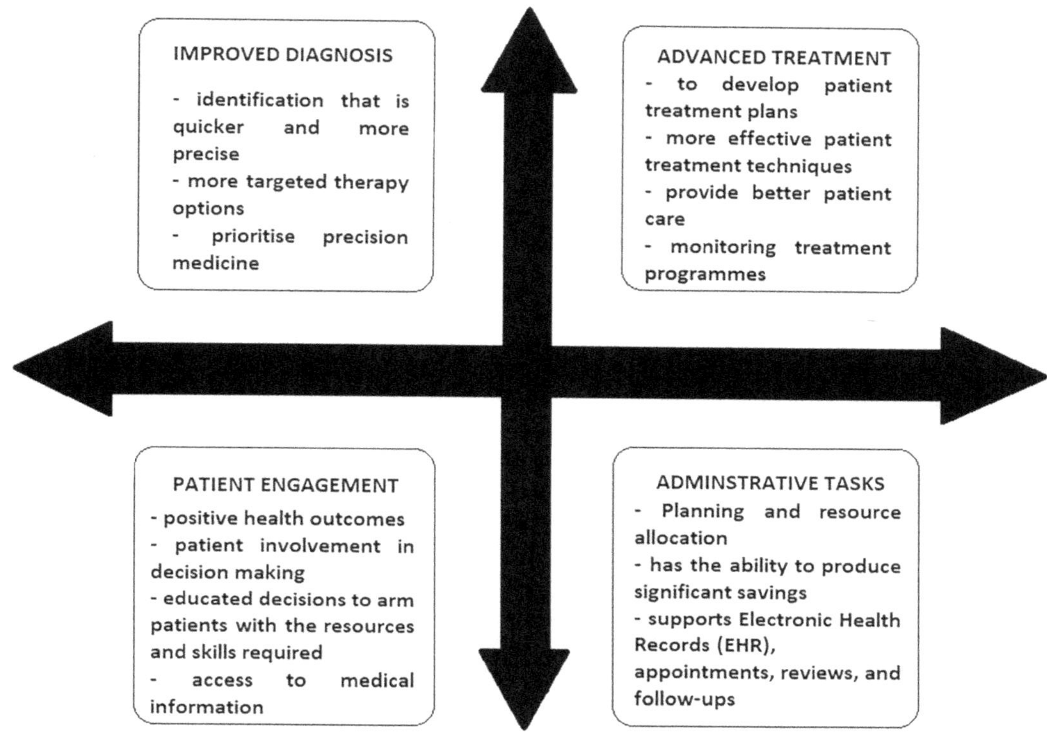

Figure 13.1 AI's effect on expectations, perception and experience.

Source: Authors'.

connected to the current situation. Customers' expectations and perceptions are out of sync, which reveals the level of service excellence [9]. When a service satisfies a customer's wants and expectations, it is of high quality [10]. Patients primarily communicate their needs by stating what people demand, like, require, and want about the care they get [11]. The needs of the patient could be seen as a call for high-standard treatment, which is something that healthcare providers and the healthcare system work to satisfy. Those who require healthcare services hope to receive excellent care, and those who are giving the care likewise have this as their top priority [12]. The EPE is discussed based on the four dimensions of patient services such as improved diagnosis, advanced treatment, patient engagement and administrative tasks shown in Figure 13.1.

13.2.1 EPE on improved diagnosis

The identification of blood-borne bacterial infections using MYCIN at Stanford in the 1970s marked the beginning of AI's focus on illness detection and therapy [13]. The practical application of these early rule-based systems was not addressed, despite the fact that they showed promise for accurately diagnosing and treating disease. They were not significantly better than the workflows of clinicians and medical record technologies, as well as human diagnosticians did not match them adequately. At some hospitals, artificial intelligence is now being tested to see if it can help with disease diagnosis. AI analysis of clinical data, academic articles, and expert guidelines may potentially help guide treatment options [14].

AI is being investigated in several dimensions like, support the diagnosis, situations like radiology and medical imaging. These programmes are still very new even if they are more widespread than other AI applications, and clinical decision-making does not yet regularly use AI. Currently, AI is being tested for usage in non-radiological applications such as dermatology and pathology, as well as for radiological oncology diagnosis (thoracic, abdominal, pelvic, colonoscopy, mammography, brain, and dosage optimization for radiological treatment). In a system that assists in scanning or analyzing stained pictures, and X-rays for symptoms of tuberculosis, COVID-19, or 27 other illnesses, AI may be applied to improve the identification of the disease. Unfortunately, only a small number of these technologies have been evaluated in prospective clinical trials. Recent research comparing deep learning algorithms to medical imaging professionals in the detection of diseases revealed that, in some applications and domains, AI is like human medical judgement [6]. AI can recognize signs of an illness more quickly and precisely using medical imaging, such as CT scans, MRIs, X-rays, and ultrasounds. Patients gain from disease identification that is quicker and more precise and more targeted therapy options. It has been advantageous to be able prioritize precision medicine, particularly the detection and treatment of cancer. Unique kinds of AI methods are employed, Artificial neural networks (ANNs) have shown more accuracy in categorizing diabetes and CVD when compared to neural networks, support vector machines, decision trees, etc [15]. An Artificial Neural Network (ANN) with Computer Aided Diagnosis (CAD) system can automate the detection pipeline accounting for accurate diagnosis, overcoming the limitations of manual methods. One such example is the study [16] where COVID 19 was detected by using lung computed tomography images. AI programme gives doctors an advantage when identifying ailments. AI offers optimism for reducing the load of diagnosis and screening on the healthcare system. According to research by the According to the National Academies of Sciences, Engineering, and Medicine, diagnostic errors are responsible for about 10% of patient fatalities. Additionally, they stated that according to an analysis of medical data, diagnostic mistakes cause 6–17% of adverse outcomes [17].

13.2.2 EPE in advanced treatment

AI is increasingly being used in healthcare to develop patient treatment plans. AI can offer more effective patient treatment techniques and monitoring treatment programmes by analyzing data from old patients [1]. AI is anticipated to have a considerable effect on numerous facets of health care, such as clinical decision-making and treating chronic conditions [18]. Despite being in the early stages of implementation, radiology, pathology, ophthalmology, and cardiology AI algorithms are making strides. The emergence of AI in the big data era can help doctors provide better patient care [19].

13.2.3 EPE in boosting patient engagement

Long regarded as the "last mile" healthcare challenge, patient engagement is probably the biggest barrier to successful treatment and good health outcomes in adherence. The more efficient and improved financial performance and customer service, the greater the level of patient engagement in their own health and treatment. Big data and AI are being used more and more to address these problems. Providers and hospitals typically rely on their healthcare practice when developing a plan of care for an acute or chronic patient. But, if the patient does not really make the necessary behavioural alterations, like reducing weight, scheduling a follow-up appointment, often, it makes no difference whether someone takes their medications or follows their treatment plan. AI-based skills can be employed for efficient personalized and contextualized treatment if greater patient involvement leads to better health outcomes. Using business rules systems and machine learning to power sophisticated interventions across the healthcare ecosystem is becoming crucially influential with health records [20].

AI improves patient interactions. One may streamline the interaction between patients and their business by giving them specialized advice and information. This might refer to giving patients information about their care and treatment in the context of healthcare. AI can also be used to suggest goods and services that would be useful to them. Teaming up with physicians under the intelligent direction of AI is one method of utilizing AI for patient involvement. This will make it easier for healthcare professionals to give patients the next-best, individually tailored actions. This information can range from medical histories to details on lifestyles. One may assist clinicians in giving patients the finest care by combining them with AI. To enable patients to make educated decisions about their health, it is crucial to arm them with the resources and skills they need. Along with the information regarding their care and treatment, this entails giving patients access to their medical records [21].

13.2.4 EPE in supporting administrative tasks

Health and social care services planning and resource allocation could benefit from the application of AI [22]. Administrative tools are also extensively used in the healthcare sector. Compared to patient care, the use of AI in this field has relatively less potential for revolution, but it still has the ability to produce significant savings. They are necessary in the healthcare industry because, for instance, typically a nurse spends 25% of their working hours on paperwork and administrative tasks [23]. Another AI method applicable to the claims and payment administration is machine learning, which can be used for probabilistic database matching. Insurers are accountable for verifying the veracity of the millions of claims. All parties involved—health insurers, authorities, and health professionals time, money, and effort by accurately recognizing, analyzing, and resolving coding problems and false claims. Through data matching and claim audits, inaccuracies in claims that fall between the cracks represent significant unrealized income potential [3].

AI also supports administrative tasks of hospitals like Electronic Health Records (EHR), appointments, reviews, and follow-ups. Electronic health records are essential to the healthcare sector since they permit data analysis spanning the entire history to the present. Also, this enhances the usage of several treatment techniques, medication, and illness management. AI can be used to interpret the records and provide information to clinicians. Algorithms can use EHR to predict the likelihood of an illness based on historical data and family history [24]. Massive volumes of data are used to train AI systems, and as part of this process, the algorithm develops a set of rules that connect its findings to the decisive diagnosis. When new patient data is presented to AI in the future, it will be capable of assessing the patient's usage of knowledge from previous data and predicting the propensity of a disorder or illness. Over the decade, the healthcare industry has produced enormous quantities of data, including information about patients, outcomes from research, and data on diagnoses. With organizations' usage of scientific techniques, they were able to work together and achieve the insight needed for successful patient treatment and efficiency [1].

13.3 METHODOLOGY

The service quality is determined by expectation, perception, and experience. These are the measures used for patient care and treatment provided by the AI. The methodology focuses on Explainable AI (XAI), the influential variable among the EPE, and Patient Care and Treatment.

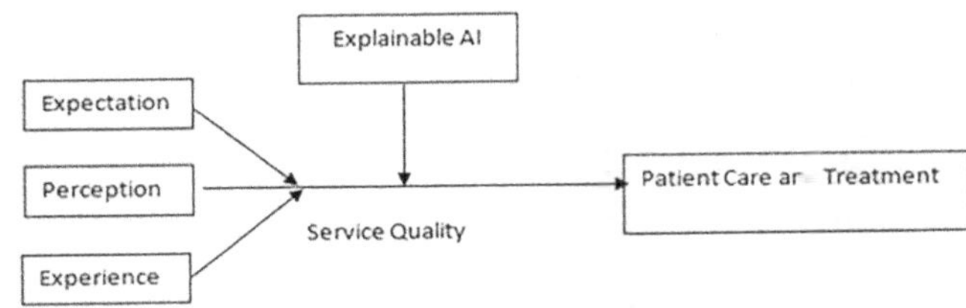

Figure 13.2 Explainable AI (XAI) influencing the EPE inpatient care and treatment.

Source: Authors'.

Figure 13.2 shows the variable XAI influencing the variables used for the service quality in patient care and Treatment. The services replaced or enhanced with AI needs Explanation to prevent bias. The challenges experienced in EPE for AI-based care and treatment are overcome by the explainable AI.

A structured questionnaire with two parts was developed by reviewing literature, where the first part represented the demographic details of respondents such as, age, gender, education, and profession, which is given in Table 13.1. Both dependent and independent

Table 13.1 The study questionnaire

EPE on improved diagnosis
As a healthcare professional, my perception of the early detection of diseases using AI is true
AI supports diagnosis
AI can predict diseases symptoms in their very early stage
In the detection of diseases, AI is like medical human judgements
AI applications are still new, and AI is not yet frequently utilized in clinical decision-making
Patients benefit from quicker and more accurate diseases detection through AI applications
EPE in advanced treatment
AI has a considerable impact on a variety of chronic diseases
AI systems can treat patients better than humans
Medical errors are minimal with the implication of AI in treatment
AI helps in clinical decision-making
Some complex decisions of patients are good to be left to AI to decide
AI in the big data era helps doctors to provide better patient care
EPE in boosting patient engagement
AI improves patient interactions with healthcare professionals
Specialized advice and information are given through the application of AI to patients
Under the intelligent direction of AI, patient involvement is improved
AI helps in making an educated decision by providing accurate information about a patient's condition
Patients can assist clinicians in giving the finest care by combining them with AI
EPE in supporting admin task
EHR, appointments, reviews and follow-ups are made easy with AI support
AI can be used to decipher the records and give the doctors information
AI can assess patients based on past data and forecasts the likelihood of diseases condition
There might be serious privacy issues in using AI for administration
With AI supporting admin tasks at hospitals, it helps in treating patients effectively
Large volumes of data train AI to develop a set of rules

Source: Authors'.

variables were measured through the second part. The questionnaire was validated through pilot study with 26 items. Twenty-three items were finally selected based on the results of the pilot study. SPSS version 26.0 was used for data analysis.

13.3.1 Sample size

The data was gathered from medical professionals (MP) and non-medical people (NMP). The valid number of respondents is 300, MP is 150, and NMP is 150, considered after pre-processing. The total number of respondents is 320, and we boosted to balance the categories and removed the redundancy and incomplete data from the survey list. Both categories equally participated in tending to all the questions, and most respondents are males. Purposive sampling technique was used to collect medical professionals' data, and convenience sampling technique was employed to collect non-medical people data. The majority of the respondents fall under the category of 30–45 years. This category of the respondent is more well versed with using technology and are more influenced by the advancement of technical facilities, which made their contribution more toward the enhancement of AI in care and treatment. The second largest group is 45–55 years, with their response showing they seek improvement in healthcare to obtain good quality service in healthcare treatments. This is an interesting factor because this category of age group is a pioneer of traditional care and treatments. Hence, from the analysis, the anticipated XAI influences the variables used for this article and is justified with the gap model.

Consistency and accuracy of the questionnaire items were tested using the reliability and validity test. The test revealed the Cronbach value of the items in the research instrument to be above the threshold limit of 0.6, as suggested [25]. It is depicted in Table 13.2, with the final 23 items after the pilot study, which supports reliability.

13.4 RESULTS AND DISCUSSION

The role of the traditional method is replaced with AI services, with the minimum access of AI in service quality, the challenges identified, and finding the improved model to prevent bias using the XAI are explained in this result and discussion session.

Figure 13.3 is the gap model of service quality between humans and AI. There are five gaps identified. We have identified the following gaps:

Table 13.2 Reliability and validity

Constructs	*No. of items*	*Cronbach's Alpha*	*AVE* (Construct validity)*
EPE on improved diagnosis	6	0.876	0.592
EPE in advanced treatment	6	0.823	0.565
EPE in boosting patient engagement	5	0.921	0.602
EPE in supporting admin task	6	0.865	0.583

Source: Authors'.

Note: *Average variance extracted.

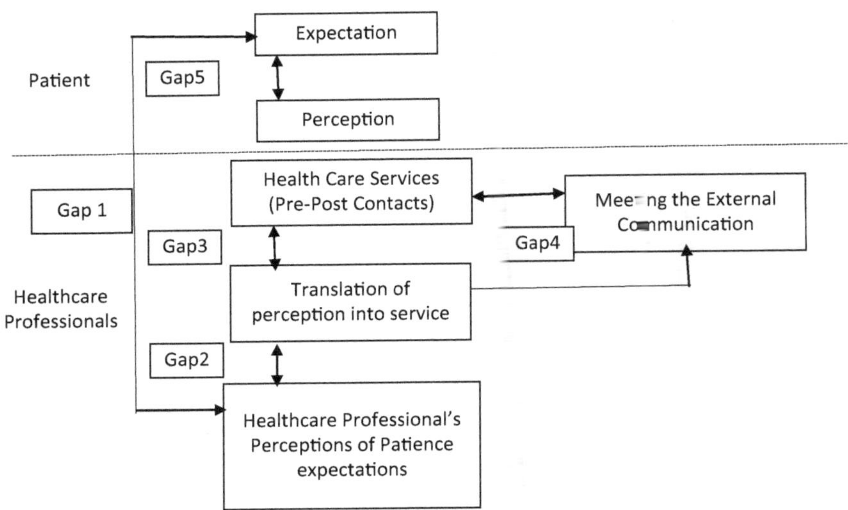

Figure 13.3 Gap model of service quality using AI.

Source: Developed by authors based on the Gaps Model of Service Quality [26].

1. The gap between Patient Expectations and Healthcare Professionals (HCP) Perceptions – less awareness and usage
2. The gap between Service Quality description and Healthcare Professionals' Perception – high description and needs improved explainable model.
3. The gap between the Service Quality description and the Service provided (Pre and Post) – satisfactory but needs improvement.
4. The gap between Service Provided and External Communication – needs explainable AI to solve the issues.
5. The gap between the Expected Service and Experienced Service – needs the full potential of AI in healthcare services.

The EPE are the key points that describe the access to the facility, waiting for a time in pre-post treatments, information about the process and the information about the patients (P), personal information maintenance, administration efficiency in running the show, communication in pre-and post-treatment to the patients and the awareness of the professionals, security for the patients and their information, satisfaction feedbacks, and ancillary services provided based patients requirements. All these are comprised of the three phases of improved diagnosis: Advanced Treatment, Boosting patient engagement, and supporting administrative tasks.

AI is used as an aiding tool for healthcare professionals in their daily work to provide service quality. The research work predicted many things among the patients and the healthcare professionals. The findings of the research will create a great impact on the society of the AI healthcare world. Based on the questionnaire, the obtained results are tabulated. Figure 13.4 shows the respondents from the medical field and non-medical fields are expecting the interventions of AI in EPE-based Service Quality.

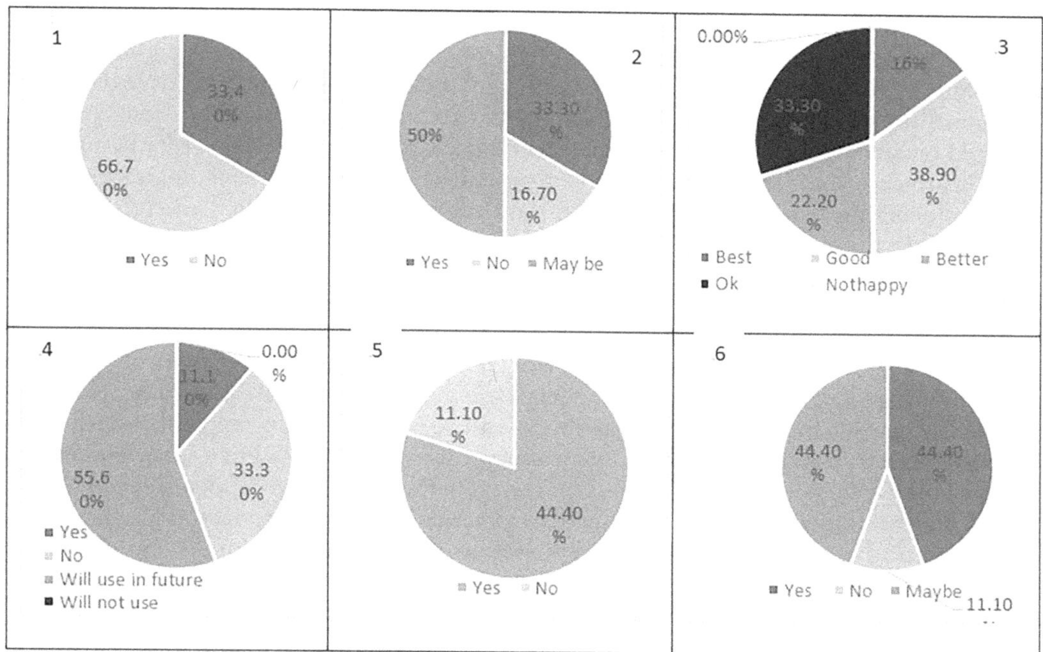

Figure 13.4 Results of the questionnaires.

***Source: Authors'* (Report generated from the survey).**

13.4.1 Percentage of the willingness to agree and to adopt AI in the EPE service quality

The percentage of people who used AI in care (*Engagement*) and treatment (both HCP and P) are 33.3% because of a lack of awareness and the fear of death. Many healthcare professionals are not aware of the technology used for the treatment, but it has been used. We may be translated to a new world and new technology but when it comes to health many are sentimental. We need someone to interact with us to console us or to explain the process when we are conscious. AI in Healthcare is a challenging task; therefore, the minimum usage resulted in the survey even for their second opinion. So, when it comes to decision-making (*Treatment*) the survey says that people are not ready to rely on machines, though it is aiding the healthcare professions in diagnosis. But the difference between agree-ness and disagree-ness is very low. So, there is high reception for adopting advanced technology for early detection and treatment with human interventions in the future.

When *boosting the service quality* using AI, there is a high chance of information threats and security issues which may arise because of myths or individuals' personal experiences. But this is possible when humans engaged in the same process. From the survey report people are not alleging the technology, there is a strong conviction that both humans and AI will suffer from security and data theft. The *Experience* of the HCP and P in the traditional service quality is to some extent. The respondents of the survey believe that the superpower which is little or more advance than humans with minimum bias will provide a satisfactory quality service. Complete adoption of AI plays a greater role in basic and advanced service quality concerning Expectation, Perception, and Experience. The result shows the maximum percentage preventing human errors by using AI.

It is advised that the government encourage public-private partnerships in the area of AI and health, support business investments in AI, enact laws and regulations pertaining to AI and health, effectively enforce those laws and regulations, develop policies addressing issues of confidentiality and privacy in AI-driven healthcare, and create a certification system for AI-based healthcare solutions. It is crucial to equip the personnel in AI in order to adopt AI-based healthcare since this will enable them to efficiently use AI systems, manage sensitive health information with care, and prevent data theft. Additionally, it is essential that any healthcare decisions made using AI-based solutions have a basis and can be explained.

13.4.2 Explainable AI in gap model

The survey shows AI can improve service quality, which is measured in terms of expectations, perceptions, and the experience of the patients and the healthcare professionals. The gaps identified in the AI gap model can be improved using explainable AI, which provides more transparency in care and treatment. It explains the human interventions and the psychological care to be given based on the vulnerability. The gaps identified among the patient and healthcare professionals, services experience and the services assured, external communication between the HCP, P, and the services, and translation of perception into the experience are demonstrating that the explainable AI framework helps the transparency (Black Box), privacy, and security (Breech and Theft), traces the experience (feedback), and improves the performance of the method used for treatment (Improved Model Performance).

From the analysis, explainable AI is needed to create more awareness and usage by providing an explanation of the diagnosis and the treatment, and an improved model for identifying the bias is considered the most significant feature of XAI, and respondents, and many researchers are satisfied with AI and believe that the XAI can improve the service quality based on EPE.

AI based treatments are efficient, but it has not reached the public well due to lack of awareness among healthcare professional and patients. Healthcare professionals are not able to elaborate on the importance and effects of AI on treatment to their patients because people are hesitant to obtain AI based treatment. This also includes issues like decision-making, data privacy, data security, and treatment. If the Artificial Intelligence integrated patient care treatment incorporates explainable AI, this solves the gaps related to AI patient care and treatment service quality among patient and healthcare professionals.

13.5 CONCLUSION

AI in healthcare is superior to human-made tools, which provide intelligence in early diagnosis, care, and treatments. Patient experience in AI care and treatment is measured by the service quality aspects such as expectation, perception, and experience. AI is used for accessing information and facilities, waiting time for acquisition, information gathering and maintenance, administration activities that are the soul of the health industry, communication between the patients and the healthcare professionals, data security, treatment satisfaction, and other services. The services produced by AI in terms of improving the healthcare industry are acknowledged by the respondents of the survey. The gap model is used to identify the gaps in patient experience (EPE) among patients and healthcare professionals in service quality to insist on the importance of explainable AI as the enhancement model in the current scenario. The proposed three different gaps are less awareness and usage among the professionals, high description, and the need for an improved explainable model. Quality service is satisfactory but needs improvement, and quality service needs explainable AI to solve the issues, which needs the full potential of AI in healthcare services. Therefore, with the findings, the service quality in early diagnosis, advanced treatment, service enhancement, and administrative tasks with AI can be improved with explainable AI (XAI) in providing transparency and enhancing the model to prevent bias. As we are turning toward an advanced AI world. if we focus on these gaps, XAI can be used for the enhancement of the healthcare industry, especially in patient care and treatment that is proved by the focus group survey report and the existing research articles. For further study, we can experimentally establish the excellence of using XAI in healthcare for an efficient quality service.

REFERENCES

1. Manne, R. and Kantheti, S. (2021). Application of artificial intelligence in healthcare: Chances and challenges. *Current Journal of Applied Science and Technology*, 40(6), 78–89.
2. Yedurkar, D. P., Metkar, S., Al-Turjman, F., Yardi, N. and Stephan, T. An IoT based novel hybrid seizure detection approach for epileptic monitoring. *IEEE Transactions on Industrial Informatics*, 20(2), 1420–1431, Feb. 2024. doi: 10.1109/TII.2023.3274913.
3. Davenport, T. and Kalakota, R. (2019). Digital Technology – The potential for artificial intelligence in healthcare. *Future Healthcare Journal*, 6(2), 94–98.
4. Secinaro, S., Calandra, D., Secinaro, A., Muthurangu, V. and Biancone, P. (2021). The role of artifcial intelligence in healthcare: A structured literature review. *BMC Medical Informatics and Decision Making*, 21, 125.
5. Rehaman, M. U. and Panday, A. (2021). Review on artificial intelligence in healthcare. *Innovations*, 66.
6. WHO (2021). Ethics and governance of artificial intelligence for health: WHO guidance, ISBN 978-92-4-002920-0.
7. ICMR (2022). Draft Ethical guidelines for application of artificial intelligence in biomedical research and healthcare, p. 7.
8. Bohr, A. and Memarzadeh, K. (2020). The rise of artificial intelligence in healthcare applications. *Artificial Intelligence in Healthcare*, pp. 25, doi 10.1016/B978-0-12-818438-7.00002-2. ISBN 978-92-4-002920-0978-92-4-002920-0.
9. Khamseh, E., Aghai, R., Baradaran Moghadam, H. and Arabi A. (2009).Satisfaction of patients about the method of providing outpatient services in Firoozgar training-treating centre of metabolism and endocrine glands clinics, Iran medical sciences university seasonal, sixth year, number one, winter; 71–74.
10. Abedi, G., Rostami, F., Ziaee, M., Siamian, H. and Nadi, A. (2015). Patient's perception and expectations of the quality of outpatient services of Imam Khomeini Hospital in Sari City. *Mater Sociomed*, 27(4), August, 272–275.
11. Reck, D. L. (2013). Can and should nurses be aware of patients' expectations for their nursing care? *Nursing Administration Quarterly*, 37(2), 109–115.
12. Abrahamsen Grøndahl, V. (2012). Patients' perceptions of actual care conditions and patient satisfaction with care quality in the hospital. Karlstad: Karlstads Universitet.
13. Bush, J. (2018). How AI is taking the scut work out of health care. *Harvard Business Review*, 5. https://hbr.org/2018/03/how-ai-is-takingthe-scut-work-out-of-health-care
14. Dilsizian, S. E. and Siegel, E. L. (2014). Artificial intelligence in medicine and cardiac imaging: harnessing big data and advanced computing to provide personalized medical diagnosis and treatment. *Current Cardiology Reports*, 16, 1–8.
15. Eren, A., Subasi, A. and Coskun, O. (2008). A decision support system for telemedicine through the mobile telecommunications platform. *Journal of Medical Systems*, 32(1), 31–35.

16. Punitha, S., Stephan, T., Kannan, R., Mahmud, M., Kaiser, M. S. and Belhaouari, S. B. (2023). Detecting COVID-19 from lung computed tomography images: A swarm optimized artificial neural network approach. *IEEE Access*, 11, 12378–12393, doi: 10.1109/ACCESS.2023.3236812.
17. Balogh et al. (2015). Improving diagnosis in health care. Improving Diagnosis in Health Care, 1–472, doi 10.17226/21794.
18. Bresnick, J. (2016). Big data, artificial intelligence, and IoT may change healthcare in 2017. Available at https://healthitanalytics.com/news/big-data-artificial-intelligence-it may-change-healthcare-in-2017 (accessed on November 2022).
19. Hsieh, P. (2017a). AI in medicine: the rise of the machines. Available at https://www.forbes. com/sites/paulhsieh/2017/04/30/ai-in-medicine-rise-of-the-machines/ (accessed on November 2022).
20. Volpp, K. and Mohta, S. (2016). Improved engagement leads to better outcomes, but better tools are needed. Insights Report. NEJM Catalyst, https://catalyst.nejm.org/patient-engagement-report-improved-engagement-leads-better-outcomes-better-tools-needed.
21. Pisarchik, A. N., Maksimenko, V. A. and Hramov, A. E. (2019). From Novel technology to novel applications: Comment on "An integrated brain-machine interface platform with thousands of channels" by Elon Musk and Neuralink. *Journal of Medical Internet Research*, 21(10), e16356.
22. Harrow Council (2016). IBM and harrow council to bring watson care manager to individuals in the UK.
23. Berg, S. (2018). Nudge theory explored to boost medication adherence. Chicago: American Medical Association, www.ama-assn.org/delivering-care/patient-support-advocacy/nudge-theory-explored-boost-medication-adherence (accessed on March 2023).
24. Hair, J. F., Risher, J. J., Sarstedt, M. and Ringle, C. M. (2019). When to use and how to report the results of PLS-SEM. *European Business Review*, 31, 2–24. 10. 108/EBR-11-2018-0203
25. Lee, S. I., Celik, S., Logsdon, B. A., Lundberg, S. M., Martins, T. J., Oehler, V. G., Estey, E. H., Miller, C. P., Chien, S., Dai, J., Saxena, A., Blau, C. A. and Becker, P. S. (2018). Machine learning approach to integrate big data for precision medicine in acute myeloid leukaemia. *Nature Communications*, 9(1), 42.
26. Parasuraman, A., Zeithaml, V. A. and Berry, L. (1985). A conceptual model of service quality and its implications for future research. *Journal of Marketing*, 49(4), 41–50. 10.2307/1251430

Chapter 14

Improved medical image captioning for chest X-rays using a hybrid VGG-ELECTRA model

J Limsa Joshi, J Christina, L Remegius Praveen Sahayaraj, V J Sharmila, and Ashwin Balasubramanian

Department of Computer Science and Engineering, Loyola-ICAM College of Engineering and Technology, Chennai, Tamil Nadu, India

14.1 INTRODUCTION

Medical facilities and technological advancements in the field of medicine are very helpful to society in terms of early diagnosis and treatment of diseases. However, with the large number of medical images being generated, doctors are facing immense pressure to manually inspect and generate reports, which can be overwhelming. Medical Image Captioning is the process by which medical images such as X-rays, Computed Tomography (CT) scans, and Magnetic resonance imaging (MRI) scans of a patient are annotated with medical diagnosis using NLP. An automatic image captioning model will help the doctors in diagnosis and thereby significantly reduce the workload of the doctors, hence saving time. Automatic medical image captioning is a growing field of research domain that is primarily concerned with developing tools and techniques for auto-rendering meaningful, accurate, and precise captions.

Autonomous production of descriptive sentences for variegated images has drawn proliferating attention and has become a primary and renowned field of research in computer vision in recent years. Captioning images requires a contextual understanding of images as well as the ability to produce precise descriptions. Image captioning requires computer vision technologies to interpret the image features and NLP tools to generate sentences from the extracted image. Hrga et al. [1] gave an overview of various image captioning techniques ranging from techniques based on templates to deep learning. Early techniques are mostly based on retrieval-based methods and template-based methods. Retrieval-based image captioning methods produce captions from a pre-existing pool of captions given by medical professionals. The retrieval-based method selects the captions from the existing pool by comparing the images and it retrieves the text of the nearest matching image. Retrieval-based methods use nearest-neighbor retrieval, text-based retrieval, semantic retrieval, and attention-based retrieval. Template-based methods focus on filling the predetermined text templates with features extracted from images [2]. Current systems also employ deep learning-based algorithms that act as encoder-decoder architecture to generate sentences.

With the recent breakthrough in hardware and storage devices, a lot of medical images are stored in hospitals and are available for analysis. Annotation and proper structural storage of these images will significantly help medical professionals by reducing the workload of manually preparing the reports.

Medical image captioning is different from normal image captioning in terms of its various factors such as limited publicly available dataset, the skewed nature of the dataset to the clinically normal data, and the complexity of the data. Medical Image Captioning also requires a high accuracy in generating the sentences making it a complex domain.

DOI: 10.1201/9781003369059-18

Chest X-ray is a frequently used radiology image and it produces images of the heart, lungs, and chest. As an example, according to Yin et al. [3], radiologists devote approximately five to twenty minutes to analyze and describe the results of a single image for one patient case. During the pandemic, this time-consuming process was further exacerbated as radiologists had to interpret over a hundred chest X-rays in one day. The pandemic also resulted in a surge in hospital admission rates, which led to incorrect and delayed reports from radiologists. This delay in diagnosis increased treatment costs. In this chapter, chest X-Ray images are considered for captioning and as most of the images appear to be similar, it is crucial to find the discriminating features and to represent those in sentence .

Hence in this work, we present a novel methodology that exploits the power of VGG-16 to extract the features from the images and the power of ELECTRA to generate meaningful sentences from the features. The first phase is to derive image feature information using VGG-16 [4], increasing the depth of the convolutional layers. VGG-16 primarily extracts the information from the image including the affected region in the chest X-Ray. In the second phase, ELECTRA is used to analyze the semantics of the image and to integrate it with features extracted from VGG-16 to generate a meaningful image description. The dataset consists of 324,400 images and is fundamentally based on the X-ray dataset of chest images provided by NIH which has around 1, 12,120 X-ray pictures that were gathered from 30,805 patients' disease datasets and is explained in section 14.3.[illegible].

14.2 LITERATURE SURVEY

14.2.1 VGG-16

Visual Geometry Group (VGG) is a modified Convolution Network Architecture that is prominently used as an innovative object-recognition model that has been prominent for multiple applications. Initially, AlexNet which was employed with a receptive field of 4-pixel stride uses a much smaller 33 receptive field with 1-pixel stride. VGG-16 has less number of parameters than AlexNet. The function of a bigger receptive field is achieved by the combination of 33 filters and 16 layers of convolution in the architecture. The network's propensity to overfit the model during training exercises is decreased by the smaller convolutional filter used by VGG. Hence these configurations were used to leverage feature extraction tasks in image datasets.

The input to the VGG architecture is an image of dimension (224, 224, 3). The VGG-16 has 16 layers with convolution and max pooling. After the 16 layers, three fully connected layers are attached to classify the images. The VGG-16 architecture is characterized by the use of 3 × 3 convolutional filters that are stacked together to form deeper layers. The model has achieved state of art results in learning complex features from the input images. The completely connected layers towards the network tail, classify the image through the features that were learned.

The VGG-16 is widely used as a base model for applications based on transfer learning methodology [3] in the arena of computer vision. Its pre-trained weights can be used as an initial point for training other models on smaller datasets, resulting in quicker convergence and increased accuracy.

14.2.2 Medical report generation image captioning models

Image captioning models are also widely used in the medical field for captioning medical images such as X-rays, fMRI, and Retinal OCT Scans [5]. Diagnostic Captioning (DC) is the process of automatically generating a diagnosis by examining the medical images of a patient availed for diagnostics. The resulting output from DC serves as supporting evidence for the clinician, as it highlights only the clinically relevant information and can improve their diagnosis. Image captioning models can also employ encoder-decoder architectures that make use of image feature vectors as input to the encoder. The encoder is a convolutional neural network in the model and the image features are extracted from the fully connected layer whilst the recurrent neural network acts as the decoder for generating picture descriptions [6].

Ivasic-Kos et al. [7] used a fuzzy-based approach for image captioning of coral images. The paper presents a novel approach for automatic image annotation that addresses the challenge of bridging the semantic gap between low-level image features and human-like interpretation. Park et al. [8] proposed a model to learn the differences between the normal and infected chest X-rays using hierarchical LSTM as well as a transformer as a decoder to generate the reports.

In vision-language learning, the objective [9] is to create models that can interpret and generate natural language descriptions for the given visual content such as images or videos. Li et al. [10] proposed mPLUG, a deep learning architecture for the vision-language learning tasks. The model was proposed to improve the computational efficiency of the existing models. It uses cross-modal skip connections to increase the efficiency. The skip connections help in skipping the irrelevant or unnecessary connections thereby effectively learning and retaining the visual and textual information. mPLUG‘s architecture comprises two distinct streams: a vision stream and a language stream. The vision stream is responsible for processing visual input and extracting visual features, while the language stream processes textual input and extracts language features. Cross-modal skip connections connect these features to enable seamless information flow between the two streams, resulting in an efficient architecture.

Wang et al. [11] proposed TieNet, a text-embedding network for detecting and reporting thorax disease from chest X-Ray. TieNet uses ResNet and LSTM decoder for multi-level attention mechanisms to extract distinct text and image features.

Yang et al. [12] introduced the MedWriter approach, which tries to estimate mental content by studying the link between functional magnetic resonance imaging (fMRI) data and semantic information of conceptualized material. MedWriter works by using the report as well as sentence-level templates for generating clinically accurate reports generation and has been a prominent application of language models. Park et al. [13] proposed mDiTag model to evaluate the difference between the normal and the patient images that contain the differences in terms of image contrast, image texture, and localized area. This information is used to generate efficient reports that suit the particular discrepancies detected. This standpoint among the transformers could be observed due to the peculiarity in the generation of feature difference vectors.

14.2.3 Language models

Natural Language Processing has made significant advancements with deep learning techniques in the past years. Language models examine large amounts of text data to build a robust system to predict the most likely next word with the support of the previous word. Language models can be broadly categorized as probabilistic models and neural network-based models.

The probabilistic language model is purely a statistical model that maps a probability to each likely sequence of words in a given language. A hefty quantity of text data is used to learn the probability distribution. The probabilistic language model can be used to foretell the probability of a particular sequence of words. Probabilistic language models are based on n-grams, where sequences of n-1 words are used to predict the nth word or the model can employ sophisticated methods such as hidden Markov models (HMM) or conditional random fields (CRF).

The neural network-based language model is a machine learning-based model that uses artificial neural networks (ANN) to learn complex statistical patterns in text data. A Recurrent Neural Network, a type of ANN is trained on a large corpus of text data to predict the probability distribution of the next word in a sequence given the previous words. This approach is used in a recursive manner to generate an entire caption for a given image. These language models can also be trained based on LSTM or Transformer-based architecture.

BERT [14] – Bidirectional Encoder Representations from Transformers is a transformer-based model created by Google. The model captures the semantic relationships between word tokens to perform tasks such as language understanding and text classification. BERT model is used to process and capture long-term dependencies between sentences. The model is pre-trained on massive text data for masked language modeling (MLM) and the prediction of the next sentence.

In the MLM-based approach, a random set of words is selected and masked in a given sentence. The model is now trained to predict the masked words based on the context of its enclosing words. The model is further trained in capturing the meaning of the words based on both their preceding and following words. In sentence-level prediction, the model is trained to predict if the two sentences are successive in the original text. It helps in understanding the relationship between the sentences in the holistic context of the text. BERT has made a significant impact in NLP tasks such as named entity recognition, text classification, and question-answering systems.

The RoBERTa proposed by Liu et al. [15] improved the BERT model by training the model against a massive and diverse corpus of text. The model addressed several limitations of the BERT model such as i) It incorporated a large amount of data from a variety of sources such as Wikipedia, web pages, and books ii) Hyperparameter tuning to improve the efficiency of the BERT model - training the model for a longer time and over larger batch size allowing it to acquire patterns that are complex in the data. RoBERTa made use of byte-level BPE as a tokenizer and an alternate pre-training scheme that allowed it to elevate its performance in generating longer sequences.

The model was further fine-tuned with one additional output layer by Delvin et al. [14]. He et al. [16] and [17] proposed DeBERTaV3, an enhanced version of BERT by replacing the mask language with replaced tokens. The authors used a novel gradient disentangled embedding sharing to further improve the efficiency.

Clark et al. [18] proposed ELECTRA, an NLP model to develop a more efficient and effective pre-training method. ELECTRA achieves a comparable performance to BERT with fewer computational resources and less training time. ELECTRA works by generator-discriminator model. The generator is trained to take an input sentence and randomly change the words in the input sentence to make it a corrupt sentence. The discriminators' role is to analyze the two input sentences and predict the original sentence or to discriminate the original sentence from that of the corrupt sentence. ELECTRA operates by corrupting or replacing certain tokens with alternatives from a small generator network. ELECTRA considerably exceeds the performance of MLM-based methods such as BERT [14] and XLNet [19]. ELECTRA has been utilized widely in sentimental analysis, modeling language, and question-answering.

The proposed model is designed in such a way taking into consideration, the critical analysis made with respect to the above-discussed language model and image captioning models. The proposed methodology uses a hybrid version of VGG16 – ELECTRA for Image captioning. VGG-16 is used to extract the image features from the chest X-ray images. The image features are then passed onto the ELECTRA for generating appropriate image captions.

14.3 METHODOLOGY

14.3.1 Dataset

Our dataset is based on the images of the processed chest X-ray dataset that is extracted from the Clinical PACS database of the National Institute of Health Clinical Centers [20]. The dataset encompasses 112,120 images of X-rays with labels of diseases from 30,805 patients. The dataset contains about 15 classes along with the description, 14 classes which include Atelectasis, Consolidation, Infiltration, Pneumothorax, Edema, Emphysema, Fibrosis, Effusion, Pneumonia, Pleural thickening, Cardiomegaly, Nodule, Mass and Hernia representing different named medical conditions and one exclusive label for "No findings". The labels for this particular dataset were created using Natural Language Processing techniques to text-mine disease classifications from the associated radiological reports. Annotations along with bounding boxes of the anomaly are also provided in the dataset. Additionally, the processed data is populated by embedding noise in the actual images to provide images of several qualities and resolutions. The final dataset consists of 324,400 images, which are then fragmented into 70% for training and 30% for testing by the random shuffle.

The dataset is prepared and formatted in such a way that the description and the unique identifier of the particular chest X-Ray are stored in a CSV file and the identifier is mapped to the name of the chest X-Ray for the appropriate training process. Table 14.1 details the disease name with the number of images.

14.3.2 Proposed architecture

The proposed architecture performs image captioning tasks using chest X-rays. Figure 14.1 shows the fundamental block representation of the methodology involved. The entire architecture comprises two main processing functional blocks which would be the pre-trained VGG-16 and the ELECTRA Component.

The workflow of the model is summarized in Figure 14.2. Initially, the training set consists of both image captions as well as input images. The images are passed onto VGG-16 to extract the features. The values generated by the pre-trained VGG-16 are sent to the encoder for generating the text embedding. The generated text captions are passed to the discriminator embedding layer for creating embedding and for further comparative discrimination. The caption that was generated is matched to the actual caption to update the parameters of the ELECTRA model. The final trained Generator of Electra will be used for generating image captions for variegated X-rays.

14.3.2.1 Data-preprocessing for chest X-rays

The images that are passed to the VGG-16 model as shown in Figure 14.3, undergo certain preprocessing steps for efficient and improvised feature extraction. The image is resized to 256 × 256. Smoothening of the image is performed using the Gaussian Blur Filters. For the

Table 14.1 Total images per disease in updated training data

S. No	*Disease*	*No of images*
1	Atelectasis	20,626
2	Consolidation	24,614
3	Infiltration	22,626
4	Edema	22,626
5	Pneumothorax	16.326
6	Emphysema	22,626
7	Fibrosis	22,626
8	Effusion	22,626
9	Pneumonia	22,626
10	Pleural Thickening	20,600
11	Cardiomegaly	19,626
12	Nodule	23,426
13	Mass	20,426
14	Hernia	21,000
15	No Findings	22,000

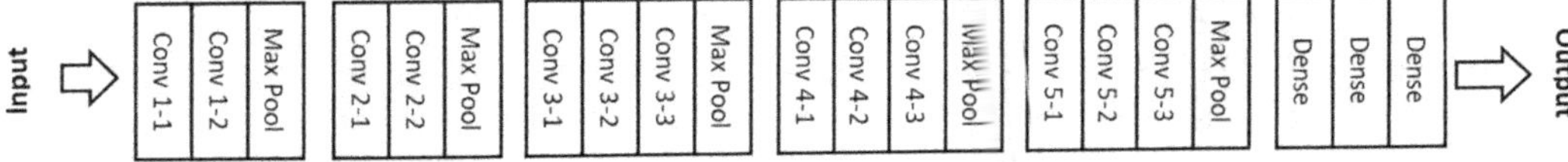

Figure 14.1 Architecture of VGG-16 network.

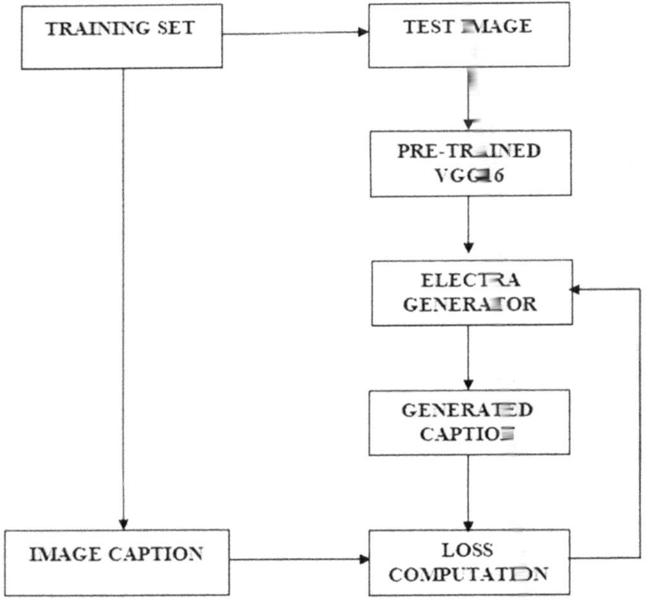

Figure 14.2 Deep VGG ELECTRA architecture.

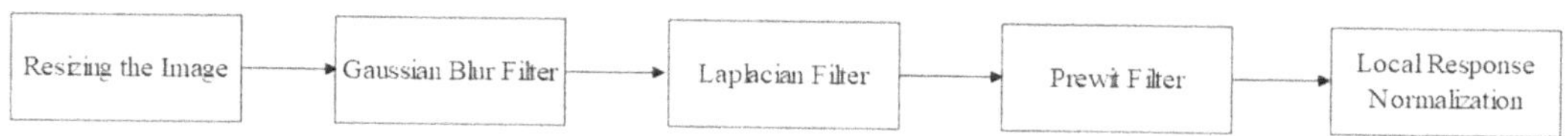

Figure 14.3 Data preprocessing for chest X-rays.

detection of edges in the image, Prewitt and Laplacian filters are made into used Laplacian filters; being a derivative filter highlights regions of rapid intensity change in the chest X-ray image. Its ability to detect edges in all directions is advantageous in this current scenario. The resultant generated feature maps from the modified VGG-16 model elevate the model performance and provide accurate feature maps. Final preprocessing steps include Local Response Normalization so that local maximum pixel values are used as excitation in the modified VGG-16 model as well as to minimize computations in the model.

14.3.2.2 Feature extraction using modified VGG-16 architecture

The original architecture consists of convolution and pooling blocks, which add up to 19 layers. The modified VGG network max pooling layers, as shown in Figure 14.4, are replaced with average pooling layers to improve the performance of the architecture. The replacement of the max pool layers is carried out since average pooling tends to take a collective average of the pixels which enables the architecture to learn the features throughout and come to a common conclusion.

For image caption generation, the features of an image must be extracted. A pre-trained model of VGG-16 is used to interpret the image content [21]. VGG series networks have three layers of convolution stacked one on top of another, with increasing depths. Reducing the volume size is treated by maximum pooling. Pre-trained VGG-16 uses pre-trained weights which aid the training process. In the process, dimensions are converted from 2048 × 2048 to 256 × 256. A dropout layer is added between the convolution layers to provide proper training. Preprocessing of the input images is performed by the VGG-16 model and the fully connected layer is removed. The feature maps that are generated by the outmost convolutional layer seem to capture all the cavities, as well as the distorted regions. Hence the feature maps that are generated by the outmost convolution layers present themselves as a vital source of information to generate a caption that explains the location as well as the severity of the disease. The feature maps are extracted directly and are passed as input to the ELECTRA to predict the caption.

14.3.2.3 ELECTRA

The architecture of ELECTRA is based on a pre-trained transformer language model that makes use of a replaced token detection architecture. The feature maps are passed onto the common max pooling layer and its results are then flattened into a single-dimensional vector. The single-dimensional vector is reshaped and padded based on the length of the input token

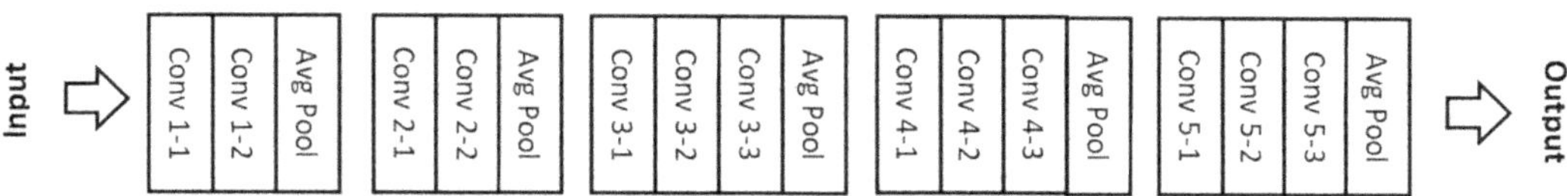

Figure 14.4 Modified architecture of VGG-16.

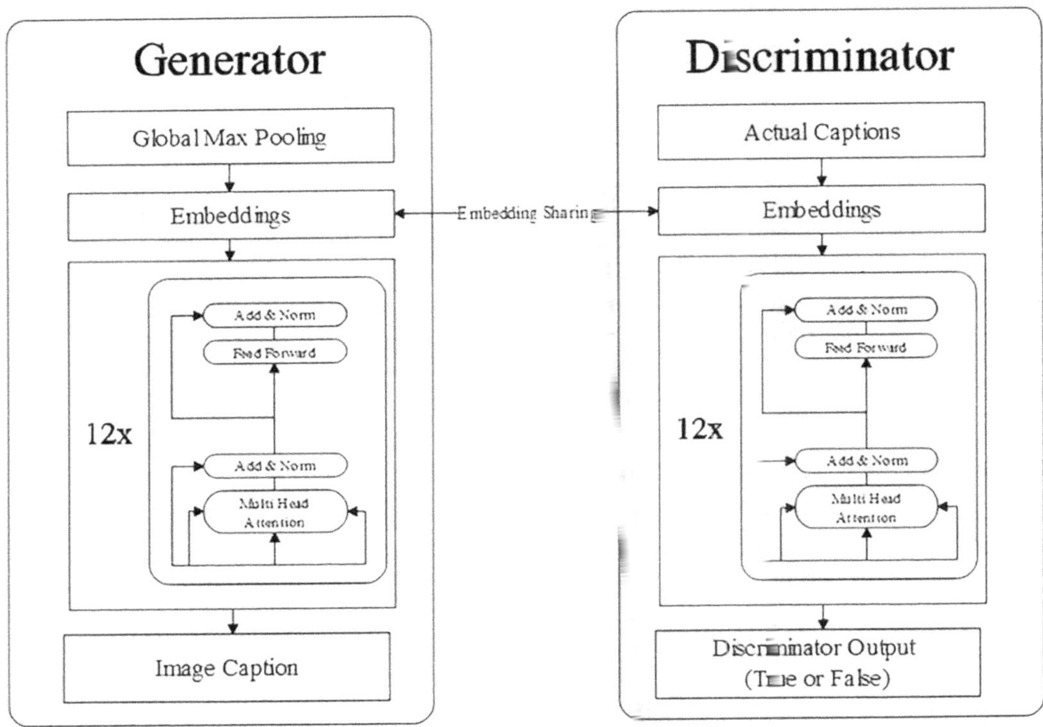

Figure 14.5 Generator discriminator architecture of ELECTRA.

embedding and is passed to ELECTRA. This vector serves as an initial embedding for the ELECTRA generator. The embedding is then used to generate full captions. The ELECTRA model is mentioned in Figure 14.5 and is trained to differentiate between authentic input tokens and artificially created tokens using ELECTRA's replacement token prediction tasks. In the input text, the actual captions of the image are tokenized with the help of WordPiece Tokenization. The tokenization is trained using the four clinical datasets from BLURB as well as the GLUE Benchmarks. Next, the discriminator network predicts if the actual tokens are the same as the tokens generated by the generator. There is no pooling projection layer in ELECTRA since it lacks a contrastive learning method [22]. This contrastive method is tuned or modified to cater to generating image captions created from the feature mappings and encodings from the feature extractor. The updated ELECTRA loss function as mentioned in the equations Eq. 14.1 & 14.2 has been tuned to take the encoded features from the VGG-16 and train its discriminator for further training and MLM loss remains the same as per the original algorithm. After the training process, the discriminator is removed from the model and the generator alone will be used for the purpose of generating the captions for the scan images.

$$L_{disc} = E\left(\sum_{t=1}^{n} -1\left(x_t^{true} = x_t\right) logD\left(x^{true}, t\right) - 1\left(x_t^{true} = x_t\right) log\left(1 - D\left(x^{true}, t\right)\right)\right) \quad (14.1)$$

$$D(x, t) = sigmoid\left(w^t h_D(x)_t\right) \quad (14.2)$$

where x^{true} *= original input string,* x *= predicted string*

The architecture shown in Figure 14.5, will have one embedding layer with ELECTRA to process the captions, replacing the token detection. The text encoder has been trained to distinguish between input tokens and tokens produced negatively by the generator network. Since ELECTRA is primarily designed for language modeling and NLP such as answering questions and classification of texts, it is trained with diverse texts to learn the significance of the medical keywords.

14.4 EXPERIMENT AND ANALYSIS

14.4.1 Experimental setup

For training purposes, the images are augmented by applying bicubic interpolation as well as vertical and horizontal flips randomly to 30% of the training dataset. All the images to be used for training and automation are resized to 128 × 128 for better performance. The preprocessed data is then used to train the VGG-16 architecture. The training took up to 5.6 weeks to reach its optimum level. The training was done with Intel(R) Xeon(R) W-1350 @ 3.30 GHz 3.31 GHz processor, 64 GB RAM, and NVIDIA RTX A4000 Graphics card.

14.4.2 Experimental results

The proposed methodology is evaluated against 324,400 images, which are segregated into 227,080 train images and 97,320 test images. In total, 14 diseases are covered in the hand-collected dataset.

Table 14.2 represents the model parameters for ELECTRA and VGG-16 architectures that are used to train the model. Figure 14.6 denotes the training plot of the entire architecture on the data set. The plot is constructed with the number of epochs in the x-axis and the discriminator loss in the y-axis. The model has been trained through 800 epochs and the loss plot is scaled to a valid limit for visualization. After the training process, the final discriminator loss was evaluated to 14.5, which signifies a proper and steady training process as well as efficient model architecture.

Table 14.2 Model parameters for the proposed architecture

Parameter	*VGG-16*	*ELECTRA*
Optimizer	ADAM	ADAM
Regularization	Stochastic Gradient Descent	Stochastic Gradient Descent
Learning Rate	0.001	0.001
Activation Function	ReLU	–
Learning Rate Delay	–	Linear
Attention Heads	–	12
Dropout	0.5	0.1
Tokenizer	–	BERT Tokenizer
Discriminator Size	–	512

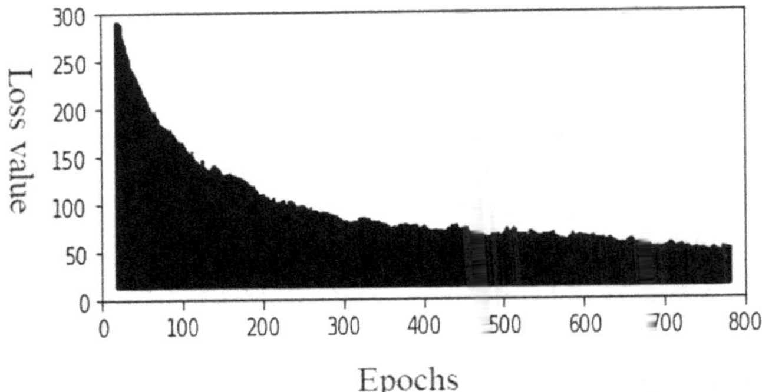

Figure 14.6 Loss curve of the discriminator.

Image captioning in chest X-rays was evaluated against the VGG16-BiLSTM, CNN-BiLSTM, and VGG16-ELECTRA algorithms. The final results are evaluated using the Bilingual Evaluation Understudy 4 (BLEU-4) Score, as well as the Recall-Oriented Understudy for Gisting Evaluation (ROUGE-4) F1 Score to define the accuracy of the prediction texts generated.

BLEU–4 is a performance measure of the quality of the machine translation output. Through the reference translations, the BLEU-4 calculates the precision of all four consecutive words in the candidate translation. The BLEU-4 Score is computed using the brevity penalty, as well as the geometric precision scores.

The brevity penalty, as well as the precision scores, are calculated as mentioned in the equations Eq. (14.3) and Eq. (14.4).

$$\begin{aligned} GA\_precisionscores(N) &= \exp\left(\sum_{n=1}^{N} w_n \log p_n\right) \\ &= \prod_{n=1}^{N} p_n^{w_n} \\ &= (p_1)^{\frac{1}{4}} * (p_2)^{\frac{1}{4}} * (p_3)^{\frac{1}{4}} * (p_4)^{\frac{1}{4}} \end{aligned} \tag{14.3}$$

$$b\_penalty = \begin{cases} 1, & if\ c > r \\ e^{\left(1-\frac{r}{c}\right)}, & if\ c \le r \end{cases}. \tag{14.4}$$

Where c = predicted length, r = target length, p = precision value for -gram

The BLEU-4 scores are evaluated using Eq. (14.5) and is used to evaluate and fine-tune the architecture.

$$\text{BLEU(N)} = \text{b\_penalty}_{*}\text{GA\_precisionscores(N)} \tag{14.5}$$

Where c = predicted length, r = target length, p = precision value for i-gram

The BLEU-4 score was evaluated to 0.54 for the testing data against the experimental parameters. Along with BLEU-4 scores ROUGE-4 F1 scores are also computed for further analysis. The ROUGE score is a commonly used metric for evaluating the summarization quality and machine translation systems. Similar to the BLEU-4 scores, the similarity between an auto-generated summary and a reference translation is measured with respect to a n-gram overlap. For the above situation, 4-gram is used, which compares the overlap of 4-grams, or sequences of four consecutive words, between the generated and reference text.

ROUGE Metric: Recall-Oriented Understudy for Gisting Evaluation (ROUGE) is a metric to compare the generated statement and the reference statement. It is analyzed by computing how much the generated image captions and reference image captions are similar. For image captioning, we use ROUGE-4 – to identify the connection of the 4 words between the reference image and the image caption that was generated. The ROUGE-4 F1 scores are computed using Eq 14.5. ROUGE4_precision is the ratio of the number of 4 grams in a candidate sentence that appears also in the target sentence. ROUGE4_recall is the ratio of the number of 4 grams in the target sentence that appear also in the target sentence

$$ROUGE4\_\_F1 = 2 * \frac{(ROUGE4\_precision \ * \ ROUGE4\_recall)}{(ROUGE4\_recall \ + \ ROUGE4\_precision)} \tag{14.6}$$

The metrics of the different models are visualized in Figure 14.7 and Figure 14.8, which interprets the idea that the proposed model using VGG16 along with ELECTRA outperforms the existing architectures such as VGG-16-BiLSTM and CNN-LSTM. A similar training strategy is applied to the other two models with similar hyper-parameter settings for proper comparative study and analyzes the trends at every interval of the training period with the help of the previously mentioned metrics.

The caption generated is "thoracic aorta is mildly tortuos" for the image shown in Figure 14.9a. For the image shown in Figure 14.9b, the generated caption is "viral pneumonia in the upper segment," and for Figure 14.9c, the generated caption is "No Findings Present in the specimen."

The training of the model is carried over by generating single-sentence captions of the anomalies that are present in the scan images. The captions can be further explained or made much more descriptive by changing the corpus and incorporating additional information in the dataset which is used for training. Further corpus text can be incorporated into the training dataset to improve performance and generate much more specific captions for the chest X-rays.

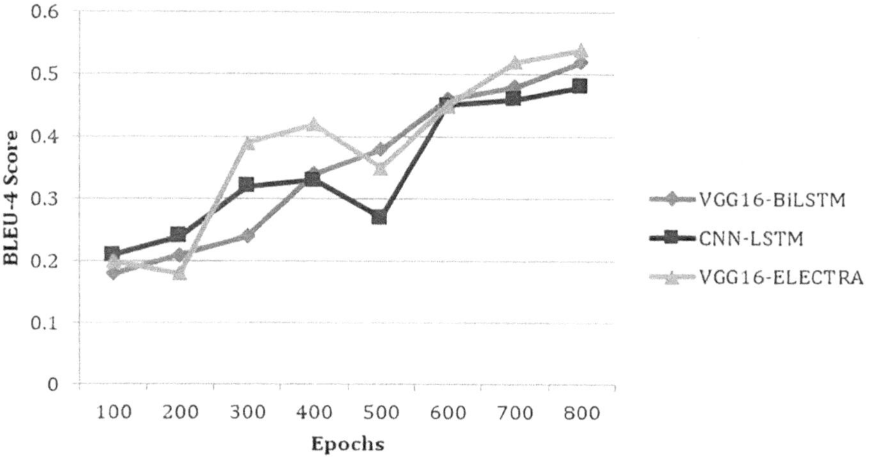

Figure 14.7 BLEU-4 curve for image captioning architectures.

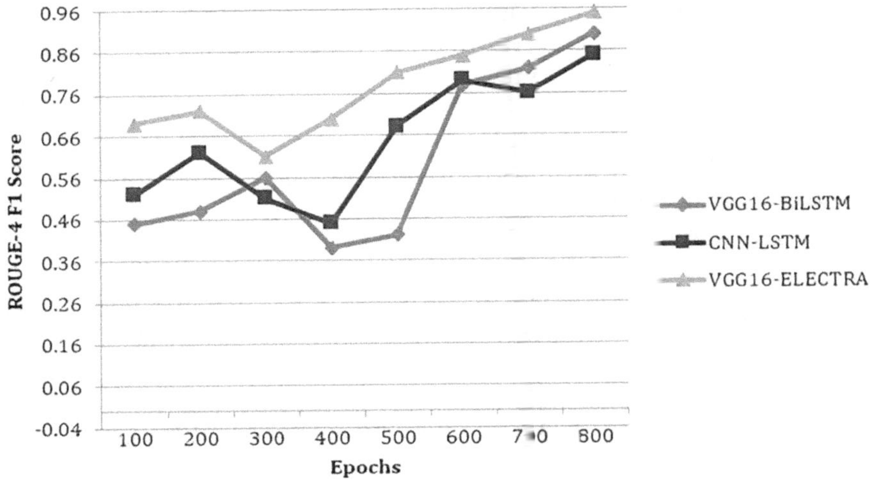

Figure 14.8 ROUGE-4 F1 score curve for image captioning architectures.

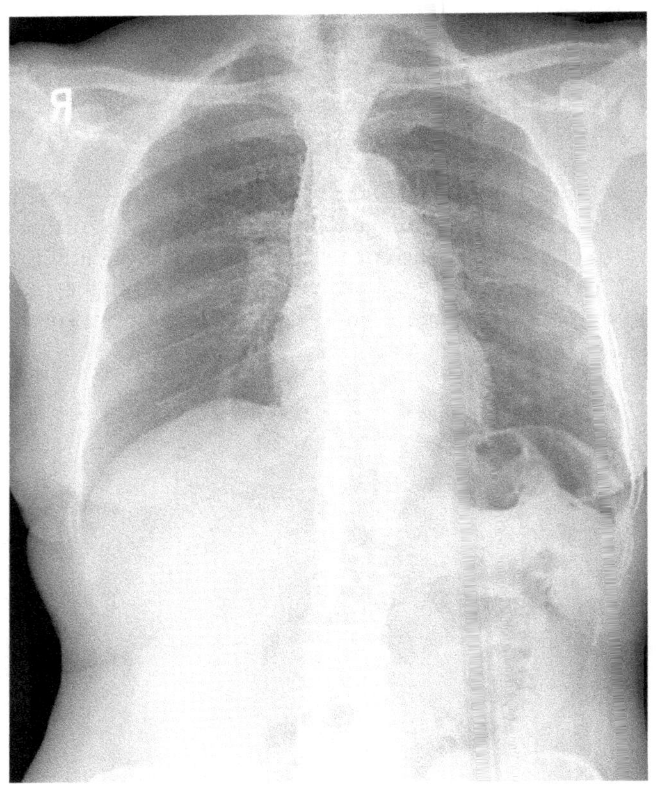

Figure 14.9a Test image-1 caption generated: thoracic aorta is mildly tortuous.

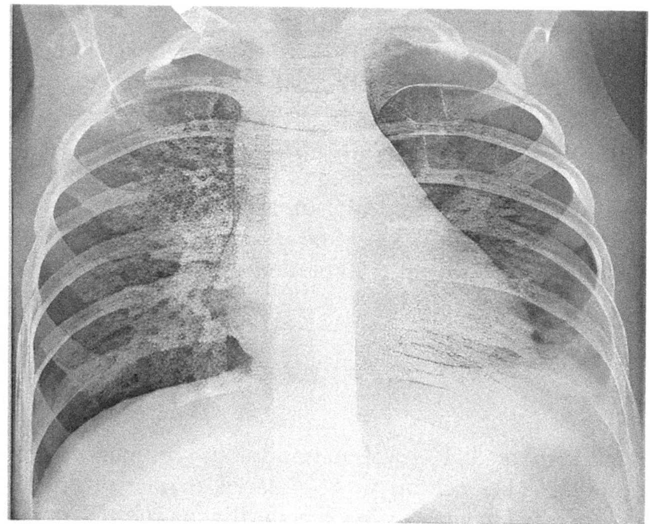

Figure 14.9b Test image-2 caption generated: viral pneumonia in the upper segment.

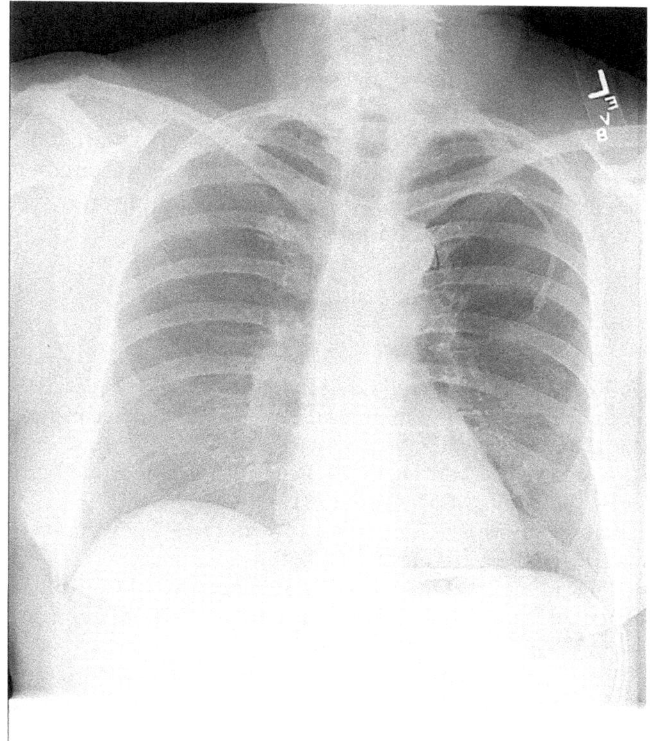

Figure 14.9c Test image-3 caption generated: no findings present in the specimen.

The previously mentioned approach can be used in multiple medical scenarios such as in the detection and caption generation of COVID cases, which would be done by articulating the core corpus with the help of the CORD-19 dataset and making use of lung computed tomography images for interpretation [23]. It can also be used in the detection and generation of medical annotations of epileptic seizures in EEG Data [24]. Preprocessing steps and feature extraction of the input scans could be altered and fine-tuned based on the requirements. Certain changes that could be incorporated in the architecture include the addition of pooling layers or modification of filters in the modified VGG-16 architecture or replacing the architecture with custom convolutional modules for feature extraction from the input images.

14.5 CONCLUSION

The proposed model employed a novel methodology of incorporating ELECTRA for medical image captioning. The method was validated against several chest X-rays for 14 diseases. The model generated image caption specifically for chest X-ray images. The model's performance was assessed through two standard metrics – BLEU 4 and ROUGE-4. The final BLEU-4 score was evaluated to 0.54 and the ROUGE-4 F1 score is evaluated to 0.95 which outperforms the existing medical image captioning algorithms. By feeding complex and varied datasets, the performance of the architecture can be improved substantially. There are certain limitations that were witnessed during the course of development such as the inability of the model to generate captions for complex anomalies as well a generate texts for new diseases. These issues can be removed by applying the active-learning approach to this model. The quality of the scan image plays a primary role in the performance of the model. Low-quality scan images lead to false-positive cases as well as predict multiple anomalies inclusive of the actual diagnoses. This model would be able to automate the analysis of large volumes of chest X-ray images, which can be time-consuming and resource-intensive for human experts, as well as reduce miscommunication.

REFERENCES

1. Hrga, I., Ivasic-Kos, M.: Deep Image Captioning: An Overview. In: 2019 42nd International Convention on Information and Communication Technology, Electronics and Microelectronics (MIPRO). IEEE (2019) 995–1000.
2. Krizhevsky, A., Sutskever, I., Hinton, G. E.: ImageNet Classification with Deep Convolutional Neural Networks. Commun ACM, 60(6) (2017) 84–90.
3. Tammina, S.: Transfer Learning Using VGG-16 with Deep Convolutional Neural Network for Classifying Images. IJSRP, 9(10) (2019) 9420.
4. Tao, J., Gu, Y., Sun, J., Bie, Y., Wang, H.: Research on VGG16 Convolutional Neural Network Feature Classification Algorithm Based on Transfer Learning. In: 2021 2nd China International SAR Symposium (CISS). IEEE (2021) 1–3.
5. Herdade, S., Kappeler, A., Boakye, K., Soares, J.: Image Captioning: Transforming Objects into Words. In: Proceedings of the 33rd International Conference on Neural Information Processing Systems. Curran Associates Inc., Red Hook, NY, USA (2019) 11137–11147.
6. Vinyals, O., Toshev, A., Bengio, S., Erhan, D.: Show and Tell: A Neural Image Caption Generator. In: 2015 IEEE Conference on Computer Vision and Pattern Recognition (CVPR) (2015) 3156–3164.

7. Ivasic-Kos, M., Ipsic, I., Ribaric, S.: A Knowledge-Based Multi-Layered Image Annotation System. Expert Syst Appl., 42(24) (2015) 9539–9553.
8. Park, H., Kim, K., Yoon, J., Park, S., Choi, J.: Medical Image Captioning Model to Convey More Details: Methodological Comparison of Feature Difference Generation. IEEE Access, 9 (2021) 150560–150568.
9. Yin, C., Qian, B., Wei, J., Li, X., Zhang, X., Li, Y., Zheng, Q.: Automatic generation of medical imaging diagnostic report with hierarchical recurrent neural network. In: 2019 19TH IEEE International Conference on Data Mining (ICDM), (2019) 728–737.
10. Chenliang, L., Haiyang X., Junfeng, T., Wei, W., Ming, Y., Bin, B., Jiabo, Y., Hehong, C., Guohai, X., Zheng, C., Ji Z., Songfang, H., Fei, H., Jingren, Z., Luo, S.: mPLUG: Effective and Efficient Vision-Language Learning by Cross-Modal Skip-Connections. ArXiv (2022).
11. Wang, X., Peng, Y., Lu, L., Lu, Z., and Summers, R. M.: Tienet: Text-Image Embedding Network for Common Thorax Disease Classification and Reporting in Chest X-Rays. In: Proc. IEEE/CVF Conf. Comput. Vis. Pattern Recognit., (2018) 9049–9058.
12. Yang, X., Ye, M., You, Q., Ma, F.: Writing by Memorizing: Hierarchical Retrieval-Based Medical Report Generation. In: Proceedings of the 59th Annual Meeting of the Association for Computational Linguistics and the 11th International Joint Conference on Natural Language Processing (Volume 1: Long Papers). Association for Computational Linguistics (2021) 5000–5009.
13. Park, H., Kim, K., Yoon, J., Park, S., Choi, J.: Feature Difference Makes Sense: A Medical Image Captioning Model Exploiting Feature Difference and Tag Information. In: Proceedings of the 58th Annual Meeting of the Association for Computational Linguistics: Student Research Workshop. Association for Computational Linguistics (2020) 95–102.
14. Devlin, J., Chang, M. W., Lee, K., Google, K. T.: Language AI. BERT: Pre-Training of Deep Bidirectional Transformers for Language Understanding. In: Proceedings of Conference of the North American Chapter of the Association for Computational Linguistics: Human Language Technologies, NAACL-HLT (2019) 4171–4186.
15. Liu, Y., Ott, M., Goyal, N., Du, J., Joshi, M., Chen, D.: RoBERTa: A Robustly Optimized BERT Pretraining Approach. In: 8th International Conference on Learning Representations (ICLR) (2020) 24–31.
16. He, P., Gao, J., Chen, W.: DeBERTaV3: Improving DeBERTa using ELECTRA-Style Pre-Training with Gradient-Disentangled Embedding Sharing. ArXiv (2023).
17. He, P., Liu, X., Gao, J., Chen, W.: DeBERTa: Decoding-Enhanced BERT with Disentangled Attention. In: International Conference on Learning Representations (ICLR 2020), Computational and Biological Learning Society (2020) 21–34.
18. Clark, K., Luong, M. T., Le, Q. V., Manning, C. D.: ELECTRA: Pre-training Text Encoders as Discriminators Rather Than Generators. In: 8th International Conference on Learning Representations, ICLR, (2020).
19. Yang, Z., Dai, Z., Yang, Y., Carbonell, J., Salakhutdinov, R., Le, Q. V.: XLNet: Generalized Autoregressive Pretraining for Language Understanding. In: Proceedings of the 33rd International Conference on Neural Information Processing Systems. Curran Associates Inc., Red Hook, NY, USA (2019) 5753–5763.
20. Wang, X., Peng, Y., Lu, L., Lu, Z., Bagheri, M., Summers, R. M.: ChestX-ray8: Hospital-Scale Chest X-ray Database and Benchmarks on Weakly-Supervised Classification and Localization of Common Thorax Diseases. IEEE CVPR, pp. 3462–3471, 2017.
21. Farhadi, A., Hejrati, M., Sadeghi, M. A., Young, P., Rashtchian, C., Hockenmaier, J.: Every Picture Tells a Story: Generating Sentences from Images. In: Daniilidis, K., Maragos, P., Paragios, N. (eds) Computer Vision – ECCV 2010. Vol. 6314. Lecture Notes in Computer Science (2010) 15–29.
22. Zhang, R., Ji, Y., Zhang, Y., Passonneau, R. J.: Contrastive Data and Learning for Natural Language Processing. In: Proceedings of the 2022 Conference of the North American Chapter of the Association for Computational Linguistics: Human Language Technologies: Tutorial Abstracts. Association for Computational Linguistics (2022) 39–47.

23. Punitha, S., Stephan, T., Kannan, R., Mahmud, M., Kaiser, M. S., Belhaouari, S. B.: Detecting COVID-19 from Lung Computed Tomography Images: A Swarm Optimized Artificial Neural Network Approach. In: IEEE Access, 11 (2023), 12378–12393.
24. Yedurkar, D. P., Metkar, S., Al-Turjman, F., Yardi, N., Stephan, T.: An IoT Based Novel Hybrid Seizure Detection Approach for Epileptic Monitoring. In: IEEE Transactions on Industrial Informatics.

Chapter 15

Diagnosing Parkinson's disease using a deep learning model based on electromyography sensors

P Padma Priya Dharishini, B R Karthikeyan, Surya Tejas V, Jash Singh, Sumukha Bhat, and G Karthik

Department of Computer Science and Engineering, M S Ramaiah University of Applied Sciences, Bangalore, Karnataka, India

15.1 INTRODUCTION

Parkinson's disorder (PD) is a major neurodegenerative disorder that is a result of the loss of dopamine and some other neurotransmitter producing neurons [1,2]. It is the second-most common disease of its kind after Alzheimer's disease. The occurrence this disease in developed countries is 1% in people older than 60 and 4% in people older than 80 [3]. This disorder is neurodegenerative, with 160 people developing the disease over 100,000 people in Western Europe, with most of those developing it in old age. Currently, the method used to diagnose the disease is mainly clinical. The most noticeable symptoms of PD include rest tremors, bradykinesia, and rigidity. As the disease progresses, non-motor complications can also be identified and worsen over time [4]. Therefore, early diagnosis of PD is very essential for a patient so that their condition can be treated to slow down the effects of the disease and plan their lives accordingly.

Electromyography sensors shown in Figure 15.2 reflect the activity of spinal motor neurons. This enables us to examine the central nervous system of a person. The activity pattern of the motor units of a person suffering from Parkinson's is extremely different from that of stationary activity under normal muscle tone in a healthy individual [3]. This shows us that there is massive potential for using EMG sensors to diagnose and monitor Parkinson's disease. It is also possible that these sensors could be used for early diagnosis of the said disease.

However, it is also found that there are certain situations where the activity pattern of that of a healthy person can be similar to that of the diseased person such as during strong and ballistic movements, dynamic training, chills due to cold and other such scenarios [3]. Building a suitable deep learning-based classification model that is trained based on data of Parkinson's disease patients can assist in diagnosing the disease in individuals accurately and effectively. The model can also be built in such a way as to exclude the above inapplicable scenarios to diagnose more accurately. Furthermore, the model can also be built to classify the four main symptoms of the disease.

15.1.1 Cause and effects of the Parkinson's disease

The Parkinson's disease mainly shows loss of neurons related to lewy bodies in many subcortical nuclei over time, leading to significant biochemical and pathophysiological changes. The deterioration and loss of nigral neurons cause lack of striatal dopamine in the body and this loss directly determines the duration and severity of the disease [5].

DOI: 10.1201/9781003369059-19

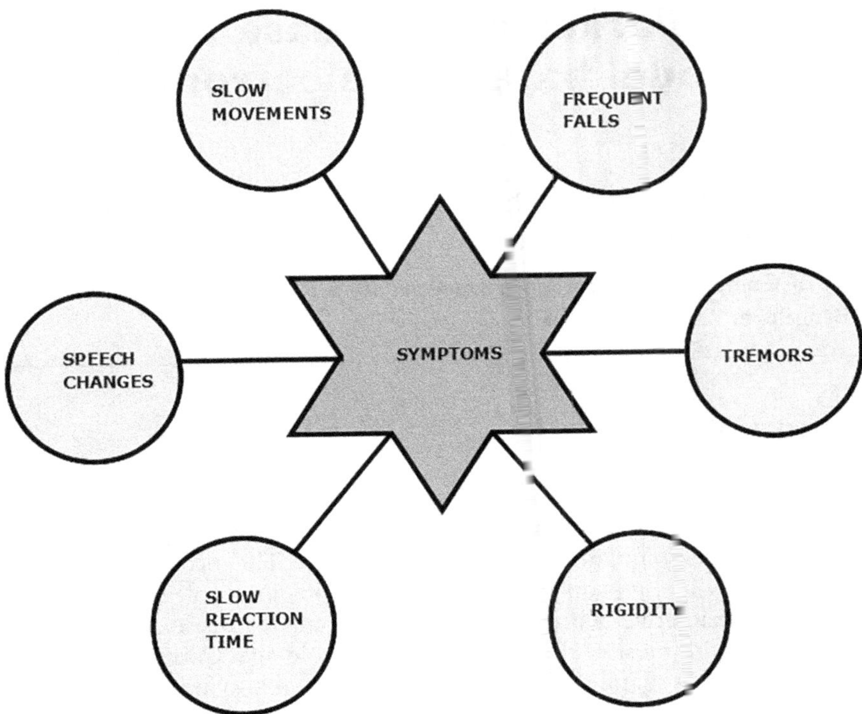

Figure 15.1 Major symptoms of Parkinson's disease.

There is also an imbalance in the dopamine receptor activity in extrapyramidal pathways. The imbalance in dopamine receptor, which is D1 in direct pathway that causes excitation and D2 in indirect pathways known to cause inhibition, produces different sets of the main symptoms unique to a patient. This means that not all people affected by Parkinson's disease display all of the main symptoms; namely, tremors, rigidity, bradykinesia, and postural instability [2], as shown in Figure 15.1. This disease has no particular specific way of diagnosis apart from assessing the patient's medical history and closely monitoring their symptoms [6].

There are many clinical signs that might display that a person might have developed PD. Change of handwriting with micrographia, reduced facial expressions, and lessened sense of smell might be a few of the notable early signs of PD. As the disease develops and progresses, symptoms such as hypophonia, drooling, and impairment of postural reflexes may manifest. Depression is also one such symptom of PD accounting to be shown in approximately 40% of the patients with PD. Voice tremors may also occur as a symptom of the disease [4].

15.1.2 The need for early detection of the disease

The disease progressively worsens the motor symptoms, making the patient more dependent, which may cause lethal falls or such situations. The worsening symptoms become a burden to the patient, the patient's family, and others around the patient. Both the motor and non-motor symptoms makes the person more dependent on others and liable to work, inducing early retirement, restrictions on certain activities and professions, and also medication and

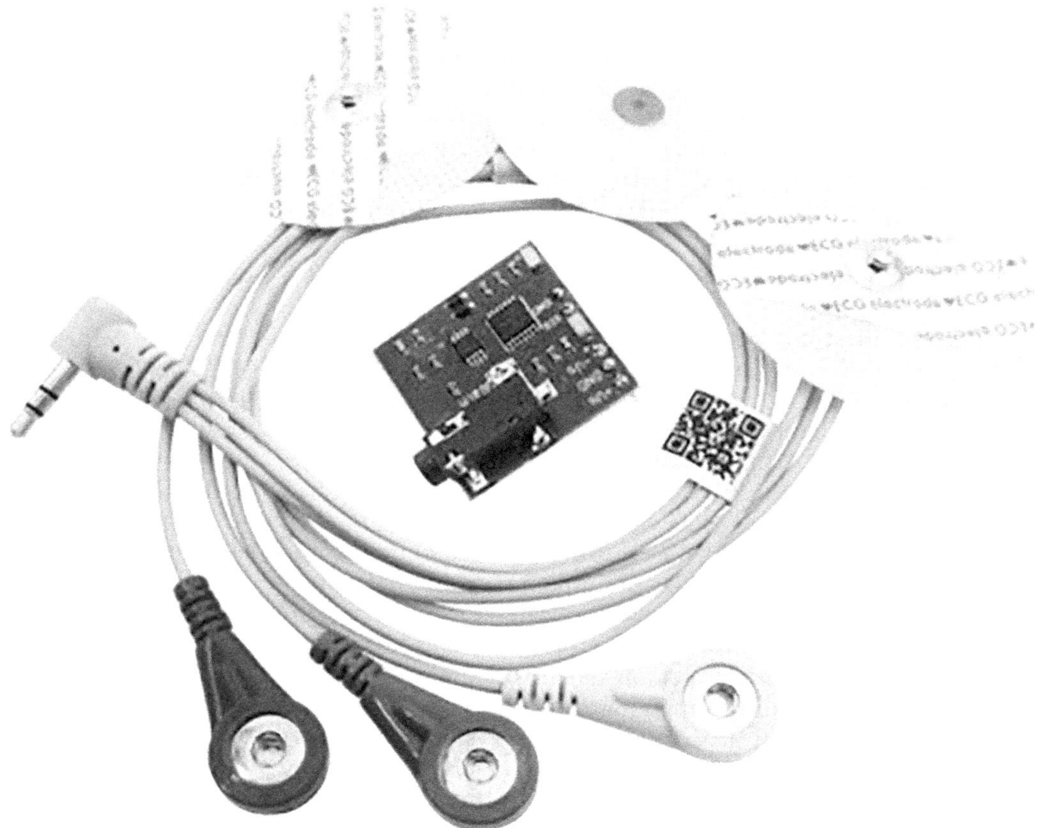

Figure 15.2 EMG sensor.

care costs [3]. Early detection of the disease not only helps the person slow down the progression of symptoms but also plans their life accordingly.

15.1.3 Current developments in the diagnosis of Parkinson's disease

Currently, diagnosis of Parkinson's disease is done using neuroimaging biomarkers and biochemical biomarkers. However, a perfect biomarker has not been developed in this field in order to accurately identify Parkinson's disease and monitor its progression. Developing such a good biomarker would aid in the identification and monitor the progression of the disease [7]. Apart from motor symptoms other symptoms of Parkinson's include depression, olfactory impairment, Rem sleep behavior disorder and other such symptoms. Besides the clinical features, neuroimaging methods such as single photon emission tomography (SPECT) and positron emission tomography (PET) are being currently implemented in diagnosing premotor PD [8]. The diagnosis of the disease is far more accurate in expert movement disorder clinics as compared to general neurologists [4]. The detection and diagnosis of the disease is highly difficult in the early stages with statistics being that only 70% of the patients are correctly diagnosed with PD [3]. Despite the various approaches of diagnosing the disease being presented, a sure-shot definitive approach is still lacking.

15.1.4 EMG sensors and diagnosis of Parkinson's

Electromyography is the process of detecting and recording the biomedical signals that are generated in a muscle during musculoskeletal contraction. The electrical activity is observed and measured when such musculoskeletal contraction occurs. During muscle contraction a potential is created at each muscle fibre known as action potential due to polarization and depolarization. The sum of all action potentials of a muscle is called motor unit action potential (MUAP). Two types of EMG methods include intramuscular EMG where needles are inserted to record the potential and the other method being surface EMG, where no such needles are required and the potentials can be measured at the surface of the limb or wherever it is to be measured [2].

Significant difference in the data recorded by EMG sensors in that of a normal person and that of a person suffering from PD can be found [2,3]. Abnormal movements can be detected easily in this manner using EMG sensors. Symptoms such as gait, tremors, abnormal posture and increased muscle tone were to return electromyography signals that are not normal. Usually, clinicians have just observed gait abnormalities and based on experience are required to assess the gait with Unified Parkinson's Disease Rating Scale. The scoring is also using on information related to the patient regarding motor and non-motor functions [2]. The scoring is divided into 5 stages based on severity. This method is, however, susceptible to human error and hence is not a definite method for diagnosis and classifying the severity. Therefore, the use of EMG sensors help to monitor the muscle actions more accurately in order to assess the patient's condition. This makes it easier for the person diagnosing. The tremors for a PD patient are rest tremors and are different from regular tremors that a normal person might have in cases of nervousness, like shivering due to cold, etc. The PD induced tremors have different results on the electromyography data based on its frequency and amplitude compared to normal tremors. EMG sensors can be used to differentiate the tremors of PD to that of a normal person for evaluation, monitoring, measuring, and identification of the tremors [2].

15.1.5 Use of artificial intelligence in the diagnosis and monitoring of Parkinson's disease

Since the regular clinical diagnosis methods of the Parkinson's disorder is not reliable enough, the use of automatic feature extraction methods such as Artificial Neural Networks (ANN) and Convolutional Neural Networks (CNN) has been proposed. Based on these propositions, methods of deep learning and neural networks have been used to detect PD more accurately, as the methods were able to recognize and analyze complex patterns better than that which can be done by a medical practitioner [9]. In the analysis and documentation, all such studies are included. It concluded the best model with the most accurate findings for each type of data collected based on symptoms. It made the analysis based on methods used on repositories of publicly available datasets of PD patients.

15.2 OVERVIEW OF PARKINSON'S DISEASE DIAGNOSING SYSTEM

A system to detect and monitor the said disease using EMG sensors is proposed. The overall block diagram of the Parkinson's disease diagnosis system is shown in Figure 15.3 along

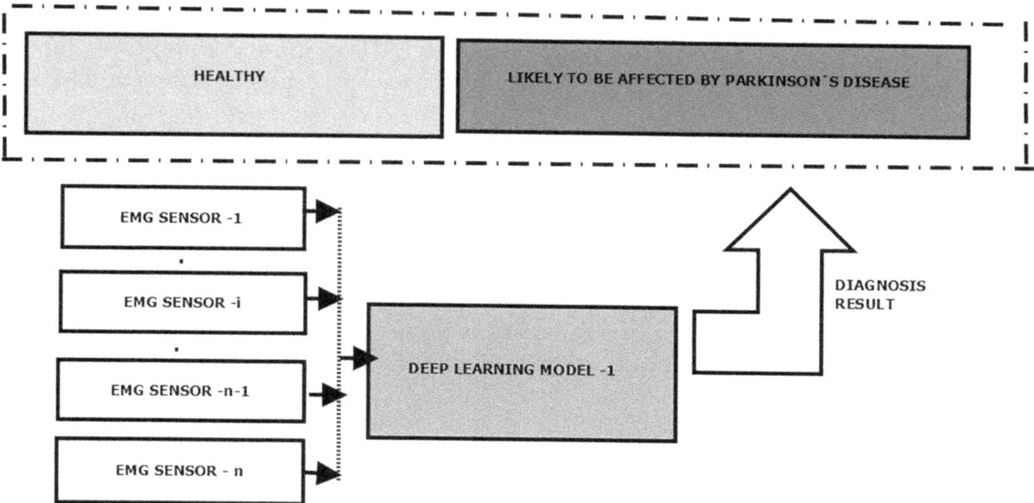

Figure 15.3 Overall block diagram of Parkinson's disease diagnosis system.

with its components, like EMG sensors and deep learning model-1. The real time data acquired from EMG sensors are stored and used as data to train the deep learning model-1 that can diagnose whether a person is healthy or likely to be affected by Parkinson's disease. Professionals can use deep learning model -2 for further prediction and prescription as shown in Figure 15.4.

15.2.1 Electromyography sensors

Electromyography is the recording and measure of electrical activity based on electrical signals generated by the body in order to facilitate motor actions of musculoskeletal

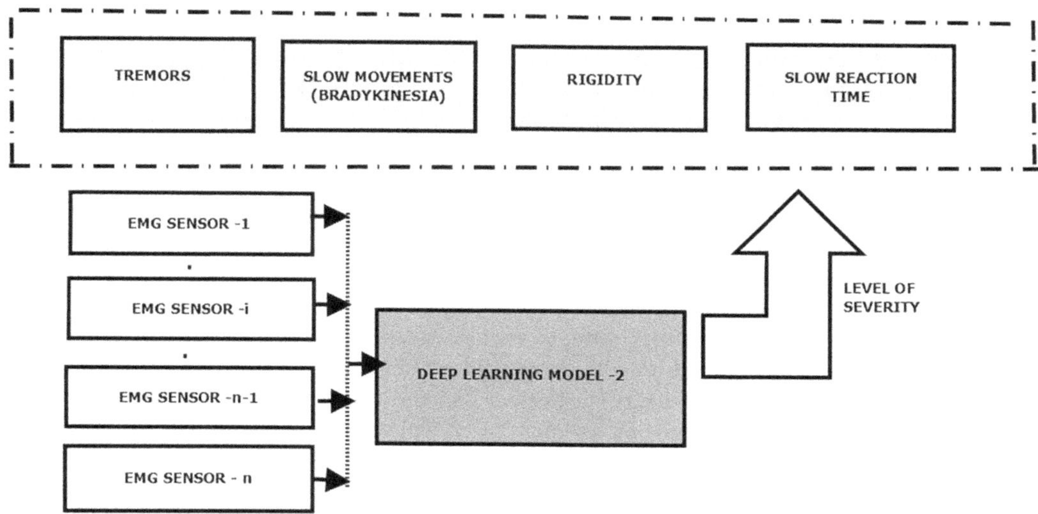

Figure 15.4 Diagnosis system used by professionals for prediction.

contraction. There are two main types of EMG sensors based on the type of electrodes used and the method. The EMG sensor can either be surface EMG or intramuscular EMG [6]. For convenience of usage and comfort of patient's surface, the usage of surface EMGs is suggested.

15.2.2 Data collection

Arduino boards are to be connected with the EMG sensors to collect data [10]. For easy and versatile coding, python language using a suitable IDE is suggested to be used to collect data. Python would also allow the processing, storage, and development of a suitable interface for data collection. The use of Arduino mega-2560 is suggested, as it provides more powerful processing in case a large number of sensors are employed.

15.2.3 Deep learning model

Deep learning model that uses the acquired datasets of a patient is to be built to analyze the motor symptoms, diagnose the disease early, and classify the symptoms. Then a report based on the classification and diagnosis is to be generated.

15.2.4 User interface

The collection of data is to be closely monitored by a professional who is to diagnose the disease. Therefore, a user-friendly and comfortable user interface is to be designed to collect data, view the report, and monitor the EMG readings.

There are two different cases possible (whether the person is healthy or likely to be infected) based on diagnosis result and four different symptom classifications and identifications provided by the Parkinson's disease diagnosing system.

15.3 RESULTS AND DISCUSSION

The professional who is performing the diagnosis has to use the user interface to record and monitor the data that will be collected from the patient and a healthy person, and the data is labelled for healthy or diseased using a suitable user interface. Further data regarding the four cardinal symptoms is collected from a person with the disease and labelled through the user interface, as shown in Figure 15.5. The interface is a medium to the professional to easily monitor the values that are being recorded in real time.

The professional should be allowed to accept the recording or reject the recording based on their personal observation and label the accepted data accordingly. This collection of data can be done via a hardware setup of the EMG sensors and Arduino board as in Figure 15.6. The collected data is stored in a suitable format (say csv).

Then the csv file, having patient data is sent to another interface such as the one in Figure 15.7, where the user is able to train and create a deep learning model based on the collected data is developed to detect if a person has the disease or not and to classify the symptoms into four main categories as mentioned earlier based on the data previously collected and labelled.

This model is to be loaded into a microcontroller with the sensors that diagnose patients in real time by collecting their EMG values. The model diagnoses if the person has PD or not

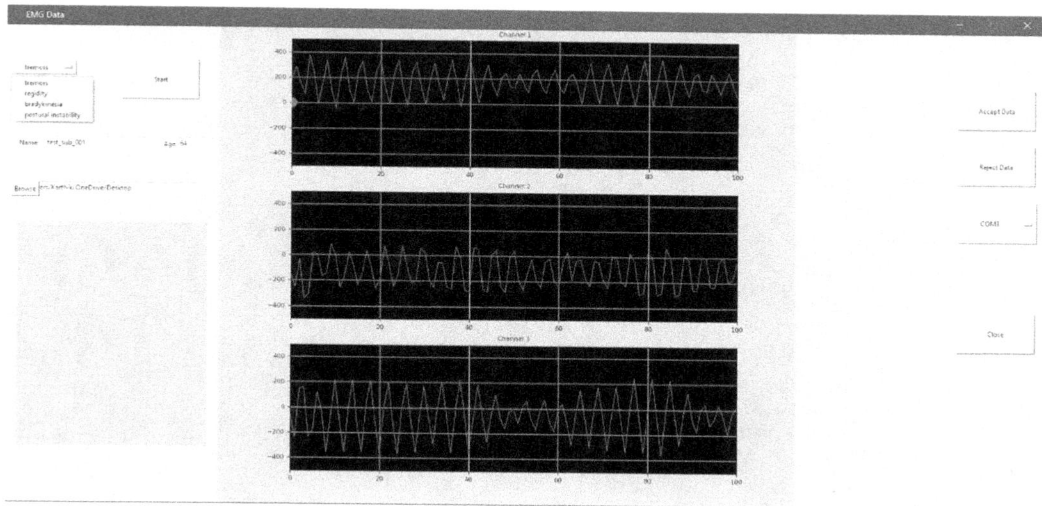

Figure 15.5 User interface to record and monitor real time data.

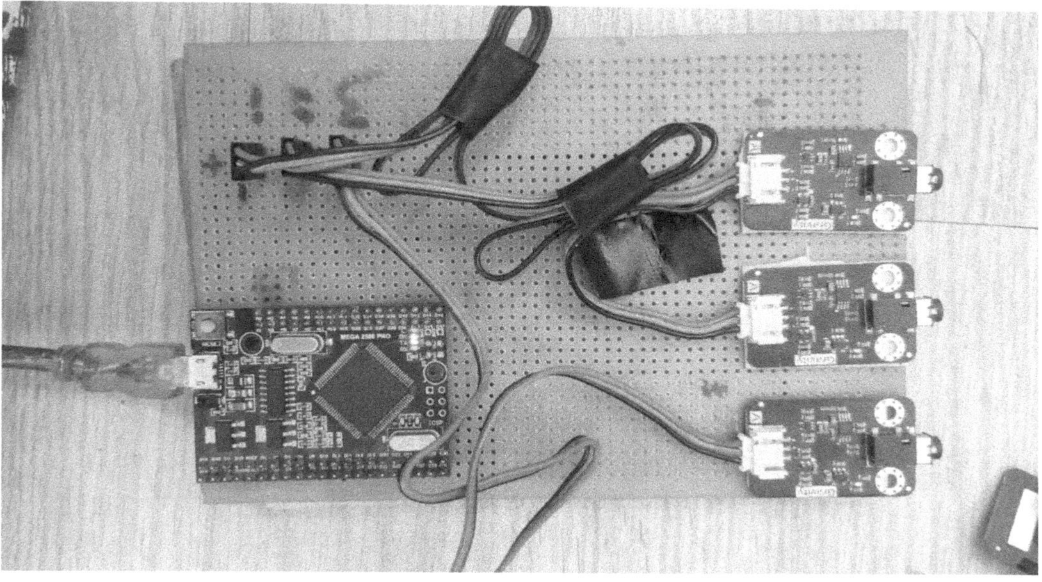

Figure 15.6 Hardware setup for collecting data.

based on previously acquired data of healthy and diseased persons. The accuracy of the deep learning model developed for parkinson's disease diagnosis system is shown in Figure 15.8.

The patient can be monitored in real time for the various symptoms and the data collected can be used by professionals for further diagnosis and predictions. Live diagnosis and classification can be done in this manner using the setup shown in Figure 15.9.

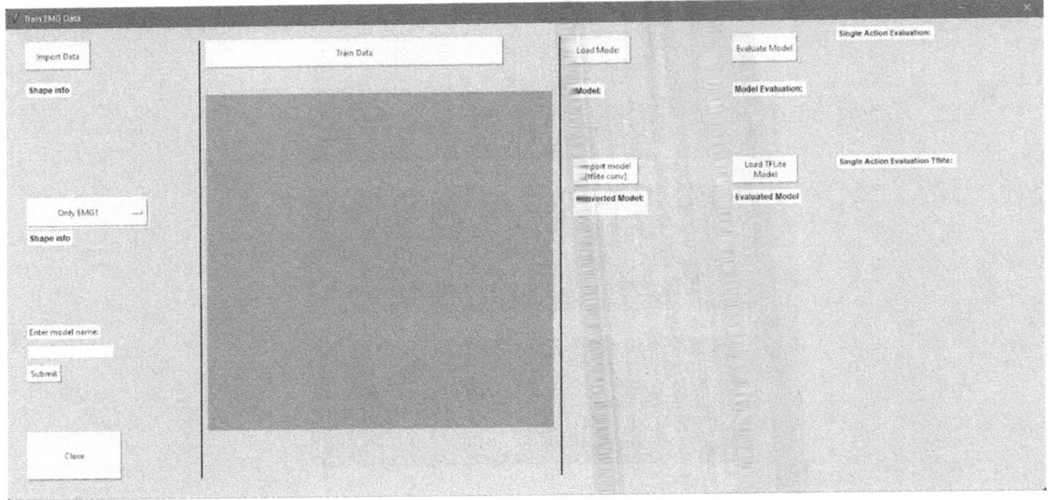

Figure 15.7 Model to diagnose Parkinson's disease.

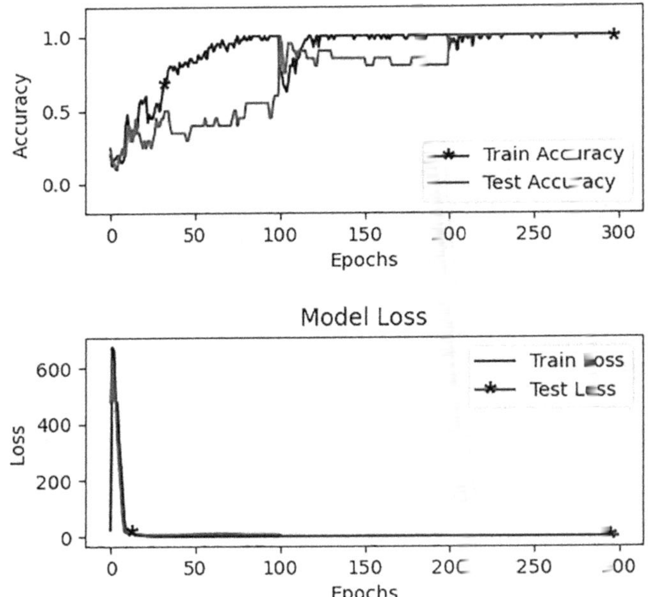

Figure 15.8 Model metrics after training.

A simple block diagram that depicts overall flow of the Parkinson's disease diagnosing system is shown in Figure 15.10. The real time data from a person is collected using an Internet of Things (IoT) setup, having an EMG sensor and an Arduino microcontroller. The collected data is stored in a .csv file and used for diagnosing whether the person is healthy or likely to be affected by Parkinson's disease.

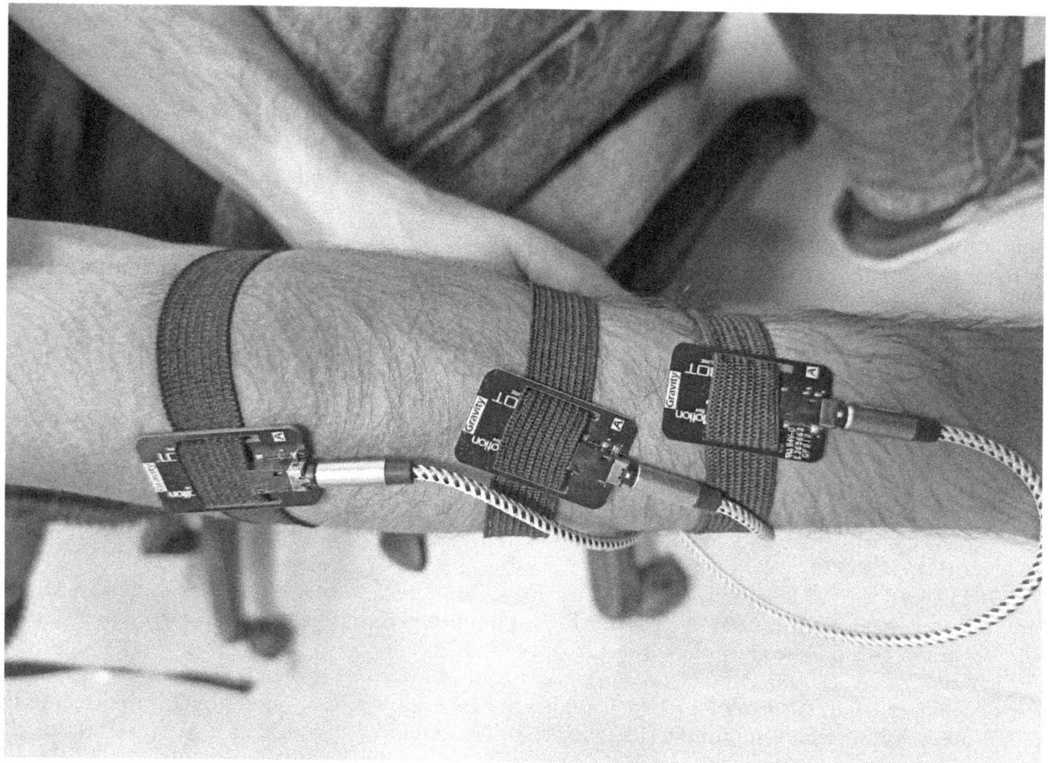

Figure 15.9 Hardware setup for live diagnosis.

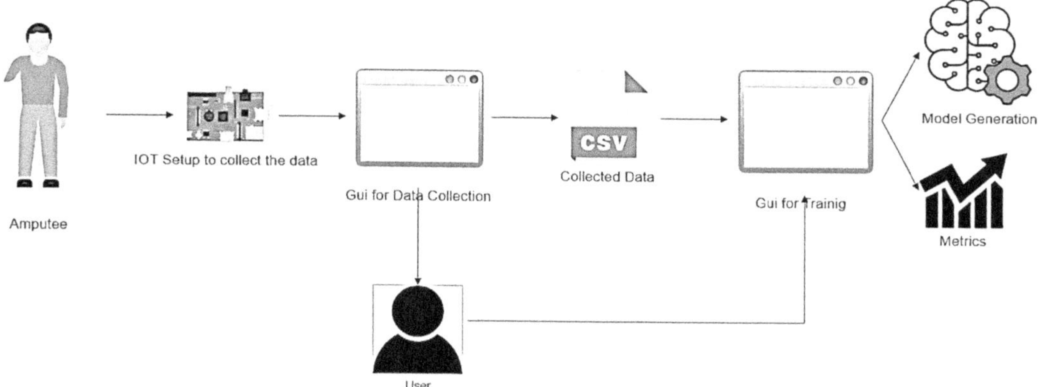

Figure 15.10 Block diagram depicts the flow of work.

15.4 CONCLUSIONS AND FUTURE WORK

The effects and causes of Parkinson's disease have been looked into to determine the symptoms of the disease and why it is important to diagnose it at the earliest stage. The current developments related to the diagnosis of the disease have been considered, and it has been concluded that there is no definitive sure-shot parameter to diagnose the disease. The current role of artificial intelligence and machine learning algorithms in the field are highly efficient and notable.

Based on the need for proper and early diagnosis of the Parkinson's disease, solutions are proposed that diagnoses the disease in an individual and furthermore can identify and classify the symptoms of the disease so as to monitor them. This monitoring enables the medical professional to assess the severity of the disease, its progression, and how effective the person's current treatment is to manage the person's symptoms. In the future, along with EMG sensors, gyroscope sensors can also be used for more precise prediction of Parkinson's disease.

REFERENCES

1. Johri, A., & Tripathi, A. (2019, August). Parkinson disease detection using deep neural networks. In 2019 Twelfth International Conference on Contemporary Computing (IC3) (pp. 1–4). IEEE.
2. Pasmanasari, E. D., & Pawitan, J. A. (2021). The potential of electromyography signals as markers to detect and monitor Parkinson's disease. Biomedical and Pharmacology Journal, 14(1), 373–378.
3. Meigal, A. Y., Rissanen, S. M., Tarvainen, M. P., Airaksinen, O., Kankaanpää, M., & Karjalainen, P. A. (2013). Non-linear EMG parameters for differential and early diagnostics of Parkinson's disease. Frontiers in Neurology, 4, 135.
4. Davie, C. A. (2008). A review of Parkinson's disease. British Medical Bulletin, 86(1), 109–127.
5. Jellinger, K. A. (1999). Post mortem studies in Parkinson's disease—is it possible to detect brain areas for specific symptoms? Diagnosis and Treatment of Parkinson's Disease—State of the Art, 1–29.
6. Adem, H. M., Tessema, A. W., & Simegn, G. L. (2022). Classification of Parkinson's disease using EMG signals from different upper limb movements based on multiclass support vector machine. International Journal Bioautomation, 26(1), 109.
7. Wang, J., Hoekstra, J. G., Zuo, C., Cook, T. J., & Zhang, J. (2013). Biomarkers of Parkinson's disease: current status and future perspectives. Drug Discovery Today, 18(3–4), 155–162.
8. Kaiserova, M., Grambalova, Z., Kurcova, S., Otruba, P., Vranova, H. P., Mensikova, K., & Kanovsky, P. (2021). Premotor Parkinson's disease: Overview of clinical symptoms and current diagnostic methods. Biomedical Papers of the Medical Faculty of Palacky University in Olomouc, 165(2), 103–112.
9. Alzubaidi, M. S., Shah, U., Dhia Zubaydi, H., Dolaat, K., Abd-Alrazaq, A. A., Ahmed, A., & Househ, M. (2021, June). The role of neural network for the detection of Parkinson's disease: a scoping review. Healthcare, 9(6), 740.
10. Arduino, S. A. (2015). Arduino. Arduino LLC, 372.

Chapter 16

Enhancing heart disease prediction with Hybridized KNN-MOPSO algorithm

R Manoranjitham[1], *S Punitha*[2], *and Thompson Stephan*[3]

[1]Division of Computer Science and Engineering, Karunya Institute of Technology and Sciences, Karunya University, Coimbatore, Tamil Nadu, India

[2]Department of Computer Science and Engineering, Graphics Era Deemed to be University, Dehradun, India

[3]Department of Computer Science and Engineering, Graphic Era Deemed to be University, Dehradun, Uttarakhand, India

16.1 INTRODUCTION

The heart regulates blood flow in the human body. The four essential tasks of the heart are (i) sends oxygenated blood to other body parts, (ii) sends hormones and nutrients to different parts of the body, (iii) carries deoxygenated blood and metabolic waste products from the body and sends it to the lungs for oxygenation, and (iv) sustains blood pressure. Any irregularity of heart functions leads to distress in other parts of the body and disturbs regular functioning of the heart, which is called Heart Disease (HD). HD happens due to narrowing and blockage of coronary arteries that controls the blood supply to the heart. The major risk factors of heart diseases are smoking, family history of heart disease, cholesterol, high blood pressure, lack of physical exercise, and obesity, etc. The symptoms of heart disease include chest pain, shortness of breath, physical body weakness, feet swollen, pressure, discomfort, etc [1].

Conventional methods of detecting HD include angiography, which has shortcomings like high cost, requires of strong technological knowledge, and can produce various side effects. To overcome these issues, non-invasive methods based on predictive machine learning models can be used. The prediction results help the clinicians in decision making and early diagnosis, which would reduce the risk of patients dying [2].

In India, the annual number of deaths from heart disease is 4.77 million in 2020, and the number of victims rapidly increases in every year. Hence, identifying heart disease early will help the patients to get the required treatment. Machine learning is an evolving subdivision of artificial intelligence. ML make the systems to learn and make predictions based on the experience. The system trains ML algorithms using a training dataset to create a model. The model takes the new input data to predict heart disease. ML detects hidden patterns in the input dataset to build models. ML techniques are categorized as Supervized Learning, Unsupervized Learning and Reinforcement Learning. In Supervized Learning, the model is trained on a dataset using labelled data that has input data and its outcomes. Data are classified into training and test dataset. Training dataset are used to trains the model while testing dataset takes a new data to find accuracy of the model. The examples of supervized machine learning algorithm are K-NN, Naive Bayes (NB), Support vector machine (SVM) and Random forest (RF) algorithms. Data mining can be integrated with the existing models to construct efficient prediction systems [3]. The performance of machine learning model mainly depends on balanced dataset and using related features from the data for training and testing the model. Therefore, feature selection is considerably important for model performance improvement [4–13].

DOI: 10.1201/9781003369059-20

The proposed model is a combination of Multi-Objective Particle Swarm Optimization (MOPSO) with KNN classifier to improve the performance over the heat disease dataset.

16.2 RELATED WORK

Akella and Akella [10] six ML algorithms like linear regression, regression tree, random forest, support-vector machine, neural network, and k nearest neighbor were tested with the performance metrics of accuracy, recall, F1 score and Area Under the Curve–Receiver Operating (AUC-ROC) and the KNN's accuracy is greater than 89% amongst other ML models.

[Kaushalya Dissanayake and Md Gapar Md Johar, 2021] authors conducted an experimental evaluation of the performance of models using six classification algorithms like Decision Tree, RF, SVM, KNN, LR, and Gaussian naive Bayes. Cleveland heart disease dataset have been applied and the relevant features were selected using ten feature selection techniques such as ANOVA, Chi-square, mutual information, ReliefF, forward feature selection, backward feature selection, exhaustive feature selection, recursive feature elimination, Lasso regression, and Ridge regression. The backward feature selection technique has achieved the highest classification accuracy of 88.52%, precision of 91.30%, sensitivity of 80.76%, and f-measure of 85.71% with other ML models.

An optimized unsupervized technique for feature selection of Multi-Layer Perceptron for Enhanced Brownian Motion based on Dragonfly Algorithm (MLP-EBMDA) has been proposed for classification of heart disease. The proposed MLP-EBMDA achieved 94.28% accuracy, precision has 96%, recall has 96%, and F1-score has 96% over UCI Cleveland Dataset.

Chi-square and principal component analysis (CHI-PCA) with random forests (RF) classifier also proposed and achieved the highest accuracy with 98.7% for Cleveland, 99.0% for Hungarian, and 99.4% for Cleveland-Hungarian (CH) datasets. From the analysis, the combination of chi-square with PCA obtains superior performance in many classifiers.

Kamencay et al. [9] presented a PCA-KNN with the scale-invariant feature transform (SIFT) descriptor in different medical images, which provides an accuracy of 83.6% with training 200 images.

Javeed [11] proposed a random search algorithm (RSA) for features selection and random forest model for heart failure detection. The random search is used for searching out optimal subset of features. Experiments are analyzed using an online heart failure database namely Cleveland dataset. The dataset contains 303 instances among them 297 instance have complete attributes information while 6 instances have missing values. Around 70–30% data partitioning method is used, and accuracy, sensitivity, specificity, and MCC are the evaluation metrics considered to measure the performance of the proposed model. The proposed model compared with other classification algorithm such as Adaboost, SVM linear, SVM RBF and extra tree classifiers. The proposed method achieves higher classification accuracy value of 93.33% on testing dataset.

[J. P. Li, 2020] this author proposed FCMIM-SVM to diagnose heart disease based on ML techniques. Fast Conditional Mutual Information (FCMIM) features selection algorithm used for features selection. Leave-one-subject-out cross-validation (LOSO) technique used to select the best hyper-parameters for best model selection. The proposed method was evaluated on the Cleveland HD dataset and has 297 instances. Standard Scalar (SS) and Min-Max Scalar have been applied to the dataset for pre-processing the dataset. FCMIM algorithm chooses features that maximum mutual information value with the target class, conditionally to the value of any feature selected before. The performance metrics include accuracy, specificity, sensitivity, MCC, and processing time is considered for evaluating the results with state of art algorithms. SVM (linear) achieved high accuracy value of 92.37%, with a computational time of 11.569 seconds on selected features by relief with LOSO validation method compared with MLP, ANN, SVM (kernel RBF), Naive Bayes (NB), and Decision Tree (DT).

More research focuses on the combination of MOPSO and feature selection. [Fei Han et al.,2021] MOPSO has been used as the feature selection technique to improve the classification accuracy on high dimensional datasets. MOPSO has been used in the grid technique to find the optimal sample and maintain the diversity of the population [14]. Researchers have proposed an improvement in the MOPSO algorithm to find the feasible solution for multi-objective optimization problems [15]. MOPSO has been used to minimize network traffic and afford an energy-efficient solution in Mobile Ad hoc Network (MANET) for determining the optimal number of clusters [16]. Cluster based MOPSO (CMOPSO) has been proposed for chemical plants to determine global-best of each particle on its cluster. Practical experiments were conducted to a hydrogen production process, which is a high-dimensional system in a chemical plant for the validation result [17]. Multi-modal MOPSO has been proposed for a problem that has two or more global solutions with a short-term memory to store each particle information for effective search space. The effectiveness of this model along with K-means clustering algorithm has been verified with 16 multi-objective optimization functions [18].

An automatic human activity recognition was constructed with MOPSO and used in game theory (MOPGMGT). Furthermore, the multi-objective clustering problem has been mapped with game theory to provide the best optimal solution without any prior knowledge [19].

From the literature, it is concluded that the use of feature selection techniques improved the prediction of heart disease.

16.3 PROPOSED SYSTEM

The KNN has been used in both classification and regression problems due to easily implementation but has a drawback of becoming slower when the data size increases. KNN classifies the data by finding the nearest neighbor for the determination of class for unknown data. KNN classification has implemented using two stages, the first stage has to find the number of instances (K) which is closest to S instance and the second stage has to choose the class of S instance from the number of instances (K). The objective of the research work is to increase the performance of KNN classifier by using multi-objective particle swarm optimization (MOPSO) feature selection methods for heart disease prediction. The main goal of this research is to improve the performance of the KNN algorithm by creating diverse training sets to generate accurate classifiers. Figure 16.1 shows the outline of the Hybridized KNN-MOPSO model.

Particle swarm optimization (PSO) has been proposed by Kennedy and Eberhart which was inspired by fish schooling and bird flocking social behavior. PSO began with the population initialization by randomly and entirely swarming for best solution in the search space by renewing the position of each particle. Each particle position has done on the neighboring particles and has its own position. PSO has considered for feature selection due to its simple implementation, quick convergence, and lower expense. MOPSO has been used for multi objective optimization problems.

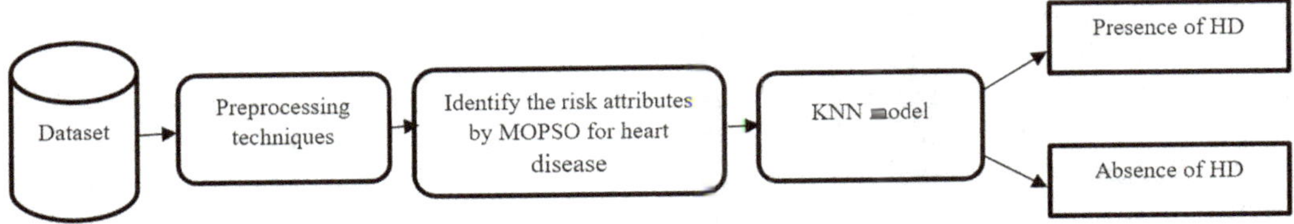

Figure 16.1 Outline of the Hybridized KNN-MOPSO model.

The proposed MOPSO algorithm consists of two steps:

- First step, MOPSO to generate diverse training sets.
  In the proposed work, each particle is represented as a training set solution with lengths of samples and features. The fitness function has two objectives of accuracy and diversity. The degree of diversity of the features is measured using the cardinality and different features selected for each training set. The best position of each particle is stored in personal memory. Each particle memory is initialized, which is the same as the initial position of that particle. The personal memory is updated if the current position of a particle is superior than the saved position in memory. The algorithm stops when the execution reaches the predefined value of 100 by trial-and-error method.
- Second step, the generated training sets is used to train and determine the number of nearest neighbors in the KNN.
  In the proposed method, the obtained solutions of the first step are used in the second step to train the KNN. Figure 16.2 shows the flow chart of MOPSO for optimal solution.

16.4 EXPERIMENTAL RESULTS OF THE HYBRIDIZED KNN-MOPSO ALGORITHM

The performance of the Hybridized KNN-MOPSO Algorithm is tested with the other ML models such as KNN, SVM, NB, LR, AdaBoost, and Random Forest based on the performance metrics of accuracy, with specificity and sensitivity using Eqs. (16.1)–(16.3).

$$Accuracy = \frac{T_P + T_N}{T_P + T_N + F_P + F_N} \tag{16.1}$$

$$Sensitivity = \frac{T_P}{T_P + F_N} \tag{16.2}$$

$$Specificity = \frac{T_N}{T_N + F_P} \tag{16.3}$$

where T_P, T_N, F_P, and F_N imply True Positive, True Negative, False Positive, and False Negative, respectively. T_P signify the samples that are predicted correctly is positive, T_N signify the samples that are predicted correctly is negative, F_P signify the samples that are predicted incorrectly is positive, and F_N signify the samples that are predicted incorrectly is negative.

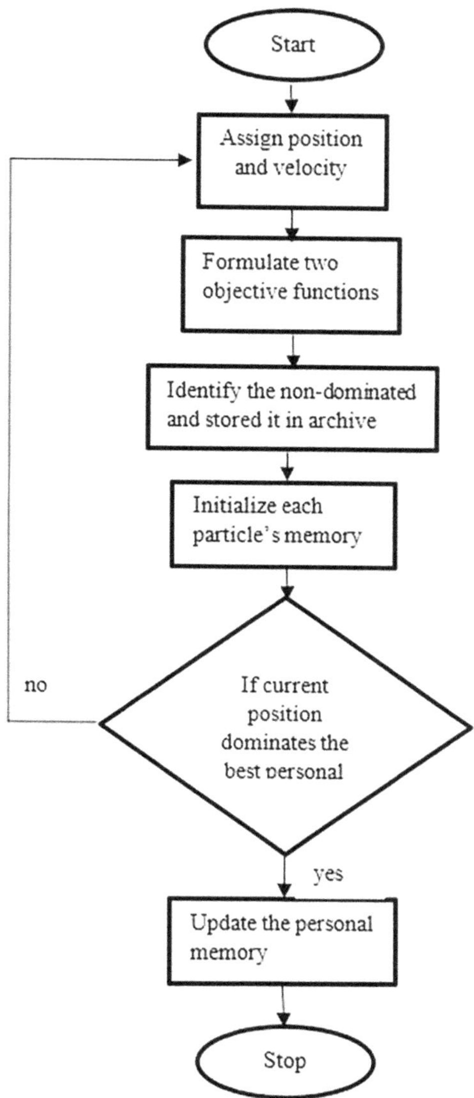

Figure 16.2 Flow chart diagram of the MOPSO algorithm.

16.5 DATASET

The UCI Cleveland dataset includes 76 attributes, using a subset of 14 features. In particular, the Cleveland database is the only one that has been used by ML researchers to date to predict heart disease, with the dataset containing 303 patient records. Table 16.1 shows 14 attribute names in the dataset and the associated range values for each with a brief description. The dataset includes 157 instances with heart disease and 126 instances with the absence of heart disease.

Figure 16.3 shows the data visualization of the dataset.

KNN classifier determine whether a person having heart disease or not by considering the given dataset. The MOPSO algorithm is used to generate accurate classifiers over training sets by producing the (near) optimal number of diverse training sets. Hence, training

Table 16.1 UCI Cleveland dataset attribute name and range values

Attribute	*Range*
1. age	age in years
2. sex	sex (1 = male; 0 = female)
3. cp	chest pain type (Value 1: typical angina, 2: atypical angina, 3: non-anginal pain, 4: asymptomatic
4. trestbps	resting blood pressure (in mm Hg on admission to the hospital)
5. chol	serum cholestoral in mg/dl
6. fbs	(fasting blood sugar > 120mg/dl) (1 = true; 0 = false)
7. restecg	resting electrocardiographic results
8. thalach	maximum heart rate achieved
9. exang	exercise induced angina (1 = yes; 0 = no)
10. oldpeak	ST depression induced by exercise relative to rest
11. slope	the slope of the peak exercise ST segment (Value 1: upsloping, 2: flat, 3: downsloping
12. ca	number of major vessels (0–3) colored by flourosopy
13. thal	3 = normal; 6 = fixed defect; 7 = reversable defect
14. num (the predicted attribute)	diagnosis of heart disease (angiographic disease status) (Value 0: < 50% diameter narrowing, 1: > 50% diameter narrowing)

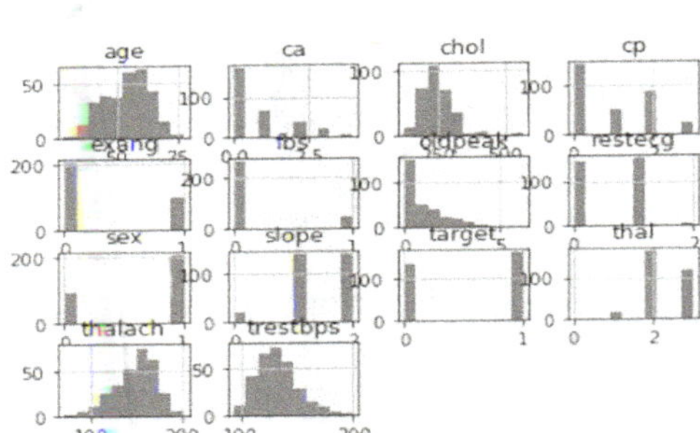

Figure 16.3 Data visualization of the dataset.

redundant and similar classifiers are overcome by determining the specific number of training sets. The parameters used for MOPSO is as follows:

The probability of each sample was 0.65, the number of particles are 100, the number of divisions are 50, the Personal and Social Best Coefficient is 2, the number of iterations is 100, the repository size is 20, the particle size is same as training size, the vmax is 5, and the inertia weight is 0.5. The dataset is divided into training and testing datasets. The data is trained by giving different features from MOPSO algorithm and also the output which is whether a person has heart disease or not. In this research work, the dataset is divided into 80% of training data and 20% of testing data.

The proposed hybridized KNN-MOPSO performance is evaluated on the performance metrics such as accuracy, sensitivity, and specificity and compared with the well-known ML models such as KNN, SVM, NB, LR, AdaBoost, and RF. Table 16.2 presented the performance metrics comparison of proposed Hybridized KNN-MOPSO with six ML models such as KNN, SVM, NB, LR, AdaBoost, and RF over the dataset. The proposed method outperformed on other ML classifiers on the Cleveland heart datasets.

Table 16.2 Performance metrics comparison of proposed Hybridized KNN-MOPSO with six ML models over the dataset

Model	*Accuracy(%)*	*Sensitivity(%)*	*Specificity(%)*
KNN	84	81.71	71.94
SVM	80	93.9	65.47
NB	77	81.71	71.94
LR	83	88.41	77.7
AdaBoost	64	68.9	58.99
RF	74	72	90
Proposed Hybridized KNN-PSO	92	94	95

Figure 16.4 shows that the proposed hybridized KNN-PSO achieves higher accuracy of value 8%, 12%, 15%, 9%, 28%, and 18% higher than KNN, SVM, NB, LR, AdaBoost, and RF models, respectively. The proposed hybridized KNN-PSO obtained higher sensitivity value of 12.29%, 0.1%, 12.29%, 5.59%, 25.1%, and 22% than KNN, SVM, NB, LR, AdaBoost, and RF models, respectively. The proposed hybridized KNN-PSO achieves higher specificity value of 23.06%, 29.53%, 23.06%, 17.3%, 36.01%, and 5% than KNN, SVM, NB, LR, AdaBoost, and RF models, respectively.

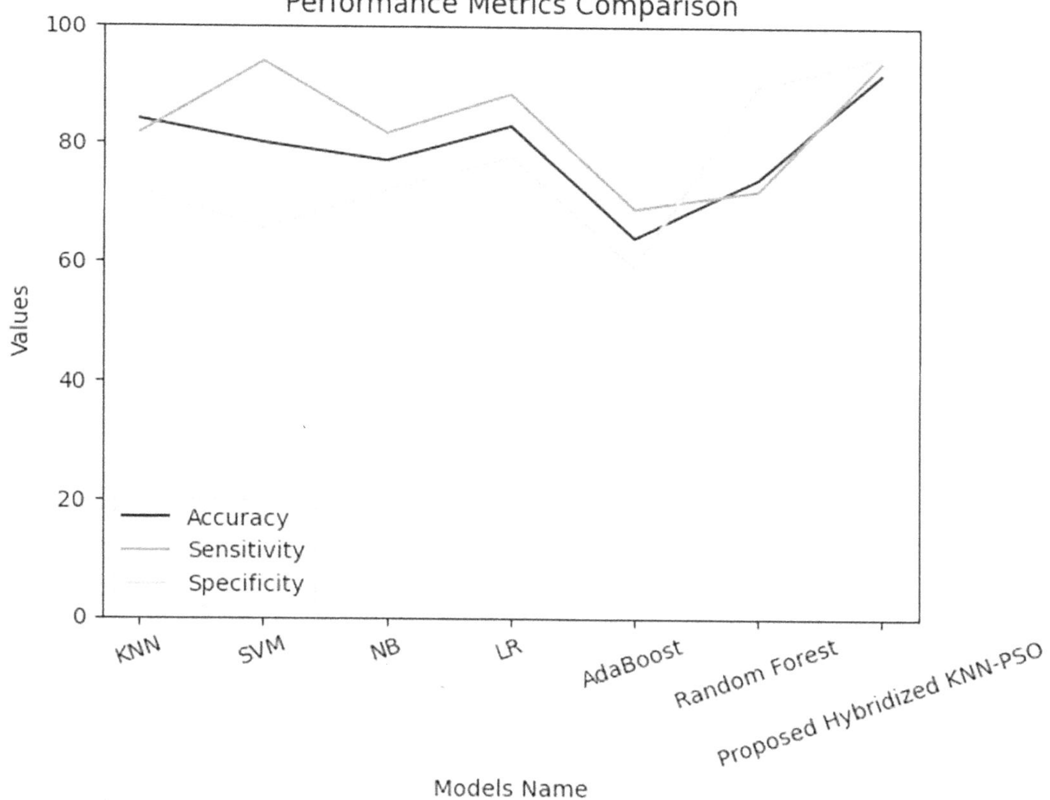

Figure 16.4 Performance metrics comparison of different ML models with proposed Hybridized KNN-MOPSO.

16.6 CONCLUSION AND FUTURE WORK

In this paper, a hybridized KNN-MOPSO is presented to improve the KNN classifier. The MOPSO optimization algorithm is proposed when considering the error and diversity objective functions, and the training sets are used to train the classifiers, resulting in the production of diverse and accurate classification. The proposed method determines the best optimal solution using a multi-objective optimization approach and reduce classification error during an evolutionary process. The experimental result analysis also proves that the hybridized KNN-MOPSO achieves highest accuracy, sensitivity, and specificity over the UCI Cleveland dataset. Comparing KNN with the proposed method, it can be concluded that the training sets generation has an important role in KNN performance. This hybridized KNN-MOPSO helps the physicians to efficiently predict heart diseases with predominant features. In future work, the result can be improved by considering large datasets, and the patient's dataset could be extended with more symptoms, which may cause heart disease.

REFERENCES

1. M. Shouman, T. Turner, R. Stocker, Using data mining techniques in heart disease diagnosis and treatment, in: Proc. 2012 Japan-Egypt Conf. Electron. Commun. Comput. JEC-ECC 2012, 2012: pp. 173–177. 10.1109/JECECC.2012.6186978.
2. I. Yekkala, S. Dixit, M. A. Jabbar, Prediction of heart disease using ensemble learning and Particle Swarm Optimization, in: Proc. 2017 Int. Conf. Smart Technol. Smart Nation, SmartTechCon 2017, Institute of Electrical and Electronics Engineers Inc., 2018: pp. 691–698. 10.1109/SmartTechCon.2017.8358460.
3. L. Breiman, Random forests, Mach. Learn., 45 (2001): 5–32. 10.1023/A:1010933404324.
4. S. Chandra, R. Bhat, H. Singh, A PSO based method for detection of brain tumors from MRI, in: 2009 World Congr. Nat. Biol. Inspired Comput. NABIC 2009 – Proc., 2009: pp. 666–671. 10.1109/NABIC.2009.5393455.
5. C. A. Coello Coello, M. S. Lechuga, MOPSO: A proposal for multiple objective particle swarm optimization, in: Proc. 2002 Congr. Evol. Comput. CEC 2002, IEEE Computer Society, 2002: pp. 1051–1056. 10.1109/CEC.2002.1004388.
6. D. Deepika, N. Balaji, Effective heart disease prediction using novel MLP-EBMDA approach, Biomed. Signal Process. Control, 72(Part B) (2022): 103318, ISSN 1746-8094, 10.1016/j.bspc.2021.103318.
7. X.-Y. Gao, A. A. Ali, H. S. Hassan, E. M. Anwar, Improving the accuracy for analyzing heart diseases prediction based on the ensemble method, Complexity, 2021 (2021): Article ID 6663455, 10 pages.
8. A. K. Gárate-Escamila, A. Hajjam El Hassani, E. Andrès, Classification models for heart disease prediction using feature selection and PCA, Inf. Med. Unlocked, 19 (2020): 100330, ISSN 2352-9148, 10.1016/j.imu.2020.100330.
9. P. Kamencay, R. Hudec, M. Benco, M. Zachariasova, Feature extraction for object recognition using PCA-KNN with application to medical image analysis, in: 2013 36th Int. Conf. Telecommun. Signal Process. (TSP), 2013, 830–834. 10.1109/tsp.2013.6614055.
10. A. Akella, S. Akella, Machine learning algorithms for predicting coronary artery disease: efforts toward an open source solution, Future Sci. OA, 7(6) (2021 Mar 29): FSO698. doi: 10.2144/fsoa-2020-0206.
11. A. Javeed, S. Zhou, L. Yongjian, I. Qasim, A. Noor, R. Nour, An intelligent learning system based on random search algorithm and optimized random forest model for improved heart disease detection, IEEE Access, 7 (2019): 180235–180243, doi: 10.1109/ACCESS.2019.2952107.

12. F. Han, W.-T. Chen, Q.-H. Ling, H. Han, Multi-objective particle swarm optimization with adaptive strategies for feature selection, Swarm Evolutionary Comput., 62 (2021): 100847, ISSN 2210-6502, 10.1016/j.swevo.2021.100847.
13. B. H. Nguyen, B. Xue, M. Zhang, A survey on swarm intelligence approaches to feature selection in data mining, Swarm Evolutionary Comput., 54(2020): 100663, ISSN 2210-6502, 10.1016/j.swevo.2020.100663.
14. K. Zou, Y. Liu, S. Wang, N. Li, Y. Wu, A multiobjective particle swarm optimization algorithm based on grid technique and multistrategy, J. Math., 2021 (2021): Article ID 1626457, 17 pages. 10.1155/2021/1626457.
15. M. Yang, Y. Liu, J. Yang, A hybrid multi-objective particle swarm optimization with central control strategy, Comput. Intell. Neurosci., 2022 (2022 Mar 9): 1522096. doi: 10.1155/2022/1522096. PMID: 35310587; PMCID: PMC8926491.
16. G. Rajeshkumar, M. Vinoth Kumar, K. Sailaja Kumar, S. Bhatia, A. Mashat et al., An improved multi-objective particle swarm optimization routing on manet, Comput. Syst. Sc. Eng., 44(2) (2023): 1187–1200.
17. S. Hong, J. Lee, H. Cho, K. Jang, J. Kim, Cluster-based multiobjective particle swarm optimization and application for chemical plants, Int. J. Intell. Syst., 2023 (2023): Article ID 5275262, 13 pages. 10.1155/2023/5275262
18. Y. Yang, Q. Liao, J. Wang, Y. Wang, Application of multi-objective particle swarm optimization based on short-term memory and K-means clustering in multi-modal multi-objective optimization, Eng. Appl. Artif. Intell., 112(2022): 104866, ISSN 0952-1976, 10.1016/j.engappai.2022.104866.
19. P. Hadikhani, D. T. C. Lai, W. -H. Ong, Human activity discovery with automatic multi-objective particle swarm optimization clustering with Gaussian mutation and game theory, IEEE Trans. Multimedia, 26 (2024): 420–435, 10.1109/TMM.2023.3266603.

Index

www.ingramcontent.com/pod-product-compliance
Lightning Source LLC
LaVergne TN
LVHW081316110826
845149LV00006B/1521